002044745

Nurses and Politics

D1578601

Also by Chris Hart:

Behind the Mask: Nurses, Their Unions and Nursing Policy, 1994

Nurses and Politics

The Impact of Power and Practice

Chris Hart

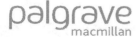

First published 2004 by
PALGRAVE MACMILLAN
Houndmills, Basingstoke, Hampshire RG21 6XS and
175 Fifth Avenue, New York, N.Y. 10010
Companies and representatives throughout the world

PALGRAVE MACMILLAN is the global academic imprint of the Palgrave
Macmillan division of St. Martin's Press, LLC and of Palgrave Macmillan Ltd.
Macmillan® is a registered trademark in the United States, United Kingdom
and other countries. Palgrave is a registered trademark in the European
Union and other countries.

ISBN 0–333–71006–1 paperback

This book is printed on paper suitable for recycling and made from fully
managed and sustained forest sources.

A catalogue record for this book is available from the British Library.

10 9 8 7 6 5 4 3 2 1
13 12 11 10 09 08 07 06 05 04

Printed and bound by J. W. Arrowsmith Ltd., Bristol

Contents

List of Tables and Figures

Tables

Figures

Acknowledgements

Friends and colleagues are now more than used to seeing me scribble down parts of conversations in meetings, pubs and restaurants or looking (more) vacant (than usual) as I try and make a mental note of something that's been said. But that is, in part, how this book was written. It was not just a matter of learning from others but the whole process of knowing them. Ian Morton thus infused this work with many of his ideas and observations about nursing and politics. The constant carer, his suggestions for Chapter 8 were invaluable and I'm eternally grateful. Discussions with Toby Kinder about the triangular model of management were the equivalent of a left foot shot from outside the box and helped shape aspects of Chapter 6. I'm grateful to Kevin Monteith for his often calm and wise advice, to John Lister and Geoff Martin for their often unwise advice over the years. Kit Opie's leftfield view is in every odd nook and cranny in the text. I blame him for the really odd ones. Eamon Pryle's overall sensibility has always been a guiding influence. Those conversations used to enliven the dull bits of Palace games – guess how many – have all been put to good use. My oldest friend and collaborator, Adrian D'Aubney, showed me how to find meaning in the debate between science and religion. He remains an inspiration, when it can be an argument for a week, laughter for a month, and a good jest for ever, a good plot, good friends, and full of expectations; an excellent plot, very good friends. My old colleagues at Lewin Road were always being tapped – often unwittingly – and now is the time to own up and thank them all, nurses, doctors, an art therapist, occupational therapists and administrator who formed the best team I have ever worked in: especially David Tracey, Hilary Williams, Candida Rosier, Angela Hughes, Kamal Gupta, Anne Boocock, Nick Clarke, Godfried Attafua, Janette Goddard, Nigel Hilton, Sheila Donahue, Brendan Thomas, Saira Razzaq, Ian Kennedy, Wendy Dyer, Kylie Draper, Leander Clynshaw, Shareen Harneker and Lucy Daniels. Writing this, I also had occasion to remember many of the wonderful nurses I encountered during different times, particularly Barbara Fisk, Barry Morvinson, Sue Ritter and Siva Govindasamy.

Special thanks are due to Dr Julia Gale and Professor Fiona Ross in the Faculty of Health and Social Care Sciences, Kingston University and St George's Hospital Medical School, as well as Chris Butler and Bernadette Hennigan at the South West London and St George's Mental Health NHS Trust for their support and that most invaluable commodity, time. Thanks also to the Liaison Psychiatry team from St George's Hospital: David (again), John Morgan, Paul Abernethie, Rachel Goulder,

Caroline Owen, Delwyn Kay, Karen Hutchinson, Jeremy Bolton, Toby Sutcliffe, Jennifer Attridge – see Lewin Road – as well as Jim Blair, Denise Bodley, Harjinder Sehmi, Trish Griffin, Edward Maliki, Maha White, Danny Lam, Sue Rush, Sue Fergy and Ian Rees Jones within the Faculty.

The chaps at Belenenses and my old, old comrades at the Maudsley Hospital are never forgotten. I have always learned a lot from Steven Pryle, always thinking global but acting local. Both Archie and Neil Lauchlan whittered on about something or other. I wrote it down and it's in here. John and Bev Mitchell provided a rural perspective. Special thanks to Jim Devine ... for many things but, most particularly, being Jim. Hamish provided welcome diversions from time to time. Richenda Milton-Thompson originally commissioned this book. Jon Reed shepherded it through the last stages with Magenta Lampson – the hardest bit of all. Thanks also to Mukesh and his team, who oversaw the production so helpfully. Special thanks to Jane Salvage, not just for writing the foreword, but for encouragement and support over the years.

Lastly but never least: to all my family – I've missed you! Brenda, Ken and Grace. My lovely sons, Nathan and Jake, were always in my thoughts as I tried to make sense of this thing called nurses and politics, and often that was all that kept me sane. I owe them about three year's worth of weekends. As for Barbara, she did just about everything except write the damned thing. This is dedicated to her, with love.

Foreword

This book aroused in me a tumult of thoughts and feelings, as it will in any reader who cares about nursing and nurses. It inevitably took me back 20 years, to the days when I was a newly qualified nurse writing *The Politics of Nursing* with my friends in the Radical Nurses Group. That book, like this, attempted both to understand why nursing continued to be undervalued, and to encourage nurses to get out from under by being more assertive and politically active.

So much has changed since then, and yet so little. Government propaganda would have us believe that we've never had it so good, and in some ways that is true. Nurses today have opportunities to develop their careers in practice, education, management, research and other avenues that few of us then dreamed of, and some even earn a decent living from it. The ten-year plan for the National Health Service appears to give nurses a central role in reforming the health system, while employers offer ever more attractive deals to recruit and retain scarce and precious staff.

Is there really anything to complain about? Chris Hart's wide-ranging exploration shows how far we have come, yet how far we still need to travel. Little has been written about nurses themselves, their place in society and in health care, as he points out; that is one reason why I felt impelled to write my book. Not much change there, then. Although the political and social landscape of the United Kingdom has changed immeasurably in the last 20 years, nursing is still an undervalued, mostly invisible profession whose grass-roots practitioners – like most predominantly female occupations – remain relatively poorly paid, patronised, and expected to shoulder ever-increasing workloads without demur. Now they are required to take on yet more responsibilities to cover for shortages of other staff, particularly doctors. As Hart's seven case studies show, many recent policy initiatives that claim to help nurses are actually fig leaves for different, wider agendas that often seem to care little for patients and even less for nurses.

Such talk is likely to have me labelled as a typical whingeing nurse, but Hart's work reinforces my belief that nurses are constantly blamed for shortcomings that are way beyond their control, and that stem from the political, cultural and organisational power structures that really shape events and behaviours. Nurses themselves are often guilty of this victim-blaming, but this book will help persuade them to look more closely at the forces that determine not only what they are paid and how they are treated, but how they deliver care and relate to patients.

Policy and politics change practice but the reverse is also true, which is where hope rests for the future. In 20 years nurses have made amazing strides forward in improving the quality of care, and in developing new ways of meeting previously neglected needs. This has come about because individual nurses have taken risks and introduced innovations, often against the odds in indifferent or even hostile surroundings. Through doing this they have learned that acting alone is not enough, and that lasting change can only come about when it is owned and enacted by the whole team.

The collective spirit that infuses excellent practice should also be harnessed, as Hart argues, for the greater good of nurses themselves. Senior figures in nursing, in the NHS, civil service, universities, professional/regulatory bodies and trade unions, have adopted a conciliatory, perhaps naive political approach that has sometimes sold nurses short. No one wants confrontation but nursing leaders have too often failed to stand up and be counted. When you consider that there are well over half a million nurses and that they are the biggest group of workers in health services, it is astonishing how easily they are pushed around.

If their organisations will not reform themselves, nurses should create new networks and local associations to fight for their rights – and the time is ripe, since an inspiring range of interconnected political movements is now emerging. Tired of sterile party politics and broken promises, ordinary people who care passionately about the state of the world are joining together to take new forms of local, national and global action. The mobilisation of opinion against the UK/US war on Iraq, for example, showed how millions of people could express their views actively even with the weight of governments against them, and no big, rich organisations to back them. Nurses can take a leaf from that book, and find new and creative ways of shaping their future; this book will inform and inspire them to do it.

JANE SALVAGE
RGN, BA, MSc, HonLLD
Independent nursing consultant and author of
The Politics of Nursing (1985), London: Heinemann

It is clear that few of the children who ride in the Mad Hatter's Teacup [at Disneyland] have read or even will read Alice, let alone the works of Mark Twain. Most of them will only know Alice's story from the Disney film, if at all. And that suggests a separation of two ontological degrees between the Disneyland customer and the cultural artefacts he is presumed upon to treasure in his visit. The Mad Hatter's Teacup is emblematic of the Disney animated film, which is itself a drastic revision in form and content of a subtle dreamwork created out of the English language. And even to an adult who dimly remembers reading the original Alice, and whose complicated response to this powerfully symbolic work has long since been incorporated into the psychic contents of his life, what is being offered does not suggest the resonance of the original work, but is only a sentimental compression of something that is itself already a lie.

The Book of Daniel, by E. L. Doctorow

List of Abbreviations

ANA	American Nurses' Association
APNA	American Psychiatric Nurses' Association
BMA	British Medical Association
CBI	Confederation of British Industry
CFP	Common Foundation Programme
CHI	Commission of Health Improvement
COHSE	Confederation of Health Service Employees
CPHVA	Community Practitioners' and Health Visitors' Association
CPNA	Community Psychiatric Nurses' Association
EU	European Union
GDP	Gross Domestic Product
GNC	General Nursing Council
HSE	Health and Safety Executive
HVA	Health Visitors' Association
INO	Irish Nurses' Organisation
MSP	Member of the Scottish Parliament
NALGO	National Association of Local Government Officers
NAWU	National Asylum Workers' Union
NMC	Nursing and Midwifery Council
NUCO	National Union of Council Officers
NUPE	National Union of Public Employees
P2K	Project 2000
PAMS	Professions Allied to Medicine
PCG	Primary Care Group
PCT	Primary Care Trust
PFI	Private Finance Initiative
PLWTU	Poor Law Workers' Trade Union
PRB	Pay Review Body
RBNA	Royal British Nurses' Association
RCM	Royal College of Midwifery
RCN	Royal College of Nursing
STUC	Scottish Trades Union Congress
TUC	Trades Union Congress
UKCC	United Kingdom Central Council

Introduction

Nurses are the largest section of the largest workforce in Europe. They are also one of the most important occupational groups in the UK. Yet despite volumes being written about their practice, comparatively little is written about nurses themselves, their place in British society, the National Health Service [NHS] or wider healthcare system. Throughout, this book refers to 'nurses'. It does not discriminate between adult nurses, paediatric nurses, community nurses, mental health nurses or any others although the text will refer to specific groups. I will also, on occasions, use the term to include nursing auxillaries, nursing assistants and healthcare assistants only inasmuch as they are involved in the work of nursing and caring for patients, work that is increasingly devalued and which, by association, devalues those who carry it out. There is a recognition, implicit throughout the book, however, that the nature of the work carried out by untrained nurses and those who have studied and been educated to apply theory to practice can be hugely different and the two groups necessarily inhabit largely different roles, even though there is inevitably an area where they overlap. Again, I will make various distinctions in the text about the differences between trained and untrained staff when appropriate. Another choice of language throughout the book will be the use of the word, patient, rather than client or user, other terms that feature in nursing and healthcare texts. This is because research regularly shows that this is the term patients prefer, even if they are healthy women attending antenatal clinics (Rild *et al.*, 2000; Byrne *et al.*, 2000). *Nurses and Politics* doesn't, on the whole, attempt to act as a 'how to ...' guide, with lots of checklists, dos and don'ts or useful tips. Perhaps that is another book. Although, in the last chapter, the book does attempt to draw its many themes towards some clear conclusions and present ideas for an agenda for change in the present and aspirations for the future, it tries to work through a series of key issues for contemporary nurses, placed in a historical context, which demonstrates that the problems nurses face today are very similar to those faced by our ancestors and, almost certainly, will still be the subject of varying degrees of angst in the coming decade. This is not to be pessimistic but necessarily realistic about the challenges facing us and those who follow in our footsteps.

The book was produced over a period of seven years and draws upon a great deal of research, including primary and secondary sources, interviews with politicians and civil servants, nurses working at all levels, and figures from the trade union movement. During this period, the extraordinary number of policies that either directly affect nurses and/or their practice has been so high that either re-writes or additional notes have been necessary in many of the chapters. Some things that seemed 'absolute' have been overtaken by other events within a relatively short timescale. This has inevitably shaped both the content and the style of the book in its aims to explore some fundamental questions about nurses and nursing. It is not a 'traditional' text book: although written for nurses to read and study, as shall be seen it tells its story in a different way and will, hopefully, be accessible to the general reader. The opening chapter acts as an introduction to nursing and nurses in the widest possible context, containing some statistical information, differences and similarities within the workforce and the politics of nurses and nursing. This is followed by two chapters that provide a summary of our history, with a special focus on crucial events in the more recent past that still impact upon us today. The first of the book's case studies is featured in Chapter 3, giving a detailed account of the occasion when nursing practice, policy and politics collided in the most vivid and spectacular way in the events that led up to and followed the clinical grading of all nursing posts in the UK. There are a further five such case studies, looking at the internal market (chosen as it gives a good account of social policy relating to health and, at the same time, suggests what may well follow if New Labour follows its plans to introduce Foundation Hospitals), NHS funding, waiting lists, devolution and local pay. These are only used to detail particular events or issues in a way that is hoped will illuminate not just the state of the road on which nursing and nurses are travelling but how and why they came to be on it as well as where they might be heading. Chapter 4 is, well, different. It tries to get behind the myths and ideologies that were used to shape nursing, as well as the aspects of our work that are unique. It looks, in particular, at the use of angels in our mythology and explores this in a new way to see if there is a deeper, less easily accessed understanding of the perception of nursing and the ambiguity towards it that can be uncovered. The chapter also concentrates on some of the religious imagery and traditions that have been incorporated into nursing while thinking about the relationship between women's work and caring, and what might constitute contemporary nursing.

Contemporary processes, influences and events that determine the work nurses do, whether that be at a national level or within their own clinical team are the focus of Chapters 5 and 6. Government policy on health and nursing is analysed in greater detail and the case studies on waiting lists and NHS funding are used to illustrate the use of smoke and mirrors that governments can use in the way in which they 'sell' policy and devise strategy. Particular emphasis is placed on attempting to understand the nature of power and how it is used in relation to nurses, who appear to be relatively powerless, while Chapter 6 concludes with a discussion about how we might think about new ways of making decisions and finding improved ways in which to manage staff and services. Chapter 7 is about the nursing unions and the problems they both face and actually create in relation to their nurse members. Chapter 8 tries to draw some conclusions about the state of nursing today, devoting space to a broad range of 'current' issues, such as nurse education, pay, the Nursing and Midwifery Council (NMC), culture and race and the relationship between stress, bullying, violence and whistleblowing. Again, although these issues are current, they have been for many years and, as the chapter develops, it tries to understand these in ways that enables the reader to think about them in a broader context. It does also put forward suggestions for an alternative agenda for change as it would have been too easy to criticise without having some ideas of how things could be different. However, it is not meant to be prescriptive. Indeed, the whole point of the book is that nurses and other readers might take the debate forward wherever they work.

Some of the changes suggested, as well as the analysis that has led to them, will undoubtedly be regarded as contentious by some. It may make for uncomfortable reading for some in positions of power and influence, be they in government, senior managerial or nursing positions, the unions, or in the increasing number of private consortia and companies that are gaining access to healthcare in this country. Yet the issues raised in the book are not about personalities, they are about institutions, ideology and systems. Some might suggest that it is not critical enough of nurses. My response to that is that there have been more than enough criticisms of nurses, with many critics focusing on issues that are actually beyond the control of the nurses under fire and failing to take into account the organisational issues which dictate and shape events and behaviours.

Despite its length, there's much that's not in this book, things that I would like to have included but which time and space prevented. The integration of health and social services, the formation of social care trusts and PCTs were all evolving as the final stages were being written. There were many details about nursing practice, the details of what nurses do in their everyday work for which room could not be found. Thankfully, they are available elsewhere. It would also have been nice to have been able to devote more space to different specialities within nursing, midwifery and health visiting, the voluntary sector and nursing homes. However, without 'lumping' all nurses together, it is the intention of this work to address the concerns of, and issues relevant to, nurses everywhere by looking at common themes. Again, while the book acknowledges that nurses are far from a homogeneous occupational group, there are many fundamental political issues that affect us all. Most importantly, *Nurses and Politics* tries to look at the processes behind the everyday events that catch the headlines, looking at context, history and particular determinants. We all know nurses are badly paid. Why? Equally, why is it that good policy intentions, like some of those put forward by New Labour in the last seven years, don't make things better in the way that was expected?

In some respects, writing about New Labour's approach to policy is like trying to make sense of a manic patient. It is not so much the detail of all that is said – there is too much and it is bewildering just to try and follow it all. One has to take a step back and judge the overall effect of its behaviour, try and see the big picture and make sense of it in its entirety. Equally, in focusing on the actions of New Labour, this is only to reflect the intentions and behaviour of the party of government. Hopefully, the reader will be able to discern how policy is formulated and power used, even though the detail is very often different from that of its Conservative predecessor. There are fairly large chunks of this book that are pretty depressing. But it has to be remembered that, for most nurses who remain in the job, at least some of the time, the job of nursing is not only rewarding but fun. Much of that comes from the camaraderie that nurses build, the bonds they create between themselves and which feeds into the relationship with their patients and the satisfaction of doing an extremely difficult job well (Radcliffe and Crouch, 2002).

Why would a book about contemporary nursing focus so much attention on the workings of non-nurses, political decision making, committees, policies, events that took place so long ago that the main protagonists are not just dead but almost completely forgotten?

All of us, as nurses, bring our own individual 'material' to the job, our own sense of who we are, of what makes us tick, our own history, influences, desires, drives and aspirations. We all have something else, however, which is 'shared history' that pre-dates our existence as nurses, and leaves us, as its legacy, an inherited imagination and mythology as well as a collective spirit, or identity, that stands at least as powerfully alongside our real history. It is this highly combustible mix that gives us a sense of who we are, as nurses, our sense of worth and value, as well as our perception of the status and position we occupy in the world in which we function.

It is in our attempts to disentangle the myths, to understand the impact of that inherited imagination, to integrate the real with the mythological and move beyond our history that nurses will break free of the oppressive elements that have constrained us and held us in their grasp for so long. If the personal is political and the political impacts upon the personal, the beginning of the political evolutionary process nursing needs to embark upon begins with each individual nurse making their own changes. In a very small way, I hope that this book may help.

1 Nurses and Nursing: The Same but Different

It's a great huge game of chess that's being played – all over the world – if this is the world at all, you know. Oh, what fun it is! How I wish I was one of them! I wouldn't mind being a Pawn, if only I might join – though of course I should like to be a Queen, best.

Alice Through The Looking Glass by Lewis Carroll

The clue is in the title. As much as it may seem heretical to some, nonsensical or irrelevant to others – or may be just a plain source of annoyance – if we are to understand nursing and its practice, we have to be prepared to develop a perspective on politics and power. Similarly, if we want to understand how politics influences nursing – which is what seems to govern the work that nurses actually do – we have to understand practice. They are inextricably entwined. Politics dominates how nurses practice and there are political implications arising out of everything nurses do. At its most obvious, politics dictates the decisions that lead to the percentage pay rise awarded – by politicians – each year. It drives the practice that emerges from policies such as those incorporated in the National Service Frameworks introduced to the National Health Service (NHS). The development of nurse-led Walk In Centres was said to have heralded a change in the role and clinical practice of the nurses working in them, but has been the subject of intense political manoeuvring since. The fact that nurses throughout the United Kingdom still run the risk of needlestick injuries, despite the existence of safe – but costlier – syringes is, again, due to political decisions made at government and local level. And if an important aspect of power and politics is about control, then controlling nurses and nursing has been a principle part of the NHS agenda since 1948, just as it was in British healthcare systems before that.

Almost beyond politics, nurses are also very much the stuff of myth. But it's not just one myth that underpins the nurses' story. Just as there is more than one history of nursing, the weighty traditions, fanciful landscapes and kaleidoscopic images are as much a part of our inherited imagination as anything that actually happened. So nurses are a surrogate for Mother Mary as well as Mary Magdalene. They are caricatured as the fragile young woman who will dutifully sacrifice herself to care for those in her charge, the domineering, fierce matron, doughty enrolled nurse, the cheery district nurse, the woman who mops the brow of the doctor on the ward and, of course, angels. Angels are everywhere in nursing mythology.

In the real world where nurses live and work, we know that they are mostly women, subject to the same external pressures as women in other walks of life, struggling to do an extremely difficult job. When it goes well, many nurses will say there is no other job like it and, despite its problems, it obviously still exerts a strong attraction and source of satisfaction for the vast majority. As we shall see later in the text, when that job is at its worst, they complain of often feeling tired and fed up, of being poorly paid, having too much responsibility, too much work, not enough respect from their managers, and of mounting stress as that work seems less and less within their control. These problems leave them irritable and restless for change. Most of all, perhaps, they will describe a feeling of being disempowered.

In the world of myth and stereotype, there was one image that, early on, was used to epitomise the 'archetypal' nurse. It is perhaps the most enduring image of all, which survived well into the early 1990s. She was portrayed as white, Anglo Saxon, well educated, heterosexual, from a relatively affluent family and working in an acute metropolitan teaching hospital. This was how nursing's hierarchy liked to project its dutiful charges. Those who lost out to its potency were the 'ordinary' nurses who fitted neither the stereotypical image nor could be placed within the mythic traditions. These might be black or from different minority ethnic groups, from poorer socio-economic backgrounds, of different gender or sexuality.

One thing that apparently bound these disparate groups together, however, was that all were nurses. But did it? Again, there's a question of which nurses we are talking about. For a flawed assumption undermines much of the thinking about nursing. Its many different groups tend to be lumped together into one, homogeneous whole, not just by the public but also in the minds of many of those working in healthcare, some nurses included. Most importantly, those involved in formulating policy not only share it but often perpetuate it. There are, inevitably, common elements to the work that are shared by all nurses but these are not always easily understood or explained. For example, all nurses are described as being in the 'caring profession' but what does that mean? Nursing 'care' is central to the work of all nurses but almost certainly means wholly different things to nurses in different clinical areas. Indeed, it's highly unlikely that nurses even fully understand the detail of the work many of their colleagues – in the widest sense – are engaged in.

Community mental health nurses would, in many cases, now have far more in common with social workers than they would with staff working on a surgical ward or an intensive therapy unit. Similarly, the day-to-day work undertaken by theatre nurses will bear little relation to the activities of a community nurse or someone involved in elderly care. There are a whole group of nurses working, almost literally, in the shadow of night duty, lost to the glare of the life and activity of their wards during the day. Most nurses still work in the NHS but an increasing number now earn their living in either the private or voluntary sectors, with different rules, expectations and approaches to practice.

The way in which nurses even think about themselves can vary greatly. Some would proudly declare themselves professionals. Others would argue strongly that nursing is not a true profession and, consequently, nurses cannot classify themselves as such. They would claim that nursing does not meet the sociologically defined criteria, with its key characteristics:

- the possession of a distinctive domain of knowledge and theorising relevant to practice;
- reference to a code of ethics and professional values emerging from the professional group and, in cases of conflict, taken to supersede the values of the employer or, indeed, governments;
- exert control over admission to the group via the establishment, monitoring and validation of procedures for education and training;
- have the power to discipline and potentially debar members who infringe the ethical code or whose standards of practice are unacceptable;
- participation in a professional culture sustained by a professional association(s). (Whittington and Boone, 1989).

If this issue, which has dogged nursing throughout most of the twentieth century, is explored within that narrow understanding, we can see that nursing is not a profession.[1] However, 'professionalism' has a much wider relevance in contemporary parlance. Professional footballers are paid, as opposed to the unpaid amateur. A 'professional foul' is synonymous with a cynical, competitiveness, originally driven by greed and money, which has infected all aspects of the beautiful game. Many behaviours and conduct in the context of work, particularly doing it well, with a sense of pride and striving towards meeting high standards, are associated with a notion of professionalism. This has nothing to do with status, training or earning capacity. Thus, punctuality may be seen as a matter of professionalism. Estate agents will talk about how their profession operates.

There are some in nursing who support Illich's view that professionalism is a conspiracy to create dependent client groups, depriving them of their right and ability

---

[1] As I support the view that nursing is not a fully fledged profession, I will generally not refer to it as such. However, there are occasions when it is politically appropriate to do so because either those individuals or organisations being referred to or discussed use the term describing themselves as professionals or nursing as a profession. I shall then use the term as they would and hope that, in so doing, this will exemplify the confusions created around the status of nurses and the complexities there are in describing the political, social and economic realities of nursing without further complicating the actual text.

to determine their own welfare and happiness (Illich, 1977). Yet, in both this wider context and peculiar to its own aspirations, professionalism remains an issue that runs like a pulsating, ideological bloodline through the body of nursing, not all of it immediately accessible, some of it inhabiting the shrouded world of symbolism and myth that hangs over nurses.

More contemporary contributors to the debate make the observation that nursing is 'essentially a practical activity, carried out by many people, qualified and unqualified, skilled and unskilled' (Holt, 1998: p 149). Nonetheless, professionalism is inextricably bound up with status and the work that nurses will do. As such, for some of those nurses most concerned with achieving it, this has long been nursing's Holy Grail. The debate about how best to invest nursing with status has been one of the factors that has effectively split nurses as an occupational group. Those who, historically, sought to advance its cause through enhanced professional status, were the proponents of longer hours, low pay, harder work, stricter discipline. They were the architects of the carefully constructed myth and the earliest of many layers of ideology which shaped the tradition of the vocational ideal, self sacrifice and subservience to a 'common good' – although, inevitably, this 'common good' was not universally seen as such. Indeed, part of the role of promoting an ideological 'professionalism' was to make the hard sell of such sacrifices not only easier but also natural, inevitable and eternal.[2] It was one which nurses' employers, whether in the old voluntary hospitals, workhouses or asylums, were very happy to buy into. Just as their contemporary equivalents have proven to now. Governments, from whichever party, and employers have always been delighted to exploit it, as can be seen by some simple examples. Early in the twentieth century, the Poor Law Workers' Trade Union was campaigning for a shorter working week. The Boards of Governors opposed this because they didn't have the money to employ more staff. Their argument, however, was that patients should not be subjected to 'unnecessarily frequent changes of nurses', that it would be harder to pinpoint 'neglect' onto individual staff members and that longer periods away from the wards would mean nurses would lose interest in their work (White, 1978: p 181). Adjusting the language to suit the time but still essentially addressing a financial issue, Frank Dobson, Labours' Secretary of State for Health in 1999, dictated that nurses, *out of a sense of duty,*

---

[2] The use of ideology 'represents a systematic set of principles linking perceptions of the world to explicit moral values. An ideology not only interprets the meaning of events but also posits the need to change or maintain the existing situation'. To maintain their power and the political system's stability, those in authority communicate various texts – e.g., ideologies, myths, doctrines, legal decisions – to members of [the system's] society, claiming them as better than any alternative (Andrain and Apter, 1995: pp 4–25).

should work for no extra money at the millennium whilst other groups of workers were being paid, literally hundreds of pounds per hour (my emphasis).

The characteristics of suffering engendered through the conditions the professionalisers sought to impose were not solely an end in themselves. There was an element of these being seen as a virtue in their own right as nursing's early leaders sought to draw on its military and, particularly, religious, origins. Contrast, e.g., St Paul's exhortation to the Galatians, 'But the fruit of the Spirit is love, joy, peace, patience, kindness, goodness, faithfulness, gentleness, self control' (Galatians 5: 22) with the qualities deemed necessary by the early nursing reformers for their new charges: kindness, patience, discipline, deference, obedience and, perhaps most importantly, 'good character' (Abel-Smith, 1960). However, beyond that lay an attempt at exclusiveness and to attract 'suitable' women into the burgeoning profession they were seeking to fashion in their own likeness (see Chapter 2).

For the more 'generalist' nurses, who argued that nursing was no different to any other occupation, where status would be achieved through earning good rates of pay and winning better conditions of service through their own efforts, the professionalisers were not just misguided but promoting a philosophy that was detrimental to nurses' best interests.

In this sense, an immediate dichotomy emerges, one that was perhaps best summarised by Trevor Clay, then general secretary of the Royal College of Nursing (RCN), during a particularly bitter period of the clinical grading dispute in 1988. Faced with growing criticism from his own members about the College's failure to support nurses who wanted to take some form of industrial action against the government's pay policy and failure to address nurses' concerns about staffing levels and workload, Clay retorted, 'We are the Royal College of Nursing, *not* nurses' [my emphasis] (Clay, 1989). Explicit within this statement was an acknowledgement that there are differences between what may be good for nurses and what may be good for nursing. Nor are these tensions easily resolved by organisations many members see as having been set up to look after nurses' interests.

The apparently more straightforward aspirations cherished by the generalists have not been without their problems. The relative failure, despite ninety years of sometimes desperate efforts, to raise nurses out of the rut of low pay, with conditions of service that are still relatively poor and the consequent low status, has left its own legacy. Nurses unsuccessfully aspiring to this particular utopia are left with a diminished sense of their own worth, a lack of confidence in their ability to influence decisions about their future and diffidence in the face of managers and the medical profession. Often they blame their trade unions and feel let down by them after unsuccessful disputes, particularly when these have been prolonged and bitter. The 1988 campaign about clinical grading is a prime example. Despite nurses averaging an increase of 15.6 per cent – one of their biggest ever, achieved after they had forced a humiliating climbdown from a then rampant Tory government – the feeling of many involved was that nurses had been conned and lost out yet again. This was especially true for the lower paid, untrained and enrolled nurses, who received the lowest percentage increases. The same was true in 1982, when the Thatcher government was forced into giving a significantly improved pay award spread over two years: however, this was seen as no victory after a year of intense and increasingly bitter struggle, falling, as it did, a long way short of the increase nurses and other health workers' originally demanded. In the pay round that straddled the millennium, both Unison and the RCN submitted evidence arguing that the position of nurses remained unacceptable, that pay was far too low, their conditions of employment insufficient to guarantee nurses' retention in the workplace and that significant improvements would have to be made if their status in society was to reflect the work they did. This evidence could have been submitted in the 1930s, 1960s through the 1980s. Contemporary prophets of doom should be reminded that there is little new in these arguments. Any cursory examination of nursing history reveals that, rather than any acute crisis, these problems are chronic and deeply entrenched.

The devaluing of nursing is not a recent phenomenon. It has always reflected on the work nurses do and their position within the wider healthcare system. As the NHS was about to be introduced in 1948, a Ministry of Health official recorded that nurses were only one step up from domestics and, with doctors firmly established at one apex of an iron triangle with civil servants and politicians, this view ensured nurses were excluded from the policy formulation and decision making machinery of the new service (White, 1985; Pettigrew *et al.*, 1988). In the years since clinical grading, however, there has been a very practical way in which such attitudes and views have prevailed upon the work of nurses in their clinical work, which has literally been devalued by managers, employers and government driving down the grades of posts awarded in 1988, refusing to recognise the worth of nurses taking on additional responsibility and extending their role without reward. The participation of nurses in management structures has been severely curtailed since general managers were parachuted in as a result of the Griffiths Report and re-organisation of 1983, with the implicit message coldly delivered that nurses weren't good enough to manage complex services. Contemporary nurses who move into managerial positions – and their numbers have increased – have, in many senses, to distance themselves from their origins and background as they move up through the structures, particularly in the area of clinical practice, which leaves few nurses feeling truly represented at a senior level within their health trust.

Even the organisations representing nurses, the trade unions and professional organisations, seem to have lost faith with their members. Although there is a sense of the 'right' things being stated in press releases and national leaders responding to situations that affect their members, there is also a growing gulf. Both the RCN and Unison seem to be increasingly aloof and unresponsive to the problems nurses are facing at the clinical coalface.

Public sympathy and support have held up but it is similar to that accorded a stricken relative or public figure stoical in the face of tragedy. 'They deserve better', people say. 'It's not fair the way the nurses are treated', is the view. But there is a degree of hopelessness and resignation about it all.

Perhaps, most of all, this is because nurses themselves seem to have lost the confidence, and maybe even the courage, to resist their fate. This has to do, at least in part, with relatively recent changes to the way in which healthcare has been re-structured and has been most notable in the broader politics of the NHS. Deciding nurses' pay awards through the Pay Review Body (PRB), rather than negotiations as is still the case with most other NHS staff, may put them in the same category as doctors and dentists – but it has only isolated them from colleagues who share the problem of low pay rather than brought the financial rewards of the medical and dental professions. The commercialisation of ancillary services has seen the loss of tens of thousands of jobs and the employment of significant numbers of people working in the NHS actually employed by private companies without the realisation of the major gains in efficiency promised or any enhancement to the culture or environment of the health service. Significantly, the vast majority of those ancillary staff would once have been trade union members, alongside those nurses who were not in the RCN. The unions were devastated by this haemorrhage of members in a variety of ways (see Chapters 3 and 7). General management, followed by the arrival of the internal market, brought a heightened business culture that was both new and alien to nurses' experience. They were managed differently, less tolerantly. And in this new 'marketplace', money did not just talk. It wheedled and whined like a psychotic whisper that won't go away, it sang out like a demented hyena. Alongside it, the even toned, rational discourse of the clinically oriented nurse was wholly drowned out. Suddenly, everything had a price, a cost code and had to be accounted for. Little seemed to be actually valued in the iconoclastic climate the new managers brought with them, as challenging the status quo and past practice became *de rigeur*; those things which were accorded value by managers were often unpopular with the nurses they were managing. The collective spirit that had proved so important to nurses at crucial moments in their history was broken as nurses' practice was individualised, they sought to cross charge one another and became drawn into arguing that their service provision to colleagues be withdrawn unless it was paid for. Making senior nurses budget holders (but, significantly, not giving them the freedom or authority to actually *manage* budgets, and thus use their resources as they think best or bring any imagination to the process) changed the ideology underpinning nursing. It became a means of getting nurses to sing from that discordant song sheet whilst tying them to practices they would not have previously tolerated. Other changes came with it. Discipline became more rigid than it had been in the history of the NHS and, in the early 1990s, oppressive 'gagging clauses' were introduced, making it virtually impossible to publicly voice concern or dissent without fear of disciplinary action, even about issues in the public interest such as standards of care or staffing levels. A succession of anti-trade union laws seriously impacted upon the unions' effectiveness. Nurse education was moving out of schools of nursing and into higher education. The extension of community care, closure of hospitals, breaking up of services and competition of the internal market created a new way of thinking. Not only were nurses 'different', they were being fragmented and were more separate than ever.

▶ The same but different

More than ever, then, when we think of 'nurses' we have to begin thinking about discrete groups under a very broad umbrella, educated and trained differently, with different working practices, skills and ideologies and often with different aspirations. Sometimes, the differences are even starker:

> Here is a riddle for you: I wear a health service uniform, I take blood, I give injections, gauge blood pressures and empty catheters. Who am I? A nurse, surely? Despite the fact that I do all of these tasks, I will never bear the title of nurse.... Why? Because I am a potential midwife – a pre-registration student of midwifery ... (Robothom, 1997).

As Ms Robothom goes on to point out, many direct entry midwives see themselves as working with essentially healthy women going through the natural process of childbirth and the shift in thinking within the Department of Health echoes this, with increasing numbers of direct access courses. However, there is still tremendous ambiguity in the political relationship between government, employers and midwives. This stretches back to midwifery's origins when working class, untrained midwives, who were often delivering babies for pauperised families, were largely discredited by the emergent medical profession. Doctors were establishing themselves as 'man-midwives' providing obstetric services to wealthier, fee paying middle-class families but needed to expand their scope if they were to become dominant. Even when the thorny issue of training for midwives – initially under the paternalistic and controlling eye of the Obstetric Society and organised by doctors – was established, there was a long struggle for reform and the development of practice which was important in beginning to define the division of labour between doctor and midwife. This, in turn, led to the hospital becoming the main site for the work of the midwife, which was to be highly influential in their socialisation.

Nonetheless, despite having elements of a shared culture and, at one time, their origins in a shared training, in more recent years midwifery has found itself relegated in comparison with nursing. Its practitioners, who see themselves as working in a semi-autonomous way, believe they have been graded lower than their work deserves. Once again, the simple politics of midwifery has seen both major parties support their arguments for improved grading when in opposition but rebuff them when in power (Gould, 1998).

Perhaps it is no coincidence that midwifery has remained a female dominated occupation. The entry into midwifery of men in 1983 has not led to significant changes and, while those entering into it cite a variety of reasons for doing so, career advancement is not high among them (Lewis, 1989). And it is one area within the wider nursing arena where men have not made major inroads into management and practice development forums.

No matter how hard done by midwives feel compared to their nursing colleagues, at least their names remained attached to the new regulatory body replacing the United Kingdom Central Council (UKCC), The Nursing and Midwifery Council. Health visitors expressed outrage that they were excluded from the title of the new body, claiming that this was only one more illustration of the government's lack of understanding about health visiting.

With far more radical origins than any other branch of healthcare, different working practices and health oriented goals, health visiting has long been on the periphery of the nursing world. Its origins had much in common with that of midwifery's, stemming from serious concerns about the rising infant mortality rate in the latter half of the nineteenth century. District nursing was developing at about the same time, and had another common link with midwifery in that one of the earliest proponents of nurses visiting people in their own homes was William Rathbone, who was uncle to Rosalind Paget, a pioneer of midwifery. It was recognised that different skills, training and attitude would be needed from those of hospital-based nurses but, in Manchester and Salford, this was being taken a step further, as a new role was developed, different to nursing and involving health education and promotion. Soon the new health visitors, drawn not only from nurses but a variety of occupations, were given a range of responsibilities, including the key task of visiting every home where a child had been born.

Despite health visiting's successes in helping to lower the infant mortality rate, vital to an imperial nation requiring a fit workforce not only at home but also abroad, being outside the hospital meant it was an occupational group that was never at the centre of healthcare and neither its model nor the attributes thought necessary for a successful health visitor were able to puncture the dominant ideology within nursing.

By the turn of this century, health visiting was seen as being stripped of its skills and knowledge base, as training courses within healthcare faculties were too short and lacked a number of the essentials to prepare future health visitors, omitting such things as child protection, nutrition and child development. With an ageing workforce, averaging out in its late 40s, there are strong fears that health-visiting skills will be lost forever.

It would be easy to understand why the Thatcher government, whose prime minister so famously declared there was no such thing as society, would have found difficulty with some of the principles of health visiting. In its position statement on public health and the role of nurses and health visitors, the Community Practitioners' and Health Visitors' Association (CPHVA), noted that concepts which underlie public health work included 'An emphasis on collective and collaborative action', as well as a 'Recognition of people as members of groups, not only as individuals' (CPHVA, 1997). This philosophy, allied to many of the components of health visiting, would appear integral to New Labour's aims of social inclusion and improving the health of the nation, which could thus be expected to support this occupational group and its work. Child health promotion and child development, child health surveillance, child protection, primary prevention programmes, working in partnership with clients, parenting programmes, working with community groups with special needs, would all seem to be essential not only to the successful care of their families but also to the stated aims and objectives of the government. And yet, in 1998, there were even proposals to shift responsibility for health visiting to the Home Office, changing the emphasis from one of social care to social control. Although these came to nothing, it is an indicator of a new government's willingness to break into nursing's increasingly unstable structures and withdraw what had long been seen as a key component of an overall nursing approach to healthcare, and revealed an insight into the internal debate about care versus social control that has been becoming more overt within government statements and policies in recent years.

The more mainstream strands of nursing have also been subject to changes almost unimaginable twenty or thirty years ago. A major part of that process has been the shift from hospital to community in the late 1980s and early 1990s. The number of hospital closures under, particularly, the Thatcher government, was unprecedented and left nurses scrabbling to keep up as they were not only finding themselves re-located outside the familiar institutional surroundings but also with rapidly changing roles.

Community mental health nurses suddenly faced a massive increase in the number of people with severe and enduring mental illness in their communities. It was clear that their training was wholly inadequate for the work they now were expected to undertake, a problem further exacerbated by Project 2000, which still did not address basic issues such as mental health assessment and crisis management or equipped nurses with an understanding of the techniques and interventions needed to take on the evolved nursing role that was now expected of them both in hospital and the community. They were also, at the time of the mass exodus from long stay hospitals, still working to different priorities, often focused on a clientele that had been referred from General Practitioners (GPs) or others working in primary care. Those people newly discharged from psychiatric institutions, with more serious and enduring mental health problems or long established mental illness, who did not engage with their community psychiatric nurse (CPN) or attend for outpatient appointments, were often then lost to services as the CPNs continued to focus on their earlier, more compliant client group and demands from GPs for a service for their patients. New nursing interventions and skills had to be developed – but not before a string of horrific tragedies had led to demands for widespread reforms. Acute mental health wards were another area where nursing suffered. Chronic staff shortages meant that often very inexperienced staff were trying to care for a group of patients who were more acutely disturbed and distressed than ever. The overall level of disturbance on the wards was only exacerbated by the rapidly shortening length of stay for all patients. Moreover, because of the pressure to make beds available for new admissions all kinds of practices, that would have been unthinkable only a few years previously have become part of every nurse's daily practice. Thus, people would be discharged earlier than was clinically appropriate, shifted from one hospital to another in the middle of the night, sent home on leave to make way for someone else to be admitted, only to find there was no bed available for them to return to. 'Managing beds' became the dominant activity rather than spending time and engaging with patients. Consequently, there was no time or opportunity to develop the skills' base and standards of therapeutic activity dropped even further.

Perhaps, this example of one factor that has influenced mental health nursing on acute wards gives a clue to how 'nursing failings' can actually be driven by the needs of the organisation at a number of levels. If nurses on acute mental health wards are working to their optimum, developing their skills and innovative practice, they will almost certainly want to keep some patients on the ward for longer periods as they help them with complex problems and behaviours that community teams, for a variety of reasons, may not be able to address. However, this conflicted with the financial and organisational objectives of almost every mental health unit in the country, which was to discharge people as quickly as possible and ensure that private beds were not used, at massive cost, to accommodate more people than the unit could manage from its own bed numbers. This financially driven set of priorities has been re-framed, of course, in the language of liberalism and progressive thinking. Most clinicians, relatives and patients themselves want to see people cared for in their own communities rather than hospital settings. Most nurses wholeheartedly buy into this philosophy but few question its financial and political context or worry about the consequences for nursing or the client group.

Work undertaken by the Sainsbury Centre for Mental Health highlighted major concerns around training, the fitness of newly qualified staff to practice and a widening gap between training and actual practice. As in so many other areas of nursing, surveys of staff and managers revealed, post-internal market, an alarming lack of co-operation between trusts (Duggan *et al.*, 1997).

Mental health nurses have, then, been subjected to as much change as any other group and there are indications that their thoughts about how they would have liked the process to have been handled are as representative as those of nurses in any other arena. Research has shown, unsurprisingly, that they would like change to have been managed more constructively and sensitively. When that change was perceived as being economically and politically driven, there was a feeling that consultation had been poor and, with a lack of middle management, they had been excluded from decision making, with those decisions being made by remote, non-nursing figures. A lack of control over staffing issues affected them and they were left in situations which undermined attempts at therapeutic work and the nurse–patient relationship. They also thought that, by being excluded from decision and policy making, they could 'never pose a threat' and were 'soft targets' if things subsequently went wrong. Interestingly, a group of mental health nurses interviewed by Peter Nolan were able to acknowledge they were poor at collaborating with colleagues from other fields of nursing but also noted the existence of inter-disciplinary tensions and jealousies (Ritter S, 1997; Nolan *et al.*, 1999). The need for better quality training that prepares nurses for the work they have to do, access to practice based research and good clinical supervision to help them whilst they do it are, unsurprisingly, constant themes.

Mental health nurses working in the community are, like their colleagues in any number of settings, having to learn to work across disciplines and with nurses from other clinical arenas. This is a 'development' which follows the planned fragmentation of services and nursing teams, as moves into the community, the purchasing of services and other major organisational changes took effect. This requires a process of familiarisation with different services and how they operate, the roles of other nurses and the perceptions and attitudes held about both their own and colleagues' work.

Invariably, there is a wide discrepancy between perception and reality, as evidenced by some work undertaken with practice nurses and CPNs. After a week long workshop, there were considerable changes in attitude about each other's work and the way in which individuals operated within their own discipline, virtually all of which were reported as favourable, particularly in relation to skill levels and, in the case of the CPN's view of practice nurses, their autonomy and relationship with patients (Nolan *et al.*, 1998). Inevitably, one of the issues about practice nurses is that they are 'in the belly of the beast', working with GPs in their practice. This has long been something of which many nurses have been wary, with the view that their autonomy and independence will be subsumed. It was certainly a major factor in community mental health nurses arguing that they should remain in separate teams, managed within mental health services. On this occasion, their arguments were supported by managers who feared that they would not be able to focus services on those with severe and enduring mental illness, whereas GPs would often seek to direct community mental health services to those who, despite having less serious mental illness, would present to general practice and often prove both time consuming and difficult to busy doctors.

Community nurses were not so lucky. Criticised in the Cumberledge Report as tending towards inflexibility in working patterns and having a poor track record of collaboration with other disciplines, they, too, also faced wider change (DHSS,

Neighbourhood Nursing: A focus for care, London, HMSO, 1986). A gradual shift in the policy of successive Conservative governments saw primary healthcare come to be even more dominated by general practice and the GP. Community nurses were drawn along in the wake of these changes, away from a holistic, public health and health promotion oriented approach. As has so often been the case, as one branch of nursing ran into trouble, another saw its star rising. With money being withdrawn from health visiting and community nursing posts, practice nursing flourished, its numbers increasing dramatically. However, this was not just about money; something else was happening. These changes reflected a philosophical change at governmental level about the nature of healthcare, from a collective, macro approach to healthcare, not just in the community but *with* a community, to an individualised, micro perspective. As GP's – long established as individualised practitioners – became fund holders and their already considerable influence grew, historical loyalties to occupational groups and working relationships within community nursing were altered (Walsh and Gough, 1997). There have been changes of a different nature under New Labour, particularly in developing the nurse practitioner's role in GP practices, and in relation to the development of General Medical Services. Yet, it is still easy to see a terminological and conceptual pre-disposition to view primary care as the province of the GP, with the nurse filling in on tasks and the parts of the role of GPs that have either been delegated or prised away to enable them to deliver other government priorities. That there is another side to this complex relationship can be seen when we examine the changes that have led to the introduction of services such as NHS Direct and Walk In Centres (see Chapter 3).

Nurse practitioners could lay claim to the title of contemporary's nursing's storm troopers, as they break new ground. Although most are now employed by GPs, their greater levels of autonomy means they see their own patients, undertake, amongst other things, chronic disease management, overseeing infection control, family planning, giving immunisations and carrying out local cervical cytology programmes. Many also have their own area of speciality, such as running asthma clinics. The UKCC, in March 2000, announced that the number of nurses recording nurse prescribing qualifications on the register rose from 2177 to 10,293 during that year.

Despite the enormous difficulties nursing has faced, in almost every sphere, groups of nurses *have* made tremendous strides forward. In mental health, nurses have developed the role of case management with new and focused interventions that have a life changing quality for people with severe and enduring mental illness, developed their role in crisis work, assessment, liaison psychiatry and the use of assertive outreach, behavioural and cognitive techniques. In intensive care, nurses have developed their role to such an extent that critics complain they could be technicians or are too close to the role of the doctor. In the field of elderly care, advances in person-centred approaches to dementia care have, again, demonstrated the scope of nursing practice in areas that once seemed so limited.

Are healthcare assistants (HCAs) nurses? At one time, the answer would depend on to whom you spoke. The RCN used to be clear that they were not. Those like Unison's Professional Officer, Paul Chapman, who championed the cause of the HCA even more than was politically necessary for his union to recruit from their number, have long argued that they are, and that it is only elitism and academic snobbery that has prevented the value of their work being acknowledged, limiting opportunities for them to have a career ladder upon which to progress, most notably into the arena of nurse registered training. Chapman takes his case even further, while at the same time looking at the practical situation facing HCAs, their trained colleagues and employers, as well as more ideologically contentious issues, stating that

> Nursing has failed to prevent unqualified staff undertaking registered nursing work without proper training or any statutory mechanisms for protecting the public (Chapman, 2000: p 28).

Such a statement places a clinical concern – that untrained staff are undertaking the work of their registered, or trained, colleagues – and then throws two significant political elements in the mix. First, 'nursing', and not nurses, has sought unsuccessfully to prevent this happening and that, by tacitly allowing the situation 'nursing' places the public at risk. This is another example of how many issues within the nursing debate need an external context. Chapman points out that 'The bulk of literature on HCAs sees them as not significant in themselves or in their impact on care but rather in comparison with, and in relation to, registered nurses' (Chapman *op. cit.*). As comes up time and again, this is linked to the notion of 'care' and whether or not that is the key nursing function.

The RCN made a political *volte face* that can only be described as astonishing, given its history in this area and attitude towards untrained staff, when its membership voted to accept HCAs into their number. As a consequence, it had to accept, by an extension of that logic, that HCAs were nurses.[3]

Perhaps the changes that have had the biggest 'internal' impact on nursing and will have the greatest long term consequences have been in the field of education. Cuts of 26 per cent in student numbers between 1992 and 1995 under the

---

[3] For the purposes of this book, it has to be acknowledged that HCAs do carry out work that overlaps with that of their trained colleagues but they cannot be considered 'the same'. To do so would fail to recognise the impact of the education and training that culminates in nurses being registered. It is not to suggest that HCAs cannot attain the same levels of education or carry out much of the work of trained nurses. Their considerable contribution to healthcare will emerge, particularly in times of major shortages of trained staff, just as has always been the case with enrolled nurses, another neglected group (in terms of pay, policy and official recognition, at least).

Conservative government, occurred while Project 2000 removed student nurses from schools of nursing attached to teaching hospitals. This immediately altered the socialisation process that had previously taken place exclusively within the nursing world, a rarefied atmosphere for students both within the school and workplace that was controlled and modified by senior nurses and nurse tutors. It was replaced by the university, healthcare faculty and student centred learning, with learners finally becoming supernumerary on their placements and the balance of clinical work and education being significantly shifted towards the latter. But it's not just the education of nurses that's been turned upside down. The world of the educationalists has become one of the 'consortium', with contracts, 'change management' (another of the Orwellian terms rolling around the NHS, which has become far too familiar to contemporary nurses and on occasions translates into being mucked about, given more work with no increase in salary and a new management structure that makes the work of the staff managed a lot less understood and more difficult). Similarly, they have seen their services 'rationalised' which, in English, means being cut and people made redundant. Those who survived are now lecturers, often lecturing in cramped conditions, with too many students to allow imaginative, high quality teaching that actively involves the student or individual tutoring and having to cram in too much course admin, marking and other work into the day.

The trained nurses mentoring the student, having been forged in a system that has gone through the revolutions of general management and the internal market, are now facing the reforms of New Labour. It can be guaranteed that almost all of them will have seen their workplace re-organised, re-structured and merged at some time in their career.[4] Some will have come through the clinical grading exercise that scarred the late 1980s. Many more will be based in community settings away from the hospital environments in which they were trained. Of course, history refuses to stand still and Project 2000 trained nurses now occupy senior positions in charge of wards and units. Another cycle is set to be completed as yet more changes are set to affect nurse education. Still further change awaits, as acts of parliament take effect, including *The New NHS: Modern, Dependable* (1997), *A First Class Service: Quality in the New NHS* (1998) and *Saving Lives: Our Healthier Nation* (1999), *Making A Difference* (1999), *Improving Working Lives* (2001) and *The NHS Plan* (2000), added to other government initiatives, such as clinical governance, new pay structures, more Trust mergers, Primary Care Groups, Primary Care Trusts and nurse consultants.

---

[4] Few nurses will take comfort from news that their perception of the inefficiency of mergers has been confirmed by research which found that they delay improvements to their services, lower staff morale and increase stress while they don't meet the financial savings targets expected. Staff often feel senior managers are ignoring their needs post-merger and that they are less involved in decision making (Fulop *et al.*, 2002: pp 246–9).

► Valuing difference or creating new elites?

The relationship nursing has with other occupational and professional groups has evolved a great deal, sometimes in relation to the waxing and waning fortunes of those groups, but, as is explored in detail in subsequent chapters, is still dominated by its deeply political connection to the medical profession. Doctors have seen much of their world challenged and change has been no stranger, even in their darkest and most conservative corners. Certainly, New Labour has exploited the many opportunities presented by the profession's abject failure to regulate itself with any meaningful sense of purpose and particularly when it has most needed to. Scandals such as those surrounding the murders committed by the GP, Harold Shipman, plus a whole series of practitioners found guilty of astonishing levels of incompetence, have presented the government with an open goal as they have sought to undermine the historical dominance and hegemony the medical profession has held in the NHS and used to resist unwelcome change. Yet, doctors still determine much of what nurses do or don't do. Considering how this happened will tell us much about the nature of nursing, why the work was shaped in the way it was, as well as how those relationships developed in the way they did. The symbiotic relationship of the nurse and doctor became even more explicit as the work of their respective groups evolved. Such is their closeness that the advent of nurse practitioners, nurse prescribing, Walk In Centres, NHS Direct and, to a lesser extent, the nurse consultant could not have happened without changes to the doctor's role.

It is typical, perhaps, of New Labour's vastly different, apparently non-ideological politics of the new millennium that, while denying nurses across the board pay rises that would bring them a serious clinical career structure, rewarding all nurses staying with the patient in the clinical arena, it has increased numbers of nurse practitioners and made real the concept of the nurse consultant. The announcement of these new posts saw the tabloids' headlines heralding the arrival of 'Supernurses' (*sic*) but many nurses greeted the decision with deep scepticism. Nonetheless, this was the most explicit attempt yet at marrying an increased status with a seriously competitive salary, albeit one that came nowhere near parity with medical consultants (see Figure 1.1). The complication, spotted immediately by nurses at all levels, was that it was another step down the road of a well paid elite that left the vast majority of the workforce a long way behind. Nurses are generally very wary of elites and have no desire to be further split by an extended system of grades.

This dislike of difference and a widening of pay differentials is, in some senses puzzling in a hierarchical occupational group such as nursing. It reflects two distinct and opposing views. On the one hand, there is a deeply conservative inability to adopt a pluralist perspective. It reflects a suspicion of embracing difference and hostility towards the opportunity for nurses, however few in numbers, to progress and become senior figures in healthcare, thus enabling them to work with

Nurse consultants	£27,000 – £42,000
Medical consultant	£48,905 – £63, 640
Discretionary points for consultants*	£2,550 – £20,365

Figure 1.1   Nursing and medical consultants' pay (2000–2001)
*Paid in addition to the basic salary.

colleagues from other occupational groups and professions as equals. However, it also reflects an alternative view, that nurse's can develop a collective identity and hold on to the aspiration of advancing as a whole rather than on a piecemeal basis. This comes out of nursing's hidden, radical tradition, with a recognition that the widening of the gap does nothing to advance the cause of the whole workforce and only further divides – and thus weakens – an already fragmented group.

The contradictions that emerge in this issue highlight familiar problems: how can the cause of individuals or sub-groups of such a diverse and disparate group of workers be advanced at the same time as the whole group? If that is not possible, should nurses relinquish their collective identity and pursue their own interests within their own discrete groups, sometimes acknowledging and capitalising upon the competing agendas of other groups of staff, colleagues and employers? That would take a cultural shift of seismic proportions, not just amongst nurses themselves but also from their representatives. The nursing unions have long fought against letting any group 'break away' from the pack, although each has sought to propel particular grades and groups on occasions when it has been politically useful. Nonetheless, when the last Conservative government was determined to introduce local pay bargaining in the mid-1990s, the unions were prepared to go to the wire to prevent it – indeed, the RCN abandoned its opposition to proposals to end its famous Rule 12, which banned any member from taking part in industrial action of any sort. This was something it had vehemently resisted in previous years, despite being under tremendous pressure to change policy, notably at the time of the pre and post clinical grading dispute.

It is of interest that the trade unions and professional organisations should so desperately want to hold nurses together within a bargaining framework, denying the differences, particularly given their lack of success in advancing the cause of the massed ranks as a whole. And it would appear nurses everywhere, whatever their background, want to go along with it, as there were no strenuous demands to abandon national bargaining and allow groups to strike out on their own. In fact, local pay bargaining is one of the few radical policies on the NHS put forward by the Conservatives that the unions were able to resist, having unsuccessfully opposed privatisation, general management, hospitals and services moving to Trust status, the introduction of the internal market and GP fund holding – although by this time the government was severely weakened and there was little managerial support for the concept (or, at least, the incredible demands upon managers' time and workload that would have gone with it). Yet, changes have been made by New Labour that would suggest that local differentials will be very much part of the future despite remaining apparently opposed to the concept of local pay and treating different groups of nurses differently, as they had been when in opposition. So no one seems quite able to decide. Nurses are different from one another yet they are the same: they should be treated equally but, sometimes, some should be treated more equally than others. Some might just be special. Looking in more detail at who – and how many – are doing what, provides some insight into the thinking behind such judgements, about the politics of the decisions. Particularly if recent historical changes are tracked.

▶ How many nurses? The numbers game

The raw politics of numbers for nurses revolve around how many staff they have in their team, how many patients they have to care for or treat, how many extra hours they have to work in a week. On the national stage, the numbers are bigger, the arguments are louder and there is not the clarity found at the clinical coalface. If a ward has five vacancies, it takes on a logic of its own, for both staff and patients; there are shifts to be covered, nurses needed for escort duties, with a need to allocate more patients to each available nurse. Only if the team is lucky, is there the problem of integrating a variety of bank or agency nurses. Within the Trust, managers may point to all sorts of complexities – about, perhaps, having to prioritise the funding of other posts, the effects of 'overspends' (rarely do managers refer to 'underfunded services' – even after the government declared in 1999, in a politically bold move, that the NHS as a whole *was* underfunded) but, nationally, it is such a tangled set of computations, claims and counter claims that what should be a straightforward, objective measurement almost becomes too difficult to unravel. Probably everyone is familiar with New Labour's reputation as the masters of political 'spin'. In the case of the NHS, this manifested as double counting the funding for new posts, announcing increases in nurse numbers twice, as if each announcement heralded more staff to come into the service. But such tactics are, in fact, nothing new. A major feature of the health debate in the 1980s was to look in detail at how many nurses were actually working in the NHS, Labour regularly charged the Conservatives with 'destroying' the NHS while Margaret Thatcher's Tories famously declared the NHS was 'safe in (their) hands'. In many respects, this was a hollow argument designed to allow political point scoring. It certainly ignored issues about the increasing number of nurses working part time or the effect of reducing nurses' hours, for instance, a policy the previous Labour government had agreed and which the Tories were obliged to implement following its electoral victory in 1979. Neither party got close to asking the far more necessary questions about what nurses are needed for, how many nurses might be needed for the work expected of them and, again, what numbers of nurses are needed in particular areas of nursing. In fact, behind the rhetoric and politicking the numbers of nurses working in the NHS actually did rise under the first Thatcher government by almost 50,000, to just under 400,000. But, when the additional 20,000 posts needed to compensate for a reduction in nurses' hours from 40 to 37.5 per week are taken into account, it was much smaller than the government were seeking credit for. The sums were further complicated by how many posts were part or full time, how many there were at particular grades, how many were students or untrained nursing staff. Because of the deployment of nurses into specialist areas, the whole equation was even more difficult to work out. Later on in the 1980s, acute shortages of nurses on children's surgical wards and ITU produced a blaze of publicity that led to major unrest in the health service, with nurses campaigning about their pay and employment, as well as the conditions restricting their ability to nurse their patients in the way they felt they should, all of which fed into the year long dispute about clinical grading. It was a blaze of publicity that would never have been generated by the chronic shortages on elderly care or mental health wards and one which failed to recognise that shortages of nurses are as old as nursing. But that's politics.

The situation in the 1990s became even more complex. With the coming of NHS trusts and the internal market, the running down of the regions and devolution of managerial authority, the availability of centralised statistics became more problematic, with Ministers suddenly – and, some would say, conveniently – unable to quantify bed losses, nursing redundancies, staff in post and the like because this was the business of the trusts and not a matter for government. Where once nursing staff were differentiated by the area they worked in, they were grouped together as 'community and hospital staff' by the Department, which is how they are categorised still.

The UKCC's annual statistics show there were 634,529 nurses on its register in the year ending March 2000, an increase of just 300 from the previous year. Prior to that, the Council had noted three years of decline. This may have been due to more people finishing their training to become trained nurses and midwives but is more likely to have resulted from a major increase in the numbers of nurses being recruited form overseas. The continued fall in nurses registered in Scotland, Wales and Northern Ireland supports this, as efforts to recruit from overseas have been far more prominent in England and it is to this country that the majority have come to work. This flow of labour has not been one way, however. Although 7383, nurses came into the United Kingdom, 5083 went the other way, the highest figure since 1990/91.

Long-term trends indicating more men on the register and an ageing force were maintained in 1999/2000. The proportion of men rose from 9.48 to 9.75 per cent, the highest ever recorded. The proportion of people on the register aged 50 and over increased from 23.30 to 23.86 per cent, also the highest ever recorded. At the start of the 1990s, 58.22 per cent of people on the register were under 40. As the decade ended, that proportion had declined to 46.46 per cent (NMC, *www.nmc-uk.org*).

Recent figures from the Department of Health show nursing numbers reaching their highest figure of the decade in 1999. However, the same figures show a steady decline in the numbers of *trained* nurses working in the NHS in England. These Department of Health statistics are broadly reflective of the United Kingdom as a whole, as confirmed by the UKCC, who reported the overall number of nurses registered had slumped to a seven-year low of 634,229. An overall fall of 3 per cent in the numbers of trained nurses since 1992 was also recorded by the Department.[5] Although it could point to a rise in unqualified staff of 8 per cent, there had, of course, been the loss of student nurses in the equation: pre-Project 2000 students were counted as part of the workforce and worked shifts as part of the teams they were allocated to, working alongside trained colleagues, but the newer students were not. Although the 1999 figures were bleak, the Central Council took some comfort in finding that fewer nurses had left the register – 21,174, compared to 27,173 the previous year, as well as with the fact that the number of newly registered nurses had risen by 10 per cent to 17,954. Apparent staffing crises and shortages of nurses are nothing new (although devastating for those nurses who are left to maintain adequate standards of care), as we shall see. However, the 1999 figures did highlight a different phenomenon about recruitment. Significant numbers of the near 18,000 nurses registering with the UKCC for the first time were coming from overseas. Around 1335 were from European Union countries such as Finland, Ireland or Sweden. Nearly 600 were from South Africa. Although there was a political outcry about the NHS being staffed by nurses from other parts of the world, as ever this reflected a lack of understanding or interest in nursing history. Ireland has long been used as a rich vein for recruitment whenever the economy there has been in trouble, as has the West Indies in the past. Indeed, nurses from both countries have been no stranger to controversy, particularly when issues about recognition, grading and promotion have come under the microscope.

The issue of race and ethnicity is another of the many 'demographic timebombs' set to explode in the face of politicians and civil servants, as it is now recognised that nearly 30 per cent of black nurses are set to retire in the coming decade. As with the rest of the nursing workforce in the NHS, black and ethnic minority nurses are an ageing group, with 40 per cent being aged over 40 (O'Dowd, 2000: p 5). In fact, well over 50 per cent of nurses, overall, are aged 35 and over and, critics of cuts in student numbers in the early 1990s were pointing to the falling numbers of females of a suitable age which meant that the government would have to recruit nearly

---

[5] The Department of Health figures for the number of qualified nurses, midwives and health visitors working in the NHS in 2002 was 330,000 or 260,000 whole time equivalents, with 33,000 healthcare assistants. This is out of an overall NHS workforce of approximately 1,166,000 people, making it Europe's largest employer. The medical and dental workforce numbers 74,000, with 26,000 consultants (see Chapter 8).

one-third of all available school leavers to maintain a steady state. This obviously creates the minor irritation of having posts available but no one to fill them, a particular problem in inner cities but also affecting different groups even more acutely. The wave of strikes and demonstrations in the late 1980s occurred in the context of vacancy levels of more than 20 per cent in London's teaching hospitals – a vacancy rate that is consistent with those of 2002.

So here we are, getting older, with more vacancies, and although New Labour are promising more staff and more students to be recruited, such plans are not so easy to enact, for even if the numbers of people necessary can be tempted to apply, there are still problems about having enough lecturers to teach them, enough placements for students to attend, with sufficient mentors to guide them through that placement. Educational facilities are already too cramped for existing numbers. If these were not enough of a disincentive, it was reckoned in 1997 to cost up to £1500 a year for a newly qualified nurse to actually get herself to work (Buswell, 1997) and the maximum earning potential for a well educated, skilled and experienced nurse staying in the clinical arena is not going to be more than £30,000 pa, a decade, perhaps, after qualification, which in no way compares to that which many other graduates could earn. Given all this, and not forgetting what many see as the most important issue of all – bursaries and payment – it's no surprise that up to 30 per cent of students won't finish their training. Moreover, Michael Walker, a Unison full time official working with students across London, stated that as few as 25 per cent may actually go on to build a career in the NHS (Revill, 1999). Given that the cost of training a student is estimated at £35,000, that's a lot of money being wasted.

The big question is whether or not New Labour's extra billions for the NHS have done enough to reverse the trend. That is not yet clear and, perhaps, it is very similar to the situation with the railways in that, having stuck with the previous Tory government's spending plans for the first two years of their term of office, it is a case of too little too late – the damage to the infrastructure of the service having been so great that, at the very least in the symbolic sense, the NHS was going to be completely derailed before the extra money and reforms could get it back on track.

▶ The discontent behind the numbers

Through all this and despite much political rhetoric, nursing is still women's work, performed by a workforce made up largely of women but managed by disproportionately large numbers of men despite positive changes in the last few years. As remarked above, the 9.48 per cent men in the nursing workforce in 1999 represents the largest number ever. But why do so many of the few go on to occupy the most senior positions? Family life no doubt plays its part. Women have babies, and thus time off or 'career breaks', from which it takes time to regain a momentum, particularly after a second birth and the likelihood of moving into part-time work. They may have to uproot and move jobs if their partner, quite likely to be the

major wage earner, switches location to aid his career development, something
a working woman cannot always do. Widely recognised factors that hold back
women's career development, such as a lack of childcare facilities, no flexibility in
working practices and an unwillingness to promote women working part-time
hours have been widely recognised by the government, but there are clearly other
issues to be considered. Some have their origins in nursing history and in the contemporary politics of nursing particularly, while others have their genesis in the
wider gender issues visible in work and society more generally. It is significant that
the careers of men in nursing were only really kick started when men were admitted into the RCN in 1960.

It is, however, particularly dispiriting to examine the results of research undertaken
by the Policy Studies Institute, which shows that men get on despite often being less
well qualified, post registration, and having less experience. Nor was it a matter of
more motivated staff making their way up the ladder – the research found that female
nurses were no less interested in career advancement than their male counterparts –
although less expectant of progress. And with good reason, for it was not only at more
senior grades that the discrepancies were noticed, but at 'F' and 'G' grades, which
women found difficult to be promoted into (Finlayson and Nazroo, 1998).

Policies such as equal opportunities may now be so well established that virtually every nurse in the country can recite them like a mantra at interview. Yet, in
practice, there is clearly a long way to go, as there are in so many other areas of
employee relations and workforce issues.

These failures go a long way to account for the high levels of dissatisfaction in
nursing. And nurses are highly dissatisfied. A survey for the *Nursing Times* in 1998
revealed that 56 per cent of respondents felt less able to meet the needs of patients
than when they had started nursing. About 59 per cent felt patients' expectations
were unrealistically high (Vousden, 1998). This survey's findings were pretty tame
when compared to those of nursing's two main trade unions, Unison and the
RCN.[6] The RCN's evidence to the PRB in 1999 showed nurses' feeling to be under

---

[6] The RCN describes itself, at different times, as both a trade union and professional organisation, depending on the context in which it is working, the way it
wishes to project itself and the argument it is putting forward. Thus, on industrial
relations issues, it is a trade union; when advancing views about nurse education it
is a professional organisation. In truth, particularly in recent years since it
renounced Rule 12 which had previously effectively barred its members from taking
any industrial action, it has straddled these contradictory positions more successfully. But, as is explored in detail in Chapter 7, the contradictions remain. Certainly,
it does have more of a clearly defined trade union role than the organisation most
like it in the United States, the American Nurses' Association, which, in effect, has
a far more circumscribed role absent of direct industrial relations involvement – and
smaller membership as a consequence. Nonetheless, for the purposes of this book it
is necessary to work with these descriptions and, at different stages, the RCN will be
referred to both as a professional organisation and trade union.

more pressure than at any time other than 1995, with more than 30 per cent strongly agreeing that they 'would leave nursing if [they] could'. 'D' grade nurses were reported to often be the only trained nurse on duty for wards with twenty beds or more – although the distinction between 'D' and 'E' grade was clearly established at the time of clinical grading as being in charge for one or more shift per week. Moreover, because of staffing shortages, nurses were also working consecutive day and night shifts to keep their wards going; the higher the grade the higher the percentage working excess hours in a week. The most pressured groups in the RCN survey were those working on medical and surgical wards, while the least pressured were nurses working in general practice.

In its evidence for 1999, the RCM claimed that 106 out of 137 maternity units were understaffed, with 57 per cent of heads of midwifery stating that staffing levels were inadequate. More than 80 per cent were still employing midwives at 'E' grade despite Department of Health guidance that they should be at a minimum of 'F' grade.

Unison found, perhaps unsurprisingly, that 83 per cent don't believe they were well paid for their jobs, even more than in the previous year. Twenty-two per cent were doing a second job to supplement their income. Seventy-nine per cent reported an increase in their workload while 90 per cent said stress levels had increased.

A more discrete survey, conducted amongst community mental health nurses (CMHNs), revealed some alarming statistics, suggesting that a very high proportion of CMHNs experienced extreme levels of stress. Forty per cent of respondents to the survey reported low self-esteem and felt others had little respect for them, often associated with unsupportive line managers (Burnard P *et al.*, 2000: pp 28–30). However, what was notable about this was that its results only echoed a number of other surveys amongst nurses both in mental health and general nursing.

What is worth exploring in a little more detail, at this stage, are the reasons behind the dissatisfaction. However, it is even more interesting to compare those reasons for more historical attitudes held by nurses in relation to their work. Surveys carried out during the period of the last two governments carry eerie echoes of a past era. The *Nursing Mirror* undertook a national survey in 1937, at the height of the first period of major unrest amongst general nurses working predominantly in London's teaching hospitals; Unison's evidence to the PRB in 1993 came after the election of John Major's Conservative government, following on the back of three successive Tory governments led by Margaret Thatcher; the *Nursing Times'* survey was carried out in 1998, after New Labour had been in power just over one year (Table 1.1).

This raises a fundamental question: if the solution to resolving nurses' grievances is as simple as many suggest, why has no one done it in the last seventy odd years? Perhaps it's worth considering who is suggesting that the solution is simple. Generally, it is the politicians – always while in opposition – representatives of nursing unions and many nurses themselves. The 'solution' almost always includes improving pay. Indeed, for some it begins and ends there. Yet, as shall be seen, political parties almost always change their tune once in power, while resolving the issues behind nurses' discontent are far from simple.

Table 1.1 Main sources of nurses' discontent, ranked in order

1937	1993	1998
Hours of duty	Managers' treatment of staff	Pay
Rates of pay	Having to compromise on standards of care	Lack of training
Petty restrictions	Staff shortages	Status
Lectures in off-duty hours	Unfair grading	Long hours
Prospects for advancement	Levels of pay	Poor staffing levels
Interchangeable pensions	Problems with patterns of working hours	Poor conditions of service

Sources: Nursing Mirror, 1938; Unison, 1993; *Nursing Times*, 1998.

Despite registering such high levels of discontent in 1998, nurses' voting intentions had changed little. Fifty-one per cent were supporting Labour prior to May 1997, the number reported as having actually voted for them in that election. A year later, the number supporting the government had fallen by only 2 per cent. Interestingly, 64 per cent of nurses said they would vote Labour in a *Nursing Times* poll conducted in January 2000 *despite* 51 per cent saying they were still considering leaving the NHS. Although there was strong support for many initiatives from the Blair government that were seen to have improved *nursing*, such as the introduction of nurse consultants, Walk In Centres, primary care groups and NHS Direct, 63 per cent perceived there had been no improvement in their overall status *as nurses* [my emphasis] (Coombes, 2000).

There does not seem to be a strong correlation between nurses' voting intentions and their contemporaneous perception of their own status and well being as a group. Politically, they have changed allegiances significantly over the past two decades, switching support from Labour to the Conservatives in the 1980s before ditching the Major government along with the rest of the populace in 1997. It's no surprise, of course, that nurses' voting intentions are going to reflect those of the country, given that there are so many of them and they are not immune to the wider political vicissitudes and concerns about political issues that don't directly affect their employment or the NHS (although it's worth noting that nurses' could easily swing seats in marginal constituencies – something no one has ever chosen to capitalise upon). However, when we later examine reasons for making political choices, it's highly questionable whether or not nurses make decisions based on their needs and best interests. It could be said that, once more, this is no different to the rest of the electorate. But maybe nurses are that little bit different, given that there is so much evidence of direct political decisions that permeate their everyday working environment. We shall see.

▶ The politics *about* nursing and nurses

What is abundantly clear is that nurses are less politically attuned, less politically involved *as nurses, about nursing* than they have been in decades. Many nurses switch off to national and local politics. This is common. People do it, whatever their job, personal, social or economic situation. But the loss of any sense of involvement in the direct politics of their own working lives is something else. Even at times when nurses were supposedly at their most 'angelic' there was a fire burning in the hearts of radical pioneers, women – for it was almost always women – who could see something that was not yet on the horizon, had not yet been imagined by their colleagues, but who had the ability to find like-minded individuals and lead nurses forward, to seek change and, most importantly, progress. Even if that involved struggle. That has not happened on any widespread basis since 1988, despite a still significant number of local disputes and campaigns, with committed nurses taking stands against things they believe to be wrong or for things they think should be happening, often in alliance with other health workers and, on occasions, users of services.

Why this is will, obviously, be the subject of the rest of this book. One viewpoint represented by Julia Fabricus is that nursing has undergone another period of profound change and, as a consequence, nurses feel differently about themselves. Prefacing her position by accepting the proposition that nursing is 'in crisis', Ms Fabricus argues:

> What is the crisis in nursing about? It can be analysed in many ways: politically, sociologically; in terms of pay, working hours, changes in the health service, changes in public expectation. Nurses feel badly used and held in low esteem I ... suggest that the crisis is primarily due to the sickness in the nursing profession and that this sickness, like many psychological illnesses, is caused by a deficit in professional *self*-esteem. Of course, no one would disagree that self-esteem in the profession is low at present, and that is part of the low morale. But my suggestion is that the low self-esteem is the *cause* rather than the *effect* of the crisis (Fabricus, 1999: p 203).

This is an interesting argument in that it supposes that nursing is in crisis, which is usually defined as a turning point (especially of disease, which neatly fits Ms Fabricus' analogy), a moment or brief period of danger or suspense. However, there's little suspense about the current state of nursing, more a state of chronic fatigue. Nor is there a sense of this being a brief period of difficulty; if one charts the history of 'modern' nursing at 150 years, nursing has been plagued with similar episodes of gloom and despondency for at least the last eighty years. These have almost always echoed past narratives, from before the First World War, the 1930s, to during and after Second World War and from the 1970s onwards. If low self-esteem is cause rather than effect, it has been present over a very long period. It is an inherited deficit. Evidence of its longevity may be seen in some of the factors described in the three surveys featured in Table 1.1. Status, prospects for advancement, the way nurses are treated, are all there with pay. But what complicates those problems is an assumption that these are there to be resolved, that is, improved upon by someone else. Government and/or politicians, managers, doctors, other nurses – someone, somewhere – will have to do something that will change this feeling. Fabricus' argument that the nursing profession suffers from something akin to depression, the remedy to which lies 'not in some kind of social Prozac ... but in psychological work by the profession as a whole', (Fabricus, *op. cit.*) then appears to have a valid point.

Something in this analysis is missing, however; in every depression there are precipitating and maintenance factors. Fabricus argues that nursing is engaged in turning away from its own special and important role. This is often referred to, almost in shorthand, as 'caring', which is denigrated alongside more academic or evidence-based interventions and seen as being inferior to the apparently curative work of the doctor. When this apparently simplistic term, 'caring', is elaborated upon, however, it can be seen as something far more complex, involving spending time with a person who is ill, distressed or disturbed by disease, injury, illness or health problems. It involves demonstrating a capacity to observe, listen and think about the patient's suffering, being able to engage them in a way that enables the nurse and patient to work towards an understanding of his or her problems, before identifying helpful ways in which these can be addressed, and also recognising that 'cure' is not always an attainable goal. Within the sterile debate about whether or not nurses should restrict their role to caring, other issues are at play. The old question about how nurses can attain status is an obvious and still important one – remembering that measures that bring status to nursing, such as nurse consultants, an extended role for nurse practitioners, do not result in the vast majority of nurses feeling better about themselves. The thorny question of professionalism, whether or not nurses can be professionals and how nurses are seen in relation to other 'professionals' also lurks beneath the surface. Alternately, does increased pay bring its own reward?

The personal and political, the ways in which nurses perceive themselves, are often separated out in such debates. Yet, the personal and political are intrinsically bound up in this analysis. How nurses feel about themselves influences how they act and how they think. These, in turn, influence how they feel about themselves. In this cycle, inherited imagination, myth, tradition and ideology are as important as actual events. The difficulty in 'owning' the dilemmas facing nurses, acting and moving towards resolving then pervades almost everything about nursing. One of the foremost influences in recent years in trying to take these issues forward has been the *Nursing Times*. Nonetheless, in trying to generate debate within nursing, even that followed in the UKCC's footsteps, who had invited sociologist and professor of healthcare, Celia Davies to make the keynote address to the Council's annual dinner on 'professionalism'. Although not a nurse, Professor Davies has long been a highly influential writer on nursing history and politics and, when the *Nursing Times* ran a debate on the subject over three issues, featuring five commentators, this was led by Prof Davies. She argued cogently that professionalism was an outdated, male-oriented garment that nurses would be well advised to discard in order that they could engage in a 'new professionalism to fit the changed circumstances ... of the end of the twentieth century' (1996: pp 44–46). Of the remaining four, only three were nurses. None were engaged in current clinical practice. The writers were all important figures in their own right, Maggie Dunn, Unison National Officer, Sue Norman, Chief Executive/Registrar of the UKCC, Christine Hancock, General Secretary of the RCN and Sandy Macara, Chair of council of the British Medical Association (BMA). All that was missing was a governmental representative. None was divorced from their own highly political agenda, quite appropriate to such a highly contentious and politicised issue and all were presumed to have something important to say – but were saying it about nursing and nurses, not as nurses. Which is, perhaps, the curse of nursing.

▶ Conclusion: nurse heroes

There is a wide variety of nurses, coming together from different backgrounds, bringing different experiences and learning distinct skills, squeezed into a system and structure that militates against pluralism and a sense of sharing. Developing and understanding a collective identity that leaves room for recognising those differences is almost impossible. Who we are as nurses, then, is a highly complex question that is not addressed by simplistic sound bites or sweeping generalisation. It is a question that needs to be considered both in terms of nurses as people and as occupants of distinctive roles. Beyond the political rhetoric, today's nurses are being trained in a new way but are an ageing, shrinking workforce. Despite New Labour's attempts to boost recruitment and new training places, they are more reliant than ever on nurses from overseas.

Yet two things begin to emerge. The first is that many, many nurses stick it out, keep coming in to work. Given some of the themes only touched on in this chapter one might express surprise that more nurses don't walk away, never to return. Even at the end of a session when nurses have described being excluded from decision making, subjected to poor management, inadequately trained, supervised and not being given sufficient opportunities to develop, the 'overwhelming feeling ... was positive, with a strong belief in the importance of healthcare and the critical role of nurses in it' (Nolan *et al., op. cit.*). This can be discerned in many other cases.

Some commentators – and, indeed, some nurses themselves, wherever they gather – suggest that this is only evidence of the whinging and whining contingent within nursing, or representative of a flawed generic characteristic in nurses that will forever relegate them to a life of subservience and subordination and makes them undeserving of anything better. Perhaps, as Fabricus and others have suggested, there is something about the perception nurses have of themselves as individuals, their sense of their own worth and ability to contain the distress and anxiety their work arouses within them. But, as I shall argue throughout this book, this notion of 'the nurse' as victim, as self persecutor, of being caught in a cycle of complaining without resolution is a political construct that is used to perpetuate a system that would be rocked to its foundation were nurses to re-organise themselves and respond in a more coherent and cohesive, confident and self consciously political way. Which means the fact that nurses are now less political in their own workplace begs much closer examination. Not in 'crisis', they face chronic problems – as well as many new ones – which have often not even been articulated properly, let alone come close to being resolved. Currently, arguments at a more strategic level tend to be *about* nurses rather than between them, something that reflects the lack of involvement nurses have in real decision making structures.

There is something else different about nurses. There is something different about their work and consequently the politics that governs it. Earlier in this chapter, the 'ordinary' and 'human' nature of nurses was briefly mentioned and it is true that nurses must – and deserve to be – acknowledged as 'ordinary' workers, the same as other health workers, carpenters, teachers, shop assistants or musicians. Yet, nurses do occupy a different place in the working classes. In work, everyone sacrifices a part of themselves for their job; the nature of work, the means by which capital raises productivity, the act of working demands it of them. Karl Marx described the act of working as, 'distorting the worker into a fragment of a man (sic).... [Its characteristics] transform his lifetime into working time ...'. But for nurses the nature of that sacrifice is different. They are people who literally touch death, listen to suffering, study the misery of the sick and the dying, and inhabit a world as confused, chaotic and conflictual as can be imagined. Going back to work every day, often with little or no support or understanding from their managers, in an environment which is now more hostile to their work than ever before, short of staff and often ill-prepared for the work, there is something essentially, genuinely heroic. That is the difference. And it is the factor that, above all else, complicates the relationship between nurses, practice and politics.

▶ Further reading

Clay T (1989) *Power and Politics*. London: Heinemann. Although this is inevitably very much a partisan view of politics and nursing, it does offer a good insight into the workings and understanding of the RCN in the 1980s.

Fabricus J (1999) The crisis in nursing. *Psychoanalytic Psychotherapy*, 13(3).

Fatchett A (1998) *Nursing in the New NHS: Modern, Dependable?* London: Bailiere Tindall.

Finlayson L and Nazroo J (1998) *Gender Inequalities in Nursing Careers*. London: Policy Studies Institute.

Hart C (1994) *Behind the Mask: Nurses, their Trade Unions and Nursing Policy*. London: Bailliere Tindall. This work is far more focused on the influence of nursing associations and trade unions on nurses and practice. Providing a more detailed historical perspective, it covers a lot of the material, events and issues that could not be included in this work.

Salvage J (1985) *The Politics of Nursing*. London: Heinemann. This seminal work offers an earlier perspective on some of the issues referred to in this and later chapters and thus makes an interesting comparison.

Useful websites

The range of Department of Health policy documents referred to in this chapter can be accessed through its website: *www.doh.gov.uk*.

More information about the nursing workforce and related statistics can be accessed, again, via the Department's website, but also via the NMC website: *www.nmc-uk.org*.

2 Past Imperfect – A Nursing History

Upon hearing that the workers of Freedonia are demanding shorter hours – *Very well, we'll give them shorter hours. We'll start by cutting their lunch hour to twenty minutes.*
Groucho Marx, in 'Duck Soup'

▶ Introduction

The old adage that to understand the present we have to know something of the past may sound trite. But the truth is often not original and, in this case, there is so much of the past that is either hidden or almost totally forgotten that it is worth the journey. Moreover, to fully leave behind the legacy of nursing's history and attendant myths, something more important than understanding is necessary. This potent mix of fact and fantasy was to have a lasting effect on nursing and nurses. By the beginning of the twentieth century, the traditions of a vocational ideal, the search for status – a search, as we have seen, still haunting nursing today – and clear parameters around the nurses' role were woven together as layers of ideology in a way that would both define and confine the work they were to do. Nursing was defined as women's work and cast in both a subordinate and subservient role. It was only in the 1980s that groups of nurses finally began to shake off their shackles in earnest and they then found themselves subjected to a comprehensive political onslaught, sometimes from unexpected quarters, that few could ever have predicted. Criticism from government, managers and sections of the press might be expected, particularly given the growing radicalism of the 1970s and 1980s. However, when such a chorus of disapproval was briefly enjoined by the nursing press, some sections of the nursing workforce and even the professional organisations then we can assume that something profound and remarkable was occurring.

One legacy of this hidden history is how often, in recent years, nursing is so poorly reported and represented in the national media. Industrial action is often greeted with announcements that this is the 'first time that nurses have contemplated such momentous steps' when, in fact, there is a significant history of such action dating back to the period immediately after the First World War, and nurses were one of the most militant groups of workers in the late 1930s. Equally, nursing's 'quieter' revolutions and clinical developments in important areas of patient care and their own internal organisation have often gone completely unreported or given scant importance. This and the next chapter will briefly chronicle some of the key events from our past, particularly the events that shaped nursing's 'modern' origins, and attempt to explain why so much about nursing and nurses' history has either been neglected or distorted.

The evolution of nursing becomes less and less of a straightforward matter as soon as one tries to trace the story of nurses and their work outside what has been the narrow confines of the majority of nursing history itself. Then the invisibility of nurses and nursing quickly becomes a puzzling reality. In 1999, health spending accounted to 6.2 per cent of gross domestic product, with nursing swallowing up a large part of that amount. Yet, one of the largest groups of workers in Europe barely rate a mention in the vast array of social policy texts, social history, political and trade union histories and, most notably, texts about the National Health Service (NHS) itself. Standard texts such as Chris Ham's *Health Policy in Britain* (1992), Klein's *The Politics of the NHS* (1989), Baggot's *Health and Health Care* (1994) and Mohan's *A National Health Service?* all pay scant attention to nurses and nursing, although they are still essential reading for anyone hoping to understand the workings of the NHS and how it fits within the wider social policy context, while Ham and Hill's, *The Policy Process in the Modern Capitalist State* (1984), offers a seminal understanding of policy models, the factors determining it and process involved in formulating and implementing policy. Astonishingly, Ham (1992: pp 44–9) recounts the events of 1987–89, from the outcry over NHS funding through until the ministerial review that led to the establishment of the internal market without mentioning nurses, clinical grading or the industrial action that rocked the Thatcher Government and forced its U-turn on funding. Even *From Cradle to Grave: 50 Years of the NHS* (Rivett, 1998) places nurses in a peripheral position in what is essentially an authorised history of the NHS. General practitioners, hospital doctors, consultants, managers and even that short-lived phenomenon, purchasers, litter the indexes and make their mark on the page just as, at one time, ancillary staff would have.[1]

If the books are right, nurses have not been terribly important in policy or political terms, just as their practice is not significant in providing care for patients. This would make sense if the things that nurses then think of as important not only were overlooked but regarded as irrelevant when looking at overall health policy and broader perspectives in healthcare. It appears mystifying unless it is understood to be a reflection of the political position occupied by nurses. Historical events cannot be divorced from the context in which they occurred. The internal politics of nursing and the systems within which nurses have worked, as well as the

---

[1] It is worth noting that one of the notable female writers on the subject, Lesley Doyal (1979), brought a different perspective to social policy and health and makes significantly more of the role of nurses than her male colleagues. These texts will feature again in Chapter 6, which looks in more detail at social policy.

way in which external events and currents have been integrated and affected all need consideration. A purely linear reading of nursing history is, therefore, doomed; it provides only a one-dimensional picture of the past, a 'traditional' history of nurses and nursing, a story of who did what and when they did it. What has been ignored or even hidden in the past is as important in helping us understand our present, as is some reflection on what has *not* happened and the reasons behind that. We are, in that respect, fortunate to have the works of people like Mick Carpenter, Monica Baly, Celia Davies, Chris Maggs, Anne Marie Rafferty, Rosemary White and many others whom I shall refer to in this chapter, all of whom have provided fine, if often neglected, accounts of nursing's past and the conditions in which it developed.

This chapter will give a very brief account of nursing from ancient Greece and Rome, through the work in religious orders in the middle ages and into the nineteenth century. It is this period that witnesses the birth of what we now understand to be 'modern' nursing and, although very well documented in numerous nursing texts, is worth a further exploration here, particularly given the importance of considering why certain events were later to be accorded such importance. The coming of the reforms that shaped nursing, including training and registration, are contrasted with the less well-recognised struggles to unionise nurses, which were pioneered in the asylums and followed by the nurses working in the Poor Law hospitals. All of these events are placed in their historical context. It concludes with the momentous events leading up to the formation of the NHS and the crucial role played by small but determined groups of nurses in fighting for the changes that played such a significant part in creating the conditions that made a nationalised health service almost inevitable.

▶ The charge of the new order: the conditions for change are established

Nursing of all types is a task that has necessarily been carried out through the ages, long before doctoring had any status or history, long before anything like a discrete body of knowledge could be identified. The term, 'nursing', actually reflects upon the act of suckling babies and the act of mothering before anything to do with waiting upon sick people. However, it is from the earliest division of labour, with men as hunters and hunter gatherers and women looking after – or nursing – the children that the act of caring for the sick begins to emerge. Nurses were mentioned in Homer's *Iliad*, where their work, though 'noble', often went unnoticed. Nursing in Roman times passed from the work of slaves to its women largely after Christianity began to have an impact and deaconesses, recognised as nurses in their own 'parishes', had an important part in the early church. Even then, they were required to be unmarried or widows. Fabiola founded what is thought to be the first Christian hospital in AD 390, leading its nursing herself. Other hospitals and hospices spread through her example and the work of friends and associates.

They housed the sick, elderly, bereaved and orphans. As the work of the hospitals grew, it was subsumed into the church, with men and women in religious orders nursing the sick as part of their religious duties.

The work of monks such as St Benedict and Casiodorus developed this further. Nursing continued to be focused into religious orders through until the second millennium, with the Order of St John of Jerusalem taking a leading role at the time of, and after, the holy wars in the eleventh century. At about the same time, secular orders began to involve themselves in nursing in small hospitals and the homes of people in their local community, although these were not as influential as their religious counterparts. However, the dissolution of England's monasteries under Henry VIII, schisms within the church and disillusionment with its practices impacted upon the practice of nursing across Europe. In England, particularly, changes to the provision of care to the sick was necessary and, after the Reformation, a number of hospitals were founded which complemented those already in existence and with a religious origin, such as St Bartholomew's in London (Calder, 1971).

By the mid-nineteenth century, however, nursing had lost its organisation and, being closely associated with women in society, was cast as work of very low status. Most of Europe was more advanced than Britain in nursing and it was a German hospital, in Kaiserwerth, established in the 1830s, that was to have a great influence on Florence Nightingale and other nursing reformers. With no clear body of knowledge or system of nursing, care would most often be provided to the sick by relatives, neighbours and friends, using skills often passed from mother to daughter, as was the case with midwives. These women were generally very poor, as were those they were caring for. The conditions in which they worked were usually shoddy and it certainly wasn't glamorous or prestigious. Given the circumstances in which they practised, it is little surprise that they had very limited success. Wealthier families were able to employ women who would nurse them and inevitably had greater choice as to who would do this.

Nursing did gain in importance within the military. Indeed, modern nursing began its rise to prominence most notably, in what has often been termed the first 'modern' war, in the Crimea, fought between Britain and Russia from 1854 to 1856, while the awful traumas of the Civil War in the United States, which took place a few years later, had a similar effect on American nursing. Radical change affected the evolution of nursing closer to home in the eighteenth and early nineteenth centuries, on the back of the social, economic and political upheaval brought about by the industrial revolution. Massive increases in the population saw large numbers of people moving into urban areas from the countryside, seeking employment in the rapidly expanding cities. However, unemployment, starvation and sickness grew equally rapidly and with catastrophic results. Out of the conditions that created a new, industrial, working class came, like Frankenstein's monster, a 'new' poor, branded by politicians, the affluent middle class and industrialists as 'feckless', work-shy and undeserving of any charity, sympathy or assistance, as well as being 'socially and economically unfit'. Such attitudes and the harsh policies that stemmed from them were justified by a form of social Darwinism and fashionable 'scientific' theories such as eugenics. It was as if there was a foul smelling infection rotting away at society's core, with a range of problems conspiring together to leave the middle classes, despite the affluence experienced by so many and the burgeoning imperial success of the early Victorian age, fearing they would be contaminated – both literally and metaphorically – by the swelling ranks of the sick and dispossessed if these were not, in some way, contained. Moreover, social and political unrest had been simmering beneath the surface for much of the eighteenth and early nineteenth centuries. Increasingly militant demands for social and political reform, wanting better conditions not just for themselves but for those they saw in even greater need, were coming from those who had found work in the new industrial heartlands, the mills, factories, furnaces and mines. Struggles for independent trade unions were closely but not exclusively wedded to campaigns for an enlargement of the vote, at that time denied to all but a privileged elite. On occasions, this conflict exploded out onto the national stage, such as when eleven people demonstrating in Manchester for the right to vote in 1819 were killed by troops at the so called 'Peterloo Massacre' or, in 1834, when six Dorset labourers were transported to Australia for seven years because they were found guilty of having taken 'unlawful oaths' for 'seditious purposes'. The crime of the so-called Tolpuddle Martyrs was to try and form a trade union. Their transportation sparked protests throughout the country, including one estimated at 100,000 at King's Cross, in London (Morton, 1989: pp 336–65).

Gradually, however, an organised working class began to emerge over the coming decades, with its own identity, demands and aims, growing in influence as a force not only in the workplace but in the wider political arena. The political unrest of the first half of the nineteenth century was fuelled by additional factors, however. Some were social, some were more specific to health, while others had aspects of both: cholera epidemics in the 1830s, 1840s and 1860s caused mass panic, but so did the dramatic increases in urban crime and a new phenomenon – at least in terms of numbers and context – madness. A very delicate social and political order was facing severe pressure, with all semblance of stability under real threat. An alternative view developed amongst social reformers that, rather than confrontation and even more austere social and political measures, steps would have to be taken to ameliorate the situation. This was not a universally popular opinion and one that was met with staunch opposition, not least from successive governments. When it came, the long sought after extension of the franchise – the right to vote – did not bring with it the great advances some had hoped for. It was, for example, a reformed House of Commons which sanctioned the transportation of the Tolpuddle Martyrs and sought to break the trade unions (Thompson, 1968: p 908). Change and social advances came in other areas, nonetheless: public health reforms were achieved, albeit on the back of the cholera epidemics, where 'the patients admitted [to hospital] were of the poorest labouring class, dirty, ill-fed, living in crowded and squalid rooms' (St George's Hospital Reports, 1864–65). This reforming process and the growing concerns about health would eventually have a direct impact on nursing as health visiting and district nursing were developed in the latter part of the century.

The tremendous resistance to change was not just ideological. There was also the cost to the nation and its economy. A limited form of welfare provision did exist, but the proportional growth in welfare demand – and cost – meant the old systems were unable to cope, particularly as they were mostly geared up to rural parish communities. As the population doubled during the first half of the nineteenth century and then doubled again before 1900, welfare spending rocketed from £700,000 in the early 1800s to nearly £7 million by the end of the century. Just as some contemporary commentators and politicians argue that, in the twenty-first century, society cannot afford our current welfare state, so their predecessors argued that spending on the poor, the elderly and sick was spiralling dangerously out of control and would drag down the rest of the economy. A compromise came with the Poor Law Act of 1834 and, consequently, the birth of a system of healthcare provision that was to have as profound an effect on nursing as anything done by Florence Nightingale (Morton, 1989).[2] It came in the form of a word that would strike terror into the hearts of the poorest in British society and, even well into the following century, would prompt a contemptuous response and dog the reputation of many hospitals that had developed out of the original buildings. It was the workhouse.

Welfare provision was, literally, to become an industry. A building programme for workhouses was established that would house the newly created destitute, the poor, the elderly, orphans and sick. Even these reforms were, however, diluted by economic and political expediency. The sick were originally to have been housed separately but, because the numbers of people with incurable or chronic illness was way beyond anyone's estimates at the time, this was quickly seen as unaffordable. The sick had to be left to suffer with the rest. They certainly had few nurses. Those they did have would have been unrecognisable to their modern day counterparts. Most of them were inmates themselves, with little or no nursing experience. No training whatsoever was provided. These pauper nurses did not receive any money. Their 'pay', such as it was, would be extra rations and clothes. Some were so frail that they needed nursing themselves, but all were portrayed as inferior in their character, agedness, lack of cleanliness, intoxication, illiteracy and promiscuity (Davies, 1980: p 85). Nurses and midwives in their own communities fared little better in terms of ability and reputation.

The pauper nurses were subjected to the same brutal regimes of labour and discipline as other inmates, designed to deter entry and reduce the overheads of the

---

[2] It is an irony that, while the work of Ms Nightingale and her followers dominate nursing history, this relatively little known branch of nursing – often reviled and widely criticised at the time – is the source to which most contemporary nurses can trace back their 'professional ancestry'.

institution. This new system of poor relief, as it was known, ensured the workhouse pauper was in 'less favourable conditions' than those of the least prosperous workers outside. With millions outside the workhouse on the verge of starvation, this meant almost unimaginable cruelties. Prison was deemed superior and preferable. Perversely, it was not uncommon for whole families to be declared destitute, admitted and put to work, no matter how degrading and senseless that work was. They would often be broken up, with the children being shipped up to factories in the North of England to work as cheap labour. Policy makers were reluctant to react to the problems of the workhouse despite growing pressure from reformers. Although it was recognised that 70 per cent of pauperism originated from sickness it was as late as 1867 that it was officially acknowledged that workhouses were turning into little more than hospitals. By 1861, just a year after Nightingale had founded her training school, there were 50,000 sick in the workhouse, often with only one pauper nurse for 120 patients. A decade earlier, there had been less than 8000 people in hospitals of any kind (Hart, 1994).

▶ The doctors take charge

Nineteenth-century Britain was fuelled by technological development and the opportunity to utilise raw materials and wealth imported from the colonies. While it was, in part, an age characterised by poverty, chaos and unrest, there was another side to it; military expansion and Britain's imperialist success saw a period of rapid expansion into world markets. Fed on this newfound wealth, came the development of rational thinking, utilitarian philosophy and the growth of science. This included an increased interest in medicine which encapsulated the hope and optimism of the ruling class, who seemed to be conquerors of all before them, particularly when it could be imagined that the intractable problems of poverty and chronic sickness were to be locked away in the workhouse. Doctors' practice was about cure. It was not provided in institutions, primarily, but in the homes of their relatively affluent patients. At the mid-point of the century, hospital admissions were still the exception although, during the next fifty years, within the hospital, the 'medical gaze' was quickly to establish a pre-eminent position. However, the pressure for social reform and the growing problems of the poor and sick meant doctors were even drawn into the workhouse. Once there, they quickly took on the invaluable role of designating who was incurable and who could be treated and put back into work. The economic drivers were far more powerful than the argument for social reform, just as creating a fit, healthy and, above all, productive workforce was a priority. These factors gave the medical profession a position of increased power and dominance.

The symbiotic relationship between doctors and nurses began to grow as doctors moved into hospitals, developing treatments for larger numbers of patients. More nurses were needed, both to carry out the doctors' instructions and also to report back their observations. An example of the practicalities of the problem can be gleaned from the hospital committee minutes from St George's Hospital in London:

> When the present system was first suggested, it was intended that the 'ward' nurse should be the responsible nurse in each ward, and should attend the medical officers in their visits and give them information as to their cases, and that the 'head' nurses should only exercise a general supervision. This idea has not, however, been carried out; and as a matter of fact, it is the *head* nurse who accompanies the medical officers in their rounds, and who is appealed to by them and answers any questions they may ask. Now it is impossible that any one person can carry the details of the cases of 52 patients in her mind at the same time. (St George's Hospital Committee Minutes, 1887)

The solution proposed by the author, Mr Pick, one of the hospital's physicians, was that a nurse should be appointed as head of each ward to be entirely responsible for the nursing of her ward. This proposal was one of a number put forward by senior doctors within the hospital to address the needs of the expanding service – although each was as carefully costed as would have happened in any contemporary hospital. He also suggested introducing two day- and one night-superintendents, an early example of how an extended, increasingly hierarchical service was born. Earlier, in 1868, the all-male committee on nursing at the same hospital had decided to appoint one superintendent of nursing. She would be 'a widow or unmarried, aged between 30 and 45', Church of England, not be absent for a whole day without the written permission of the board (and who would have to give written permission for any nurse to leave the hospital), while earning a salary that must not exceed £100 per year (St George's Hospital Committee Minutes, 1868).

The service was also being separated out on grounds of class and privilege, with affluent patients receiving far better treatment. Doctors also wanted more and 'better' nursing, requiring still more nurses. The desire to have a better class of young woman filling that role became a key factor. It corresponded with the desire of nursing reformers to give nursing greater legitimacy and status. Immediately, this was a cause of conflict and complication, contradiction and compromise. For although there was, on some issues, a shared agenda for change, the nursing reformers did not agree with everything the doctors wanted. Nor did all nurses.

To begin with, there was the matter of control. This was a complex issue: nurses had no role in the management or decision making within the Voluntary Hospitals, just as they did not within the Workhouse. The nature of their work was dictated by the doctors and their practice. Policy, such as it was, was made by boards of governors and hospital management committees. However, the expansion of the work undertaken by doctors made it inevitable that so, too, would the work of nurses, which meant nurses would have an opportunity to say more about the organisation and running of the institution. The struggle for control was only just beginning and the nursing reformers were ready and willing to take it up.

▶ The future takes shape – the coming of the reforms

It is widely accepted that the work of Florence Nightingale and a small band of nurses had been highly influential in reducing the appalling death rate of casualties in the Crimean War. Her reputation from the war, her energy, zeal and background readily identified her as a key figure in the process of reform. Although untrained herself, she used her pre-eminence to raise £45,000, a fortune in those days, through a national appeal. This was ploughed into a training school, opened at St Thomas' Hospital, in London, in 1860. Although, behind the scenes, the new school was beset with problems, including high drop out rates of students, a revolution was taking place.

In fact, so much of Nightingale's early work and 'achievements' are shrouded in myth – some of it of her own making – it is very difficult to disentangle them and make a clear judgement. Nightingale's modern day critics, perhaps being drawn into responding to the way in which events in her life have been appropriated and mythologised by organisations and some of nursing's hierarchy, often fail to recognise the significance of some aspects of her work in its historical context, judging her – inevitably poorly – against today's political, social and economic standards. Those who have spent sufficient time and space sifting through the differing accounts and evidence, such as Ann Summers (1988), Dingwall *et al.* (1988) and Baly (1986) are well worth reading, as they reveal the complexity of relationships, politics and pure chance that contributed to the development of early nursing reform in relation to Nightingale. However, there can be no doubt that, for good or bad, she really was one of those crashing through a political brick wall in the mid-nineteenth century when she played her part in the process of establishing a unified system of nursing, with its own hierarchy, rules and ideology, whose members were loyal to one another. Nightingale and the other women involved believed that the strictest discipline possible was the thread that tied the service together.

As senior nurses were taking on a managerial role, actual nursing duties – notably, the care of the sick – were becoming the priority, taking the place of the domestic duties and amalgam of things previously prescribed for them. Not only were nurses observing patients on behalf of the doctors, they were beginning to interpret their observations.

It was in this necessarily changing world that the so-called Nightingale reforms made their impact. The details are in some ways less important than the subsequent re-telling of the Florence Nightingale story – one that still pervades the consciousness not only of nursing but still holds a place in British history that is as familiar yet foreign as tales of Nelson's victory in death at Trafalgar or Wellington's triumph at Waterloo but, ironically, distanced from the Charge of the Light Brigade, the other event so closely associated with the Crimean War.

The training school at St Thomas' Hospital instituted a one year training, based on principles of rigorous discipline, supervision, character building and loyalty. It followed on from King's College Hospital, which was training pupil nurses from 1856 and St John's House, where training for nurses took place under the guidance of a clergyman in priests' orders (Abel-Smith, 1960: p 19). Nightingale's school – although rarely visited by the grand dame herself – also provided an understanding of hospitals as institutions, with a need for sound administration, improved hygiene and infection control. An impact on organisational structures resulted, enhanced as Nightingale nurses were sent out to capture the position of matron in hospitals, spurred on by their mentor to pursue an improved position for nursing within their own institution as ruthlessly as she was at a national level. The success of this strategy was in its limited scope: it was not about subverting or challenging the medical hierarchy's right of practice, curative role or overall authority over the patient, nor the lay administration in the financing and running of the hospital itself. Rather, it was to establish a nursing 'department', with its own hierarchy, an objective broadly achieved by the end of the nineteenth century.

The struggle for control now focused on training and who would prescribe this. Would it be doctors or nurses? The outcome was that, although senior nurses were involved and were instructing nurses in their nursing duties, training was framed entirely – and circumscribed – by medical practice, subordinating the role of the nurse to one of a male, medically dominant model. The knowledge imparted was sufficient to allow nurses to act as informed assistants but did not match that provided to doctors themselves.

This was not entirely without cost for the doctors for, even these limited changes, coupled with other reforms, meant a further change in the balance of power was inevitable. Nurses were interpreting what they saw and ward sisters beginning to translate what doctors wanted as a result of observations and delegating tasks. Doctors, however reluctantly, were having to rely on nurses to be successful in their treatment of patients.

▶ The battle over registration

'Suitable' women, i.e., middle class, educated and well bred, were now being attracted into nursing, but still in insufficient numbers. Nightingale was convinced that this was not a major concern: she believed 'character' was the key to good nurses and women from different economic and social backgrounds could be moulded and trained. Part of this involved inculcating the 'new' nurses with the ideological values, ethos and aspirations of the dominant class. Nightingale's opponents on the issue of 'breeding' and background eventually stumbled because there were simply not enough middle-class women willing to come into nursing and they failed to understand the simple – but highly political – overriding preoccupation of the medical profession, hospital management committees and government, which was to have sufficient numbers of nurses, whatever their background. They also wanted an occupational group which would subordinate itself to the wider needs of the 'service', as defined for them.

The modern nurse was not the elite to which some had aspired then, but was considered an advance on what had gone before. She was caring, feminine, nurturing, disciplined, trustworthy, clean and of 'good character'. In this, she could be strongly contrasted with her predecessors, the 'Sarah Gamps' and 'Betsey Prigs',[3] caricatured as poor, foul mouthed, dishonest, promiscuous drunkards.

There was some truth to the dreadful image attributed to the older, untrained nurses, who, despite their alleged faults, still worked in hospitals, workhouses and lunatic asylums. Yet those like John South, a St Thomas' Hospital based surgeon, wrote in 1857 that standards were nowhere near as bad as depicted, defending the character and integrity of the nurses. He was not alone in his view but the net effect of the overriding criticism was to justify pushing them out in favour of the more newly trained nurses to pave the way for change. In order to do this image was even more important to promote if money and influence were to come the reformers' way and they were to get the necessary support for their plans.

The pace of change was rapid. It was not, however, a peaceful or simple path that was followed. Aided by philanthropists such as William Rathbone, Nightingale was able to place trained nurses, under the control of one of her matrons, Agnes Jones, into the Brownlow Hill Institution, a workhouse in Liverpool. Gradually, despite the opposition of 'vested interests', 'public prejudice' and 'timid administrations', Nightingale and others, such as Louisa Twining, were able to bring change even to the workhouse, with Nightingale sending out stinging rebukes to those who thought paupers undeserving of good nursing care. However, the major battle focused on whether or not nurses should be registered. It was a thirty-year long struggle which split nursing down the middle. The argument for better, less variable standards of nursing and midwifery was becoming well established, aided by the training schools that were following on from the St Thomas' example. However, the case was now being put that not only should anyone wishing to call themselves a nurse or midwife be trained but also have their name held on a central register. Doctors had been doing this since 1858.

Those who said that training was, in and of itself, sufficient were not helped by the considerable inconsistencies still existing into the latter part of the nineteenth century, when it ranged from one to four years. Although Florence Nightingale had

---

[3] These older, poorer, untrained nurses took their name from Dickens' memorable creations in *Martin Chuzzlewit*.

initially actively sought lower-class women for training, the St Thomas' school later set up a 'fast track', one-year training for 'Lady Pupils' who actually paid to be trained. It was women from this group that then went on to become Nightingale's 'stormtroopers' in the nursing reform movement.

There was also a lack of consensus about the content and quality of the training itself, although it was still not mandatory for a practising nurse or midwife even to be trained. There was no way of distinguishing between trained or untrained, good or bad nurses. Most important for proponents of registration, they saw no status for nurses while this situation remained. Registration would determine who was fit to practice; protect the public from poor or bad nurses; regulate practice and behaviour by exerting formal standards of discipline; set national examinations and minimum standards of entry for training and fees for both. It would also facilitate accreditation of hospitals and their training schools.

Another agenda was also being played out. The main advocate of registration was Edith Bedford Fenwick, herself a former 'lady pupil'. It was, ironically, this group, whom Nightingale had groomed to push through change, who now rejected their mentor's notion of creating competent, practical nurses, trained on a course that was within the understanding of a 'country girl'. The issue, as is so often the case in nursing, was far from simple. It might seem elitist to believe registration would improve the character of the women who went in for nursing while wanting to benefit the 'richer classes' both into letting their daughters become nurses and let themselves be nursed. However, for Bedford Fenwick, speaking at the turn of the century, 'the nurse question [was] the woman question', and became part of the wider feminist struggle to win the vote (Abel-Smith, 1960: pp 60–2). Conversely, Nightingale thought registration would greatly damage nursing, primarily because of it being tied to examinations, which she believed could not reveal the true competence of a nurse and would become a distraction from the woman's personal qualities when being considered for selection and training.

In pursuit of her cause, Ethel Bedford Fenwick set up in 1887 one of the first nurses' associations, the British Nurses' Association, later the Royal British Nurses' Association (RBNA), proudly claiming to represent nursing's elite – even though one-third of its ruling body was comprised of medical staff.

The year 1896 saw the formation of the Women Sanitary Inspectors' Association, which was eventually transformed into the Health Visitors' Association. Registration was an aspiration here as well, but being a relatively new group of workers with no difficult historical legacy, notions of a trained workforce sat more easily alongside the type of collectivist, radical ethic that was evolving among sections of the nursing workforce in the Poor Law hospitals. The traditions and efforts of the nurses working in the most adverse conditions in workhouse infirmaries, as well as the asylums, were ignored. These were not the right sort of nurses for Bedford Fenwick and her followers. The RBNA's proposals for registration would have meant nurses not being paid any salary, paying to take exams and be registered – it would have excluded nurses working in Poor Law hospitals and asylums. Anyone not registered would have been prevented by law from practising. The relatively small workforce that would have stemmed from such proposals would undoubtedly have status and been in a strong position to negotiate its position within the wider field of healthcare – one of the major concerns of those in the medical profession opposing it.

In fact, the medical profession was torn. It wanted to have suitable nurses to assist medical practitioners. The benefits of having better trained nurses were recognised by more enlightened doctors. Both sides of the nursing divide on this issue had cultivated strong alliances with medical colleagues. Yet, within the more conservative circles of the medical profession, strong resistance remained to the developing nursing hierarchy. Moreover, registration would weaken their position in other important areas – notably financially. For example, registered midwives would inevitably impact on doctors' practice, where a guinea was charged for each birth attended. District nurses would also affect the business of rural GPs (Cowell and Wainwright, 1981).

Midwives were, in fact, the first group after doctors to be registered but, when registration was attained in 1902, the issue was largely fudged. All practising midwives with one year's experience and 'of good character' were admitted to the initial register. This was a reasonably well circumscribed group, however, unlike nurses who were growing increasingly disparate and fragmented. The RBNA unsuccessfully sponsored a succession of parliamentary bills through to the beginning of the First World War, never really able to address the fundamental flaw at the heart of their argument: from where would the numbers of the 'right sort of women' they wanted to form the nursing workforce be found? This was the principle reason the government opposed each bill put before it, recognising that placing a limit on the recruitment pool of women able to enter into nursing would place even further strain on an already stretched service. Even since the early days of the St Thomas' school, the numbers of probationers, or student nurses, dropping out of their training was averaging at a rate of about 30 per cent, with a third of those being dismissed for a variety of offences, including disobedience and a lack of sobriety (Baly, 1987). The task of building up a workforce capable of meeting the demands being made of it was arduous and beset by internal differences and external pressures.[4]

---

[4] It is another of the anomalies of nursing history that this dropout, or 'wastage', rate, as it is often referred to, has rarely changed, even though nursing leaders and politicians periodically pick up on it, denounce it as scandalous and demand that 'something must be done', as we shall see in subsequent chapters.

A growing trend towards philanthropic gestures and liberal reform is often placed at the heart of the social progress of the latter part of the Victorian age. However, closer examination reveals more practical necessities underlying many of the changes. The discovery that 30 per cent of the applicants to fight in the Boer War were medically unfit prompted public outrage and alarm in official circles (Davin, 1978). As well as a need for fit young men to fight its wars, Britain also needed more young men to colonise its expanding empire. These factors were among those that had paved the way for public health reform and incidentally advanced the cause of health visitors and registration for midwives. War, in those circumstances, could be good for mothers and babies on the home front. Indeed, it was another war that was to propel the issue of registration for nurses and improved standards to the top of the political agenda.

Little over fifty years on from Nightingale's rise to prominence as a result of the Crimean War, the First World War highlighted the chaos and inconsistencies of a service that had no national framework, organisation or co-ordination. With insufficient numbers of trained nurses, untrained volunteers, female and male, had to be enlisted. They worked alongside trained nurses in Voluntary Aid detachments (VADs), a system administered by the British Red Cross Society. Partly as a means of trying to address this chaos, senior nurses and members of the medical profession working with the British Red Cross Society decided the time had come for a new nursing organisation and formed the College of Nursing Ltd in 1916. Its main objectives were to establish better training and a uniform curriculum for nurses. In addition to this, its founders wanted the College to be the organisation that would approve training schools and maintain a national register of nurses – exactly the aim of Mrs Bedford Fenwick's RBNA. Unlike the RBNA, however, the College was a coalition of nurses, doctors with hospital committee members, the key difference being the involvement of the latter group. This, as well as the fact that it enlisted the support of most of the training schools, put the College in a powerful position in the maelstrom that was becoming nursing politics.

The government recognised that something more had to be done to organise or regulate nursing as a result of the problems thrown up by the First World War. This was one of the reasons it shifted its position on registration. There were two other – perhaps even more compelling – reasons that had nothing to do with nursing itself but everything to do with the wider social changes in the country: the first was the acknowledgement that, after years of resistance, women had defined for themselves a new role in society during the war years and were going to have to be granted the vote. Given that nursing was almost wholly a female occupation, nurses were suddenly going to have significantly more political power. The second was that the trade unions, for the first time, were finding success in organising amongst nurses.

Between the years 1910 and 1914 British trade unions had become caught up in a conflict with government over pay and working conditions 'which took a revolutionary course and might have reached a revolutionary conclusion' (Dangerfield, 1966: p 196). In 1912, a phenomenal 38 million working days were lost in disputes involving over 1 million workers.[5] The asylum workers had set up the first health workers union in Britain in 1910 and the Poor Law workers, including nurses, had done the same in 1918. The asylum workers undertook their first strike that same year, fighting for the right to wear their trade union badges. Giving in on registration was preferable to losing nurses to the trade unions or, even more worryingly, the emergent Labour Party. However, the nursing organisations were hopelessly split about how – and, most importantly by whom – registration should be managed. With no means of bringing the RBNA and College of Nursing together, government ministers ignored their best instincts and were irretrievably drawn into the affairs of nursing. In so doing they wrong footed the nursing organisations, who had assumed that one of them would be successful in administering the new system of registration. Finding the RBNA and College of Nursing irreconcilably divided, and with members of both Houses of Parliament having decried the motives of both camps for wanting control of any formal organisation, the government set up the General Nursing Council (GNC) as a new body to maintain a register of nurses and approve training schools. It also reserved significant authority for itself in matters of nursing policy.

Many of those opposing registration feared it would so narrow the field and intakes of new nurses that it would soon become a political and administrative albatross. The Act of Parliament was passed in 1919, probably the only time that the chronic, underlying problem of nursing shortages was masked. This was, in part, due to the large numbers who had been recruited into the VADs. Matters were not helped when the new GNC replicated nursing's existing divisions. It was made up of lay members, doctors and sixteen nurses, the majority of whom were matrons or ex matrons. The College of Nursing had nine members on the Council. There were only two nurses from Poor Law infirmaries and none from the asylums. With the GNC dominated by College members and their supporters, the minority, led by Mrs Bedford Fenwick, were vociferous nonetheless. Nurses had managed at last to successfully follow in the footsteps of the doctors – but not all other professions – by having their own registering body. But they had also institutionalised their differences in their ruling body. Whatever the rights and wrongs of registration as

---

[5] Compare this with the apparent collapse in industrial relations in 1979, when a 'mere' 30 million working days were lost or 1992, after several pieces of legislation restricting the power of trade unions, when 500,000 days were lost, in both cases from a much larger workforce. By 1997, the number had fallen still further, to just over 300,000. Repeating history, inasmuch as the number of strikes has increased following the election of a Labour government – despite Tony Blair's continual claims that New Labour has broken such patterns – 800,000 working days were lost in the first nine months of 2002 (Garavelli, 2002).

it was perceived in the years before and during the First World War, the legacy of that particular struggle was to resonate through the subsequent decades. One of the most profound aspects of that is the simple, stark fact that there never have been sufficient registered nurses to match demand.

▶ Unionisation – nurses take on a different struggle

In some respects, registration was also about what to do *with* nurses. Primarily, inasmuch as it was the agenda for nurses anywhere, it was for those working in voluntary hospitals, particularly the large London teaching hospitals and particularly those nurses working in senior positions. It may have been an issue for nurses elsewhere but they had other things on their mind as well.

The anxiety of government, nurses' associations and hospital committees about nurses becoming unionised was not misplaced. Again, the reasons behind nurses' decisions to join the union lay in their roots, or history. The Poor Law nurses, those working in what were now Poor Law hospitals or infirmaries and which had previously been known as workhouses, had been stigmatised by caring for the poor and incurable in much the same way as were asylum attendants, literally locked away with their charges, within the growing number of insane asylums being built across the country. Perhaps because of this hostility and the nature of the work, as much as their social background and economic class, both groups developed a far more collectivist tradition.

Ironically, many of the innovations to nursing practice and reforms later attributed to those nurses working in the voluntary hospitals actually originated in the Poor Law hospitals and, even before then, the workhouse. The voices of Nightingale and Louisa Twining were far from alone in calling for reform and the transition from a makeshift service provided by increasingly overwhelmed pauper nurses to Poor Law nurses came with the arrival of paid nurses imported from the voluntary hospitals. Nonetheless, they too soon fell victim to the reputation of their predecessors, despite carrying out similar duties to those of the ward sisters at St Thomas' Hospital, including domestic duties, attending upon the sick and administering medicines (White, 1978). That they were also among the early groups pioneering nursing people in their own homes did not earn them much in the way of kudos either.

Although they were now being joined by women who had received a formal training, many of the remaining nurses working in the Poor Law hospitals were there only because they were desperate to earn money. In the asylums, the situation was even worse, since the work there was even more despised. Not only were the inmates branded as feckless and undeserving, but the staff were widely believed to be 'idle and disorderly' (Nolan, 1994). Just as had been the case with the workhouses, the growth in asylums was associated with the 'progress' of the industrial revolution and their number multiplied as did the numbers of unemployed and in poverty, although at an even greater rate. Again, there was a fear amongst the middle classes that they might be 'infected' by the insanity of the poor and destitute. Thus, the building of the asylums was not just about treating madness; more, it was about isolating and excluding society's most difficult and problematic. Such behaviours and conditions were quickly medicalised. Doctors declared that insanity was not the result of demonic possession or people suffering from some form of spiritual malaise (Foucault, 1961). In so doing they gained influence and power with the promise of understanding and cure. However, as the number of inmates mushroomed with no cure in sight, that optimism faded and the external economics of funding large institutions became paramount in determining events inside them, a policy that was complemented by a laissez faire attitude to the asylums themselves and, again, justified by the same social Darwinism that had determined the fate of the poor in the wider society.

There was already a long history of asylums by the nineteenth century, with Bedlam being the most famous. There had even been an age of apparent enlightenment, during the seventeenth century, when Pinel had famously unchained the Paris 'lunatics' after the French Revolution, treating them with 'the restraint and kindness that sickness deserves' and Tuke had established a humane and relatively liberal regime at his York Retreat (Miller, 1962: p 304). Although the extent of the success and, indeed, just how enlightened life was in the institutions, has been disputed in some texts, there can be no doubt about the oppressive regimes that evolved in the late 1800s. Science and rationality were increasingly dominating social and economic life. Yet, the asylums were paternalistic, class ridden, authoritarian and built around a perverse moral code that ruled that, for the wealthy, educated and elite, a system of rewards and incentives would provide suitable motivation to improvement, while compliance and co-operation from the poor and powerless – including the inmates and attendant – could only be elicited by a system of repressive rules, punishment and fears. In this, the asylums did no more than mirror the society that spawned them.

As the expected rates of 'cure' did not materialise the focus shifted. Care was mechanistic, aimed at maintaining cleanliness and tidiness, exercise, good conduct and occupational work. The asylums developed farms and small industries as means of supporting themselves financially. This often meant medical superintendents hanging on to their best workers, regardless of their mental state.

These changes also had implications for the role of the attendants. As had occurred in hospitals, the increased number of patients meant more nurses were needed. Given that the wages were the approximate equivalent of the lowest paid agricultural workers and domestic servants, and their strength was seen as much of an asset as care or compassion it was perhaps no surprise that this was usually seen as the work of last resort for men who had previously been unemployed. Recruitment and retention were inevitably a problem. With few female nurses and fewer still from educated or wealthy backgrounds, there was little demand for reform from the workforce. However, training was initiated, in Scotland in 1856 (where a number of innovations in practice were pioneered), and some psychiatrists did attempt to replicate the changes taking place in voluntary hospitals without relinquishing control over practice in the asylums. Indeed, the first form of any nationally recognised training occurred in the asylums, with examinations for nurses and attendants being established by the Medico-Psychological Association (MPA) in 1890. When contemporary mental health practitioners refer to the 'medical model' of psychiatry, they may well not realise that for many years this was, in fact, virtually the only model and was made central to nursing practice more than a century ago, as doctors monopolised the training of asylum attendants to an extent that did not occur in any other sphere of nursing. This was done through a handbook written in 1885 for attendants by doctors and sanctioned by the MPA. The so-called 'red book' described the work of the nurse and attendant and was the basis of the nurses' training and practice, remaining in use, in updated forms, until 1978 (Nolan, 1994: pp 63–4).

Through a similar process to that which occurred in the general hospitals, nurses and attendants started making observations of patients and then interpreting them. They gained ascribed power outside the prescribed hierarchy of rules and procedures. It was, however, a relatively small concession, for if the institution was to have its effect within the framework designed for it, the staff had to be subordinated as much as the patients. Conditions were exceptionally harsh and authoritarian. All staff – married or unmarried – had to live within the institution, usually in rooms adjacent to the wards, with working days of 10–14 hours. Attendants would have one day off per month when they were allowed out of the asylum; male and female staff, as with the inmates, were segregated and marriage was only allowed with the permission of the superintendent. When inmates escaped, attendants could be charged with the cost of their recapture and financial penalties existed for the loss of keys and other rule infringements.

Even though training did infiltrate this closed world, no other group of nurses wanted asylum workers on the same register with them. Mrs Bedford Fenwick's RBNA was the most vociferous in this but Henry Burdett, the spokesperson of the Hospitals' Association, believed, 'No attempt should be made to get ladies and gentlemen i.e. persons with gentle upbringing, as attendants' (Carpenter, 1980: p 135). The MPA did maintain its own register of nurses and attendants and the asylums started to recruit trained – female – nurses from Poor Law and voluntary hospitals to try and improve standards. This move was resisted by the male attendants who rightly feared that they would lose their jobs, find their wages undercut or at least see themselves disadvantaged in terms of promotion.

▶ Women take a different lead

Lacking the hope that sprang from the work of reformers, asylum workers sought another route to improve their lot, which was similar to their outcast cousins in the

Poor Law hospitals. The first attempts at forming trade unions, in the 1890s were ruthlessly frustrated by the employers. The Asylum Workers' Association, run by matrons and doctors and with similar objectives to the RBNA (although not supported by it in any way) lacked staff support and was eventually overtaken by the National Asylum Workers' Union (NAWU) in 1910. Nurses in the Poor Law institutions followed suit in 1918, forming the Poor Law Workers' Trade Union. In both organisations, nurses allied themselves with other health workers, rather than the nurses' only approach taken by the College of Nursing and early Associations and found themselves the victims of bitter attempts at suppression by their employers, the major cause of the NAWU's first strike at Bodmin in 1918.

There were other differences. In their early years, these unions were radical and often took the cause of their patients as part and parcel of their demands for better conditions. Poor Law nurses were caring for the poorest and most vulnerable from their own local communities and gradually some amongst their number did much to expose the scandalous conditions their patients found themselves in; these were not patients who had been selected and nor would they be discharged because they were incurable. Indeed, such people were actually taken in from the voluntary hospitals. The asylum workers, meanwhile, became embroiled in a series of disputes across the country, fighting for more pay and a shorter working week.

Often these disputes were led by female nurses and the gradual decline in female membership of NAWU from the late 1920s coincided with its growing conservatism. However, a decade later it was not only women working in the asylums and old Poor Law hospitals, which came under the control of county councils in the 1930s, but also those from the major London teaching hospitals, who finally confronted their employers. Their anger was about the still appalling working conditions they had to endure, low pay and the staffing shortages that had worsened since the immediate post war period when registration had occurred.

This was the point at which, however tentatively, nurses dared to turn away from the tradition of the vocational ideal, the suffocating discipline and blind loyalty that had been demanded of them by their leaders. For the first time, a trade union was formed exclusively of nurses working in major teaching hospitals. This was the Association of Nurses and it had broken new ground by confining itself to recruiting nurses only. Amongst the trade unions and Trade Union Congress (TUC), supported by the Labour Party, there had been strong political agitation to see a shorter working week and minimum wage introduced, but these were always resisted by an alliance of government and hospital employers. A 54-hour week was not uncommon at the time; discontent with this was matched by unhappiness at a whole raft of petty restrictions and a code of discipline that was being seen increasingly as both overly rigid and unnecessary.

Not only were shortages of trained staff extremely serious, there were still approximately one-third of all probationers, or student nurses, dropping out of their training each year. Having taken a profoundly pragmatic position to beat off the RBNA in the debate about registration, the College of Nursing was now actually advocating an even longer working week and less pay. Growing unrest throughout 1936 and 1937 was the major factor in the formation of the Association of Nurses. It played a pivotal role in articulating nurses' anger and leading them in their unwillingness to accept the status quo – even if it meant coming into confrontation with the employer. Facing mounting unrest by nurses, the Conservative government of the time setting up the Athlone Committee to investigate the reasons behind the shortages, with a remit to look at nurses' terms and conditions. The Committee discovered that the patchwork system of independently funded voluntary hospitals – increasingly reliant on charitable donations – was in financial and administrative chaos. The local authorities, which now ran the old Poor Law hospitals were similarly ill equipped to run their services. Neither could afford to pay nurses a decent wage or employ sufficient numbers of nurses to staff the wards.

The Athlone Committee ultimately recommended a national system of recruitment and training and a national mechanism to set levels of pay and conditions of service, with a framework to facilitate trade union representation. Although it was not spelt out as such, it was inevitable that this would mean having a nationalised health service, a long cherished ideal of the nurses involved in the campaigns, the trade unions and the Labour Party, which was now a serious player in national parliamentary politics (Hart, 1994).[6]

The Committee's work was interrupted by the Second World War, but a chain of events had been set in motion. State intervention was becoming inevitable. The Rushcliffe Committee took up the issue of agreeing national pay scales for nurses and trade unions, as well as professional organisations, now had a seat at the negotiating table. The Royal College of Nursing (RCN), as it had become in 1939, had to reverse its position on pay and hours, falling in line with the trade unions; the government had, for the first time, to fund an increase in nurses' wages while also recognising the new entity of the enrolled nurse as a means of tackling the shortage of trained staff. The Liberal peer, Lord Beveridge, was also completing his report into welfare provision. The way was being paved for the arrival of the NHS.

Labour was swept to power in the general election of 1945. Its overwhelming parliamentary majority was actually the first working majority it had ever enjoyed and, able to claim genuine public support, it set about implementing a programme of reform the likes of which had never been seen before. The Bank of England, transport, electricity and gas, the coal, iron and steel industries were all nationalised. For the first time, the trade union movement had a direct corporate relationship with the government. The Conservatives had refused to implement the recommendations of the Beveridge Report in 1943 and, when Labour set about

---

[6] See Chapter 7 for a fuller description of the extraordinary events during this period.

enacting a National Health Service Bill in 1946, vehemently opposed them. In this, they were joined by the medical profession, whose opposition was actually a lot more difficult to overcome. With Beveridge as the architect, it was left to the new Minister for Health, Aneurin Bevan, to take on the mantle of stonemason and carve out the new service. Through the prolonged negotiations that took place between him, his civil servants and the medical profession, Bevan was forced to, as he eloquently put it, 'stuff the consultant's mouths with gold' by sanctioning financial merit awards no-one else in the NHS would be entitled to, retaining private beds and preventing doctors becoming salaried state employees, as well as providing them with separate negotiating arrangements and the best employment rights by far of any occupational group in the new service. Moreover, in the process they had placed themselves in a unique place at the heart of a policy making triangle, with politicians and civil servants (Haywood and Hunter, 1982; Morgan, 1992; Hart, 1995).

The views of civil servants and hospital management committees when it came to nurses were slightly different. Nurses were 'one jump away from domestics' and held in 'obvious contempt' (White, 1985).

In some respects, this set the tone for the first few decades of the NHS. Nurses had been as instrumental as anyone in paving the way for the new service and were essential to its success. Yet, they had not been given anything like the authority to match the responsibilities that were being laid at their door. In the very early years, their work barely changed. Perhaps remarkably, some appeared to pay scant attention to the momentous change occurring around them. In some cases, this was clearly political: in the St George's Hospital Gazette, e.g., the only reference to it can be found in an article by Sir Ernest Graham-Little MP. An ex-physician at the hospital, he wholeheartedly supported the British Medical Association's (BMA) opposition to the Beveridge Report, calling it 'the first open attack on the medical profession', then turned his attention to the NHS Act, 1946, 'an expression of the purest socialism' (St George's Hospital Gazette, January 1948). This was not meant to be a compliment. There is only the barest mention of it in the hospital's committee minutes. More surprising is the lack of reference to the new service in the minute books of trade unions of the period. Until then, however, nurses had been deliberately focused into their own hospitals, receiving little or no information about what was going on elsewhere, with little opportunity to develop any understanding of the wider issues affecting nursing or make comparisons with their own work or workplace. They were still shaped by an ideology that was designed to inculcate a tradition of vocational ideal characterised by subservience, loyalty and obedience, with initiative curbed.

For others, it was different. Avis Hutt, like Thora Silverthorne, a woman who combined her nursing with communist beliefs, had supported radical struggles including the Republican cause in Spain and the anti Fascist marches in London's East End, even when it threatened her own employment, and campaigned tirelessly for a national health service. For her, like so many who had campaigned for it, the sense of triumph was almost overwhelming. As Nurse Mary Witting wrote in the *Nursing Times* on 3 July 1948:

> The great principle has been accepted. Never again need any of us suffer disease through lack of money. Let us be proud that a country still poor after a war has taken this courageous step. It will be responsible for its sick without question, because on the health of each member depends the health of the community. We are part of the service. This is a great time to be alive.

▶ Conclusions

Behind the mask of the traditional history of subservient women applying themselves to a vocational ideal, lies a hidden story of struggle, hardship and a very different type of sacrifice than that usually portrayed. It is almost uniquely a women's history as nursing was established as women's work. The origins of nursing in religious orders was, ironically, augmented by the work of nurses in wartime. The most significant progress in the development of 'modern' nursing took place in Europe, with the hospital at Kaiserworth being a big influence on Florence Nightingale. As nursing took shape, so an organised working class was emerging, pressing for economic, social and political reform, with trade unions becoming established despite fierce government opposition. The industrial revolution had already brought great change and the need for greater welfare and healthcare provision was becoming irresistible. Medicine was establishing itself and the demand for more and 'better' nursing was inevitable. The brutal exploitation of nurses in asylums and the workhouse reflected prevailing social and political attitudes, as well as the treatment of those they were caring for, society's poorest and most vulnerable but the search for the 'suitable women' who would deliver a new form of nursing was never realised – there simply were not enough middle-class, well-educated young women from what was seen as the correct background who were available, willing or able to do the work. Nonetheless, the expansion of the hospital allowed nurses to become involved in the running of the institution at various levels and for nursing to evolve its own structures, hierarchy and organisation, based on new ideologies and using carefully cultivated myths and doctrines to define itself and exploit the existing gender relations and role of women in society to create a malleable, subservient workforce in such a way that their own needs were never even articulated.

The interweaving of a complex variety of factors thus combined to forge a healthcare system that was growing in a piecemeal way, with nurses central to its success but far from at its centre when it came to decision making and shaping its evolution. It was partly driven by altruism and well intentioned, liberal reformers but partly due to more malign influences that saw it as a means of legitimising the prevailing political structures and of ameliorating the potential social and political unrest of the period. Economic and ideological controls were thus key issues.

The debate within nursing moved on to one about training and education and then, in pursuit of internal control, to include registration. Irrevocable splits were opening up in nursing. These were not, however, the result of dominant personalities. It was a battle of ideas, of imagination and vision; there were also conservative and vested interests to be protected. Ironically, government was drawn in to resolve it and, despite attempts more than a century later, never to escape from having overall responsibility again.

Gaining in confidence and power after the First World War, the trade unions organising in health were defining a different agenda, with nurses at their forefront. They were increasingly radicalised until, in the early 1920s, they suffered major setbacks at the hands of the employers. Yet, a series of remarkable women had, again, picked up the torch by the mid-1930s and were articulating a different inherited imagination than that of the matrons, doctors, hospital committees and boards of governors seeking to control them. Their radical campaigns had a liberating effect that reverberated throughout the healthcare system of the time, then struggling with a growing funding crisis and staffing shortages. The women who led the Association of Nurses, the Guild of Nurses and other nurses' organisations played a significant part in creating the necessary changes that led to national structures of pay, education, conditions of service and identity that were integral to the recognition of the need for a nationally organised health service and a new era for nursing.

▶ Further reading

Abel Smith B (1960) *A History of the Nursing Profession*. London: Heinemann: the first of the great works about nursing history, it is still required reading.

Allen P and Jolley M (eds) (1982) *Nursing, Midwifery and Health Visiting since 1900*. London: Faber and Faber.

Baly M (1987) Nightingale Nurses: The Myth and the Reality. In: Maggs C (ed) *Nursing History: The State of the Art*. Kent: Croom Helm.

Carpenter M (1980) Asylum nursing before 1914. In: Davies C (ed) *Rewriting Nursing History*. London: Croom Helm: as well as Mick Carpenter's chapter, virtually all the other chapters are worth reading for a richer and broader understanding of nursing history, particularly for the way in which they eschew the 'great men and women' perspective of the subject.

Carpenter M (1988) *Working for Health*. London: Lawrence and Wisehart: an authorised history of the healthworker's union, COHSE, this utilises some excellent primary source material to give a detailed account of the role of one of the key trade unions in nursing history.

Carr EH (1961) *What is History?* Harmondsworth: Penguin: although this has nothing to do with nursing, it offers a fascinating critique of the writing of history and the factors that determine it.

Dingwall R, Rafferty AM and Webster C (1988) *An Introduction to the Social History of Nursing*. London: Routledge: again, despite its age, still required reading for anyone seeking a deeper understanding of the subject.

Morton AL (1989) *A People's History of England*. London: Lawrence and Wisehart.

Nolan P (1993) *A History of Mental Health Nursing*. London: Chapman & Hall.

White R (1978) *Social Change and the Development of the Nursing Profession*. London: Henry Kimpson.

3 Nurses in the NHS – from Being 'One Step Up from Domestics' to Clinical Militancy

We want the full percentage pay rise we are asking for. We also want to ensure that there will be no more cuts affecting patients. Enough is enough.

COHSE nurse, reported in the *Evening Standard*, 20 February 1988

▶ Introduction

The National Health Service (NHS) was often described as the jewel in the crown of the 1945 Labour Government. It was one of the instruments with which the post war Labour Government – and many of the people who had voted for it – hoped it would transform British society. Nurses were at the heart of the new service, at least in terms of numbers and their importance in delivering healthcare en masse to an eagerly waiting population. While for some, its arrival was a case of 'carry on nurse', with the transformation from the unwieldy collection of local authority and privately run voluntary hospitals something that passed without any great fanfare or fuss, for others it was a time for great celebration, the culmination of years of campaigning and the opportunity for old aspirations to be realised. At its heart, however, the NHS contained a series of contradictions that would inexorably combine to create an implosion that would play a major part in a redefinition of the entire healthcare system. These were inherent in nursing's structures, its dearly held aspirations and the ambivalence of both the medical profession and hospital management committees towards nurses and nursing.

This chapter explores key events affecting nursing within the NHS. These include the establishment of the Whitley Councils, the system designed to provide a national bargaining framework for nurses and all other health workers employed within the service, with the exception of the medical profession. The nursing organisations were vying for superiority within these while nurses were trying to develop their clinical role. Gradual change came in both spheres. The cultural, social and economic revolution heralded by the Beatles gradually infiltrated the corridors of the nation's nurses' residences as nursing practice moved away from task orientation to the nursing process. As the 1970s progressed, industrial relations became the key issues affecting the health service and this chapter attempts to understand why. The 1980s only saw more conflict as, first, nurses and other health workers came into direct confrontation with the government, with nurses going it alone only five years later. Clinical innovations were now coming faster than ever before but the government's agenda was wholly different, concerned with containing costs and introducing new managerial structures. As shall be seen, what was actually a more fragile consensus around the role and nature of the NHS had already snapped. Again, space prevents detailed examination of most of these. The intention is not to provide a detailed account of events but give a flavour not just of a rediscovered history but also a wider focus and context for particular problems nurses faced that will, hopefully, benefit the reader and show the patterns and principles that are so often exemplified in decisions on matters about nursing that affect nurses.

The issues surrounding the implementation of the new clinical grading structure in 1988 are presented as a case study because it is a classic example of how policy, politics and nursing practice have collided. This period witnessed a direct and momentous confrontation on a national scale between nurses and government that went far beyond pay: it was also about the very nature of the work that nurses thought they should be doing. It is a fascinating story in itself. Most importantly, however, it was perhaps the key event in a thread of interconnected policy decisions during the late 1980s and early 1990s, the consequences of which had the most profound effect on nurses and nursing and are still with us today.

▶ Not all is rosy in the Garden of Eden

The views of the civil servants and hospital management committees, coupled with the manoeuvrings of the doctors and the lack of power nurses' organisations had in shaping policy, had an immediate impact on nurses in the new service. Given that the problems about training, organising and paying nurses had been one of the most significant factors in necessitating a change to the healthcare system, little was done to re-organise or adjust the nursing structure. Seen as a homogeneous group, when they were far from that, no attempt was made to introduce any social system that might bring some sense of coherence to the new, enlarged nursing workforce. With Whitley Councils being set up as the new bargaining machinery, both nurses and their organisations were being squeezed into a straitjacket with no room to establish a pluralistic tradition. And the Nurses, Midwives and Health Visitors Council was, from the outset, the scene for new rivalries that would prove as destructive as the old ones that had been perpetuated by the College of Nursing and Royal British Nurse's Association (RBNA). The biggest of the new trade unions solely representing staff in the NHS was the Confederation of Health Service Employees (COHSE). It had been formed from an amalgamation of the unions representing healthworkers in the county council hospitals and those working in the mental hospitals, both groups of workers bringing with them a tradition of fighting for improved pay and conditions as the best way to represent their members, very much in keeping with other trade unions such as the National Union of Public Employees (NUPE). The professional associations, of which the Royal College of Nursing (RCN) was by far the largest and most powerful, were intent on pursuing the goal of status through adherence to the vocational ideal. Instituted within the NHS bargaining framework was a fundamental philosophical difference and ideological faultline that would prove a powerful hindrance to nurses.

Unlike most of the trade unions, the RCN was not affiliated to the Labour Party, which meant that it didn't donate any money to the Party, didn't have members on its ruling national executive and had no formal links with it. Nonetheless, it was determined to be recognised as the dominant nursing organisation with the Labour administration and Ministry of Health. Its success was measured by the fact that College members accounted for eighteen out of the nineteen nurses sitting on the new regional boards and that it had twelve seats on the Whitley Council compared to COHSE's four.

Despite the initial hopes and warmth towards it, the NHS was already running into problems. Britain was paralysed by its war debt – particularly to the United States, which terminated its lend lease programme early into Labour's period of office, rendering the country virtually bankrupt. The hypothesis that improved healthcare would rapidly improve the health of the nation, thus enabling lower expenditure, was quickly proven to be wrong as the NHS went over budget and unsuccessful attempts were made to reign in expenditure, even though all benchmarks of efficiency in patient treatment and care were showing dramatic improvements and many previously fatal diseases were being conquered. Within a decade, the number of full time nurses had risen by 15.9 per cent and part time nurses by 54.1 per cent (Webster, 1969). But by then much of the original idealism had been tainted.

The principle of free healthcare for all had been sacrificed as soon as dental charges were applied. Bevan, the charismatic Welsh Health Minister, a figurehead for radicals within the Party, had resigned from the Labour government, which was itself then cast into the political wilderness after the 1951 election, not to regain power from the Conservatives until 1964. Nonetheless, an apparent consensus held in the NHS throughout that decade and the 1960s. The NHS was a 'good thing'; it was certainly popular and, despite some rumblings about the drain it was having on the national economy, was adjudged by most political commentators to be effective at what it was supposed to be doing. The existing model was not, in actuality, that different from what had gone before. The medical profession had secured its position at the centre of the new service. The hospital had been secured at the centre of National Health Service provision.[1] The voluntary hospitals – of which many had faced an insecure future because of serious financial problems – were now the cream of NHS hospitals, with London's teaching hospitals occupying the most prestigious positions, followed by those in other metropolitan centres, with this prestige attracting the lion's share of funding. The old local authority hospitals, now brought under the control of the NHS, were still associated with their Poor Law origins and seen as second rate by many local people who were expected to use them.

Nor had nursing practice changed much. It was essentially task allocation, the system that had evolved out of the way nurses were organised into a distinct occupational group. The essence of the work the nurses had to do was simple: provide care to a large number of patients within a particular setting. So the ward sister, or nurse acting on her behalf, would allocate individual nurses to take everyone's temperature, measure and record blood pressure readings, exchange empty for used urine bottles, change dressings, bathe patients and so on. The nurses would work their way down the ward, washing people or organising them for baths, then make all the beds. This 'industrialised' or 'production line' nursing meant that the work was both carried out anonymously and could be carried out by anonymous individuals, especially students, who would spend relatively short periods on the wards. Reviewed extensively in the 1940s, this method of practice was supported by the RCN's Horder Committee and, although criticised by the Ministry's Wood Committee, continued. There were differences in what nurses of different grades would do, reinforcing the hierarchy that held the system together. The elaborate dress code also played a part in this, with differing hats for nurses of different ranks, different coloured belts and dresses, all of which were used to denote the status of nurses within their own occupational group. These social constructs were not simply a remnant of nursing's military heritage; along with the petty rules, traditions and codes of behaviour and conduct, they were also a means of keeping at bay the intense physical and, in particular, psychological discomfort that arose from being in such close proximity to the sick and the dying. This social 'glue' was of immense importance and never fully appreciated or understood until Isobel Menzies' groundbreaking work, originally published in 1960, which peeled away the process like an onion and explained how these defences against anxiety shaped the structure and work of the institution, creating a dysfunctional environment

---

[1] An integral part of Bevan's early plans were for local government involvement in managing health services. Innovative health centres, symbols of the aspirations for a primary care based service, were to have been built all around Britain as a key feature of a new service, fundamentally different from the hospital led services that had dominated healthcare since the latter part of the nineteenth century. Financial constraints had meant that not a single health centre had been built by 1950, although the government had not been able to afford to build any new hospitals either.

when the displaced anxiety would be 'acted out' in ways that did not allow the participants to resolve the difficulties they were both grappling with *and* creating. (Menzies, 1970). Changing the method of practice without attending to the psychological consequences was to have ramifications few could have imagined.

Little progress was made in terms of nurses gaining more 'professional' status in the NHS. This should have offered the trade unions a great opportunity to advance their cause – except that they were not making much better progress on pay and conditions' issues. Although the situation was infinitely better than had existed pre-NHS, the first dispute within the NHS came within its first year, when student nurses in COHSE waged a successful campaign for improved wages. As the years progressed the centralised bargaining system utilised through the Whitley Councils became bogged down in bureaucracy. There were ten different councils, with management and civil servants on one side of the table facing combinations of fifty-five different unions on the other. Nurses and midwives had their own council but also had wider issues about terms and conditions settled through the General Council. On the crucial issue of pay, despite the fact that often bitter negotiations went on, the councils could only make recommendations to government and annual pay rises were not automatic. A cycle developed, with several years of healthworkers securing no pay rise at all or one below the rate of inflation, followed by a larger increase to appease health workers' growing anger. Consequently, twenty-six out of a possible fifty-three major settlements had gone to arbitration by the late 1950s (Klein, 1989).

Another significant change had resulted from the RCN's acceptance that there would be a second level nurse – the enrolled nurse. After many years of staunch opposition to such a development, they had done a complete political about turn. This was predicated on the recognition that, if it was to maintain a close relationship to the Ministry of Health, it would need to accept that containing cost was fundamental to the future of the NHS and that arguing for a trained workforce made up solely of registered nurses was not justifiable or for 'the good of the service'. 'The good of the service', 'the needs of the service' or 'the common good' were used as a mantra for justifying all sorts of policy decisions that would have been very difficult to sell to junior nurses, especially as nurses were so far out of the decision making loop. And when the policies were even more potentially problematic, for instance keeping pay artificially low compared to other occupational groups like teachers or police officers or cutting back on services, 'the needs of the service' was translated into 'the needs of the patient'. Even when the actions were patently not in the interests of either nurses or patients. That senior nurses colluded in this process, as did the nurses' organisations, only made this harder for junior nurses to resist.

▶ Revolution at the bedside

Thus nursing moved forward into the mid-1960s in a state of unease with itself, its employers and the anonymous figures making decisions that affected it. Outside the health service, the world was rapidly changing, with social, cultural and, above all, economic revolutions sweeping the western world.

Labour was back in power. Trade unions were flexing their muscles, the young suddenly had disposable income and the revelatory changes in communications had opened up seemingly endless opportunities. Moreover, the culture of deference was being thrown off at every turn, perhaps symbolised most potently by the outright opposition of so many young people to the Vietnam War. For the metropolitan young at least, sexual repression became a thing of the past, hair lengthened, skirts shortened and Britain was transformed from a vision of gloomy, post war black and white to one of primary colours. Organised religion was losing ground to Eastern and more esoteric philosophies as people adopted a more questioning attitude or looked for more immediate gratification. The use of hallucinogenic drugs (estimated to have been used, during the late sixties, by 'several millions of the brightest young men and women of their generation') created a shift in perception unlike anything experienced at any time in the past (McDonald, 1994). While Britain's youth was awakening to The Beatles' *Sergeant Pepper*, Bob Dylan, Andy Warhol and The Rolling Stones, the nation's nurses were still locked up in hospital nurses' homes, expected to behave like nuns, earning less than shop assistants.

Change forced its way in as the dwindling thread of consensus *within* the NHS finally snapped. There were already nurses influenced by the work of the American, Hildegard Peplau. The influence of the nursing process was also being felt from across the Atlantic. Amongst those nurses who were receptive to these new ways of practising were those who still hoped for greater status for nurses through improved standards of care, professionalisation and improving the education nurses received. These 'professionalisers' had largely been marginalised even within the RCN as its most senior nurses had allied it with government, managerial priorities and the 'good of the service'. Now, with the general explosion of creativity and yearning for change, they were able to tap into the wider social and economic changes occurring, trying to create a more intimate, personal relationship with the patient, taking a more holistic approach to nursing care. The nursing process matched the evolving agenda of the professionalisers, as nurses carried out their own nursing assessment, prescribed nursing care, implemented it and then evaluated the results. Doctors could not prescribe this nursing care, managers could not give direct instructions or make pronouncements about it. Now there were no intermediaries between nurse and patient. The nursing process brought them together completely – whether the patient wanted that or not. And there was evidence that not all patients did, particularly those from working class backgrounds, who found it woolly and intrusive (Dingwall *et al.*, 1988: pp 217–19).

The nursing process, in the way it individualised care and the nurse's role gave the impression of nurses breaking with the cloistered confines of the past, defining their work and, on a grander scale, something of the future of nursing. It also reflected another side of sixties change. Corporations were getting bigger and more powerful.

The manufacturing of consumerist goods was changing from the older methods of mass production and sameness to one of specialised products that emphasised an impression of 'choice', non-conformism and individuality. Marketing these goods and exploiting the new communications media increasingly insinuated business into the fabric of everyday life. Consumerism was a relatively new capitalist phenomenon: it had shaped the nuclear family and was now focusing on the individual – particularly the young – as its ideal market. Society was beginning to give way to the individual consumer and the private relationship was beginning to assume a far greater importance, as reflected by the growth of psychological groups, cults and therapists, especially in the United States, whose corporations were drawing upon the work of psychoanalysts to influence their design and marketing strategies.

The nursing process was finding its way into practice in the late 1970s but unexpectedly failed to make the desirable impact its advocates expected. Status did not increase, hospitals were not rushing to introduce individualised care and, worst of all, many of the nurses expected to implement it were indifferent or, at worst, antagonistic. This reflected the third broad grouping of nurses that had emerged in post war nursing. All three were, in their own way, of equal importance and had varying degrees of influence and power at different times, depending on their connection to external forces and wider political agendas. At best, there was an uneasy tension between these groups and, at worst, they would be in direct conflict with one another.

The 'professionalisers' sought greater status through higher educational standards and blending the art and science of nursing. Primarily, this group was working in education or occupied senior positions within clinical practice. It rarely had direct responsibility for the maintenance of the service. Professionalisers sought innovations in clinical care and to create working practices that would give nurses greater autonomy. As nursing progressed and their agenda began to bear fruit they were the nurses who gravitated towards education, centres of excellence and clinical nurse specialist posts.

The 'managerialists' were nurses who wanted nursing to achieve power and status through taking a place at the decision making table, with heads of other occupational groups, notably doctors and hospital or service managers. It was to the service and these disparate groups, as well as nursing – rather than nurses – that the managerialists aligned themselves. Inevitable to this position was the need to negotiate and, as part of that process, make compromises. One of the best examples was the decision to support the introduction of a new grade of trained nurses in the shape of the enrolled nurse. The problem for the managerialists was about whether the compromises were worth the gains they were able to make. One consequence was that senior nurses inevitably tested the loyalty of both sides of their nursing workforce and, much later, at the time of the introduction of general management, when that loyalty and practical support was needed it would not be there.

The 'generalists' were the vast number of nurses, often working in unglamorous settings, away from the major teaching hospitals, who saw nursing as, if not just another job, then an occupation that was deserving of a salary comparable with similar groups and decent conditions of service. They believed that traditional, industrial, means were needed to achieve progress. Largely the inheritors of the legacy of the Poor Law nurses and asylum attendants, they had more of a collectivist tradition and a greater level of scepticism about the vocational ideal. Less interested in the professionaliser's agenda and more loyal to their own grades than they were to their managers or the service, it was to be sections of this group that would gradually exert more influence after the quiet, clinical revolution of the 1960s and early 1970s.

▶ Modelling change

On one level, change was gathering pace. The nursing process was being introduced into hospitals up and down the country – at least on a policy level. In practice, as well as the reluctance of nurses expected to adopt it, the progress of the new way of nursing was also sabotaged by suspicious managers. Ill thought out in its implementation, much of what had made it a valuable experience in the United States was either lost or did not fit the culture and tradition of British nursing. Yet the appetite of supporters for change had been whetted. In many places where it was a success, the nursing process took root as a 'bottom up' exercise, championed by nurses in individual clinical settings long before it was even written about in the UK nursing press. Once it had found its way onto the pages of the nursing journals, it not only made further progress but was expanded upon by nursing models which explored the nurse–patient relationship in even greater depth, as well as the balance between physiological and social systems and goal setting (Royle and Walsh, 1992: pp 2–11).

These developments brought with them more pressure on the nurse. Greater individual involvement brought with it greater responsibility and, eventually, accountability. Yet there was still no increase in prescribed authority or status. Nurses were also much more in touch with their patients on an emotional level. Swapping the protective layers provided by task allocation for the intensive, detailed nursing of a much smaller group was to take its toll.

However, many of the same influences that had produced change within nursing and the NHS also saw the *external* consensus surrounding the service snap. The increased radicalism of the general workforce, as well as an end to a reliance on tradition and deferential attitudes inevitably, if more slowly, found their way into the health service. In part, these were accelerated by the adoption of more a business-like approach from managers in the 1970s. They were expected to manage on tighter budgets as the economy faced greater pressure, changing the culture within the NHS from one of job security, consensus and stability, to one of increased competitiveness in much larger, more anonymous district general hospitals that had been likened to 'health factories'. Equally, the unions recognised they had to try to deliver on the promise of substantially improved pay and conditions.

That the charge into a new era of industrial relations should be led by the medical profession should come as no surprise, given the British Medical Association's (BMA) record of antagonism to Labour governments in the NHS and its record as the most demanding of all health service trade unions, particularly when its members interests were perceived to be under threat. And lead the charge it did, in 1972, with a work to rule to defend its members' right to treat private patients in NHS beds, a move which brought the other health service trade unions into direct confrontation with the then Labour government. At the same time, attempts were being made to get more work from fewer staff, leading managers to introduce incentive bonus schemes for ancillary workers. This meant the unions had to recruit large numbers of stewards to represent members locally and actually undertake the detailed negotiations involved in the process. Hospitals, where the vast majority of NHS staff, nurses included, still worked were being transformed into a hotbed of radicalism, to the point where there were so many disputes that industrial relations was suddenly defined as, 'The problem for the health service' (Haywood and Alazewski, 1980: p 28).

There had already been a relatively minor pay dispute involving nurses in 1970. In 1972 over 100,000 ancillary workers answered their unions' call for a one day strike in a dispute over increased pay, a shorter working week and longer holidays. Although they achieved only a fraction of their initial objectives, the strike made ancillaries important. Management negotiations with them increased. Ancillary stewards and branch secretaries were representing large numbers of nurses in COHSE and NUPE, carrying with them the lessons learned from their own industrial action. Low pay for NHS workers was still a source of major discontent and, by 1974, even the RCN, which for so long had fought a rearguard action against increasing nurses' pay for fear that it would attract the wrong sort of woman into nursing, was dragged into the new arena, threatening mass resignations of its members as part of its 'Raise the Roof' campaign. COHSE went further still, under pressure from its own members, embarking on a substantial campaign of industrial action, recruiting significant numbers of general nurses for the first time as a result. The national bargaining machinery, in the shape of the Whitley Councils, having been one of the stumbling blocks to conflict resolution in the first place, was completely unable to accommodate the changed climate. Industrial relations were in a state of freefall.

The first major re-organisation of the NHS, in 1974, had been initiated by Labour, planned by the Conservative government which replaced it and then actually implemented by a successive Labour administration. This effectively ended the role of the matron – in the twentieth century at least – but strengthened nurses' position as consensus management at strategic, as opposed to operational, level was introduced. However, the reality of medical syndicalism (which beautifully describes the way in which the BMA operates – as a form of trade unionism that seeks to secure power for its members), was unchallenged as representatives of local consultants and GPs were given the right of veto, ensuring the balance of professional power was undisturbed. Moreover, it was widely accepted that what doctors' representatives promised 'in committee' would not necessarily be delivered by doctors on the wards (Klein, 1989).

Unsurprisingly then, the re-organisation failed. First, because it was unable to please local vested interests by providing a local system for genuinely resolving difficulties and disputes. Second, it did not give central government what it wanted, which was control of how policy was applied and allocated funding spent. Instead, it was even more bureaucratic and complex in structure than what had gone before.

There was no clear pay structure for all participants to work within and no government had yet managed to develop a coherent pay policy. This wasn't helped by the fact that nurses were hopelessly divided both internally and from other health workers. There were also mounting funding problems on the horizon which were certainly not going to ameliorate an already deeply frustrating system. An example of this was in the findings of one committee of inquiry in the late 1970s, that different managements had, at separate times, threatened to close two thirds of Liverpool's hospitals (Bosanquet, 1979). The Labour Government of 1974–79 had only been able to secure a loan from the International Monetary Fund by guaranteeing to make stringent public expenditure cuts. It also agreed a 'social contract' for keeping wage rises down with the trade unions nationally. The main impact of this was felt in the public services, while industry and the private sector were able to find ways of softening the year on year pain that went with it. £5 billion was lost from public spending in less than two years, added to the £1.2 billion cut by the Conservatives immediately prior to Labour's election victory in 1974 (Lister, 1988).

Further conflict became inevitable – the scale of it, however, was wholly unexpected. The now infamous 'winter of discontent' of 1978–79, a widespread programme of industrial action by a number of trade unions, including those representing health workers from hospitals up and down the country, is almost universally linked to the victory of Margaret Thatcher and her Conservative Party in May 1979. Those health workers had endured major cuts in services, increased workloads and already low levels of pay that were effectively worsening year on year. The attempt by the government to impose a 5 per cent limit on any increase, far 'below' the level of inflation, was the last straw. The ensuing dispute impacted most keenly on the public sector. The NHS attracted some of the worst headlines, with healthworkers – nurses included – accused, often wrongly, of such acts as turning away cancer patients from outpatient departments and stopping food deliveries to hospitals. A return to work was eventually negotiated on the back of a commission being established to conduct an independent review. Ironically, the Clegg Commission, which conducted the review, recommended a wage increase of 9 per cent – paid up by the new Tory Government, despite its rhetoric about the dispute and trade unions (Mohan, 1995: p 142). Nonetheless, rhetoric turned to reality as the new government made 'control' of the unions an early priority. Until then, post war legislation had been largely favourable to the labour movement, apart from Ted Heath's Industrial Relations' Act in 1970. Now, with public support and union membership declining, a whole raft of hostile legislation was to be passed.

The most bitter of all NHS disputes, however, occurred in 1982. Again, the issue was pay. The Conservative Government had no official incomes policy dictating wages for public sector workers like nurses. Nonetheless, each pay settlement was below the level of inflation and nurses were in direct confrontation with the government less than three years after the 'winter of discontent'. It was a dispute that demonstrated nurses' growing strengths but, even more pointedly, their overwhelming weaknesses. During the eight months it lasted, the unions had been able to mobilise a march of 120,000 health workers and their supporters in the September of 1982, held days of action up and down the country that affected an estimated 1500 hospitals, saw members of other unions risk jail as they campaigned on health workers' behalf, and held the public's support throughout 'in the largest display of working class unity and solidarity since the general strike of 1926' (Carpenter, 1988: p 378). But little progress was made in negotiations.

Unity amongst the various union officials representing the different disciplines within the NHS was stretched, particularly as those who had relatively small percentage of the workforce had equal say with the biggest. The leaders' demands and tactics were more conservative than those demanded by their members. Most significantly, the health service unions were hopelessly split (Hart, 1995). Trevor Clay, the RCN's general secretary was urging further negotiations with the government when the Trade Union Council (TUC) affiliated unions had rejected this outright, believing there was nothing new to negotiate about. The RCN membership had also rejected the current offer from the government about which Clay wanted to negotiate (Nursing Mirror, 14.7.1982; 1.9.1982; 22.9.1982). With the unions unable to agree how to prosecute the dispute further after the September national day of action, it was already faltering; the Conservatives exploited these divisions and uncertainty and tempted the College to the negotiating table. From that moment, the dispute was doomed.

The government offered a two year deal that didn't match the unions' demands but was an improvement on previous offers. It also split nurses off from other health workers and the negotiating process by agreeing a Nurses', Midwives' and Health Visitors' Pay Review Body (PRB), similar to that for doctors and dentists. The dispute effectively ended in December when COHSE voted to call off its industrial action at a special conference. No decisive action had taken place after the momentous September demonstration.

The interpretations of the outcome of the '82 dispute were as, if not more, important than the reality. The NHS unions had taken on the 'Iron Lady', Margaret Thatcher and her government. While they hadn't won an outright victory, they had forced them to the negotiating table because of their industrial action and won concessions. They had held together an unwieldy coalition of forces with reasonable success. Both because of her fear of a repeat of such a strategy and nurses' role in it, Thatcher had been forced to offer something that would dent its control over pay settlements for the largest group of workers in Britain – the PRB. Nurses had finally come of age as an industrialised workforce, proved their muscle and established a brand new tradition for themselves that would see their transformation to a group that could achieve status through steadily improving pay and conditions.

That was one way of looking at the outcome. Another was to suggest that the contradictions inherent within the nursing workforce had always been lurking just beneath the surface, destined to sink the ship of unity long before it sailed into port, flags flying. When they did, and the RCN signified a willingness to re-negotiate, this undermined the unions' strategy and health workers throughout the NHS were doomed to accept a settlement that had been within their grasp months earlier and would not have led to the nurses being irrevocably split off through the PRB and everyone's cause irretrievably weakened.

The RCN and, in particular, Trevor Clay, could be seen as hero or villain. Going back to the table was either inspirational, given the faltering state of the dispute and increasingly acrimonious atmosphere within the trade union camp, or self-serving and treacherous, selling out the fundamental principle of trade unionism, that of solidarity.

It was a turning point for nurses, even though the implications could not have been fully seen or understood at that historical juncture. Having been united with other health workers on the key issues of pay and conditions, they were now separated on pay, which was to be determined through an entirely new process. The nurses' own representatives, their trade unions and professional organisations, with the management/government side, would submit evidence to the PRB. This independent body would then recommend an award. The rub only came at the final stage of this process – for the recommendation went back to the government, who then decided whether or not to implement it.

The RCN hailed this as a victory for its 'common sense' approach to trade unionism, its willingness to negotiate; this was partnership between government and the workforce, taking the element of conflict out of nurses' pay and finding new solutions to old problems. For the leadership of COHSE and NUPE which, between them, had the vast majority of non RCN nurses in their membership, the issue was far more tricky. Given that the PRB was a reality, they had to sell to nurses it as a victory – and they did ensure their own, untrained, nursing auxiliaries and assistants were covered by the PRB, against all out opposition from the College, who argued that this brought non-nurses into the review process – but at the same time placate their ancillary and other non-nursing members, who perceived nurses as, yet again, being treated as a special case.

Perhaps because of this, they certainly did not trumpet the offer of the PRB as a consequence of their own radicalism in pushing forward their industrial relations agenda, seeking to establish a fair system for achieving significant improvements in what they saw as the key indicator of nurses' status, their monthly salary cheque.

Nurses drew their own conclusions. COHSE was always the biggest rival to the College in the NHS, being solely a health service trade union. Although NUPE, as a general public sector union, had more members, it had far fewer in health than COHSE, with a smaller percentage of these being made up of nurses.[2] COHSE's membership peaked in 1982, with nurses switching unions in order to be able to participate in the industrial action. It declined after that until its demise in 1993 (when it merged with other unions to form Unison) apart from a brief revival during the campaign of 1988. The RCN, meanwhile, went from strength to strength, its membership soaring by 80,000 to a declared 300,000 in less than a decade.

In the year before the health workers' dispute, the Tories' popularity had sunk to an all time low and Margaret Thatcher been polled as the most unpopular prime minister since Second World War. Unemployment had more than doubled to 2.5 million. Two events reversed this and ensured the domination of a Conservative agenda in politics for a further fifteen years: victory in the Falklands War in 1982 and, one year earlier, the formation of the Social Democratic Party which split any effective parliamentary opposition in two. It was to be a turgid time for the unions as a whole. The Miners' strike of 1984–85 and printers' dispute at Wapping in 1986 signalled an end to an era of industrial trade unionism that had lasted more than a century. In the NHS, ancillary services were handed over to the management of commercial companies as the government embarked upon its so called 'privatisation' crusade in the name of efficiency and cost cutting. Not only did the ancillary staff find themselves either losing their jobs or having to accept vastly reduced pay, holiday and sick leave entitlement, but the unions lost thousands of members as the companies refused to recognise them or placed sufficient pressure on staff to stop them remaining as members. Moreover, this was only after sustained campaigns to stop the government and the expenditure of hundreds of thousands of pounds as well as immense effort on the part of local, regional and national officials. Many activists who had been ancillary workers were lost.

Services were also being, at best, re-organised or, at worst, cut back. Again, the unions were in the forefront of campaigns to stop the most excessive of these measures but, as many of these cuts did not affect nursing staff, again, the RCN was left free to concentrate on other things, which it was doing to great effect.

---

[2] The whole problem of accuracy in union membership is dealt with in more detail in Chapter 7. There are no accurate historical records of nursing membership in either of these unions, but we can make certain deductions from general trends and contemporary records. Prior to the formation of Unison, given COHSE's numerical advantage in nurse membership, I will focus on that as representatives of an alternative vision to that of the RCN for the sake of simplicity.

The attitude of COHSE members to the PRB remained ambivalent and there were regular attempts from members at its annual conference to get the union back into a negotiating framework. These were all defeated as first David Williams and then Hector Mackenzie, its general secretaries during this period, were able to point to better pay increases for nurses than other health workers were achieving and improvements on pre PRB years. But nurses were, nonetheless, falling behind yet again in the pay stakes as the government played its nap hand and refused to implement the PRB's recommendations in full. By the latter part of the 1980s, the cuts affecting other parts of the service were also impacting on nurses. Given that nursing had been so conservative, generally, for most of its history and that, only a few years earlier, the National Union of Mineworkers, the most powerful trade union in the country had been ripped apart at the hands of a Thatcher government that had gone on to rampage its way to its third successive electoral victory, it might seem remarkable that, not only were nurses ready to confront government for the third time in a decade, but were prepared to do this on their own. Yet that was just what was about to happen – with one difference. It wasn't just about pay this time. It was far more personal than that. Clinical militancy was about to make a brief but momentous appearance.

▶ Case study 1: The 'clinical grading dispute' – the interface of practice, politics and policy

The quiet revolution at the bedside was in full flow by the mid- to late-1980s. Primary nursing had been developed from the nursing process as a model to put nurses in the driving seat of patient care. It brought with it an even more finely honed concept of 24 hour responsibility for the primary nurse, whose care plan was to be followed by colleagues even in her/his absence, coming out of the four key components to this new form of nursing: responsibility, authority, autonomy and accountability (Ersser and Tutton, 1991). There was also a far greater administrative and time burden than had existed with the old kardex form of notekeeping, as nurses documented their own care plans – often negotiated directly with the patient – a detailed history and, in some cases, a nursing diagnosis sheet. This placed the nurse even further at the apex of the patient's care. The detailed knowledge the primary nurse could develop about the patients they were nursing gave them a natural, if ascribed authority and, as a consequence, genuine status in the multidisciplinary team. New structures were needed for the primary nurse to communicate not only with fellow nurses but also the rest of the team, doctors included. Now even the nurses' hierarchy was subverted, as senior nurses were effectively bypassed. The recognition that many people were, in effect, facing incurable medical conditions, or would require long term care even after surgery, gave even greater legitimacy to a form of nursing that allowed its protagonists to get on with their work more autonomously. Perhaps it was these more subversive effects that meant that primary nursing never received widespread central or managerial support, or even that given the nursing process. It was inevitably widely promoted by the professionalists and educationalists in nursing. Far from universally adopted, it nonetheless remained a framework that gave nursing even greater legitimacy. With a new system on the horizon for educating nurses that would finally see students as supernumerary, have more stringent entry requirements and academic standards throughout the training, it looked as if the professionalists' star was firmly on the ascendant. Yet these advances in the role were still not delivering greater authority across the board while greater responsibility and workload, as well as the more intense, personalised relationship with patients, had brought greater, almost intolerable, increases in the levels of stress.

The 1980s also saw nurses even further established as the core of the NHS, forming 51 per cent of the NHS workforce (although they received only 45.4 per cent of the NHS pay budget even after the pay awards of 1988 and 1989). More than 80 per cent of nurses were still working in hospitals. The dramatic bed closure programme that was to re-shape the NHS, most notably in London and other major cities, was already underway, with a significant rise in the number of day cases and inpatient cases being treated. They would go on to rise by 90 per cent and 40 per cent respectively in a decade by 1990. The length for inpatient stays was, however, decreasing at an equally dramatic rate and the sum total of these changes was that the workload of the average nurse was estimated to have increased by 37 per cent from 1962 to 1984 and doing so far faster towards the end of the decade (Observer 10.1.1988; Carpenter 1991: p 45).

The *NHS Management Inquiry* was a relatively tiny document given its grand, though somewhat anodyne title. It had been authored in 1983 by Sir Roy Griffiths, assisted by a small team. None of them had any direct experience of working in the NHS. The report proposed introducing general management into the NHS and was to have a revolutionary effect on what nurses could and could not do, from having enough sheets to being managerially accountable to non-nurses for the first time in decades. It paved the way for nurses to become budget holders – but, significantly, not managers, meaning they had responsibility to ensure their wards or units did not spend more than allocated but not how that money might be spent. Tiers of nursing management were lost as general management percolated down through the NHS and a new culture was being created, with business practices, terminology and attitudes gradually becoming commonplace. These changes were, often surreptitiously, resisted by nurses and other health workers. The unions and professional organisations waged major campaigns against the principle of general management and some of the initial plans implemented by the new managers – usually involving programmes of cuts – but ultimately to little avail. The problem Sir Roy's critics had was that the entire health agenda had virtually been hijacked by the New Right (see Chapter 5). Faced with the question of what they would do as an alternative, no one was able to mount a coherent argument and, even if they did, given the ideological nature driving the change, it was not being listened to.

That this far reaching report, with its blueprint for the most radical re-organisation of the NHS in its history, was written by the boss of a supermarket chain was just another of the cruel ironies of the period. Nurses were barely mentioned in it, despite figuring as the major casualties of its implementation, however unintentional. Its most famous quote, nonetheless, invoked Florence Nightingale, suggesting that, were she 'still carrying her lamp through the corridors of the NHS today she would almost certainly be looking for the person in charge' (Griffiths, 1983). Within a few years of The Griffiths' Report being implemented she probably would have been looking for the exit. Many nurses were.

The continued problem of the 'wastage' rate among student nurses was now compounded by serious problems recruiting and retaining trained nurses. Shortages were most acutely felt in critical care and highly specialised areas of nursing. Thirty-five per cent were dropping out of RGN training in the mid-1980s, with 30 per cent of trainee enrolled nurses. More worryingly, even before that, the number of new students had fallen by 30 per cent. In some parts of the country trained nurse vacancies were running as high as 20 per cent. As relatively senior nurses left the clinical arena, their absence and the loss of their experience had not only to be contained by their less experienced successors but also managed for whole ward teams.

In 1987, just months after the Tories' landmark electoral victory, a baby died in Birmingham, awaiting treatment because of a shortage of suitably trained nurses. A succession of similar stories followed, creating the aura of a cash related crisis. The arguments about health service funding had gathered pace during the decade, and more information about the inequalities of regional funding was surfacing. In an age when consensus was meant to be a thing of the past, a new one was emerging, one that even many managers signed up to – surprisingly perhaps, given the accusations of managerial appointments that were increasingly politically motivated – of demand outstripping resource. By the beginning of 1988, newspapers were still reporting horror stories, with doctors saying young children and other patients were either waiting unacceptably long periods or even dying because of nurse shortages. This seemed to legitimise the nurses own sense of deepening grievance and, for a while, it looked as if, having started to express that grievance, there would be no stopping them.

Into this simmering cauldron, the government threw a new ingredient that would quickly have it boiling over. The catalyst was the leaking of the news that it was planning to scrap the special duty payments paid to nurses working late shifts, nights and weekends. Within days, thirty-seven nurses, all members of NUPE, staged a 24 hour strike. Although criticised by the *Nursing Times* and suffering the outright condemnation of the RCN, they were hailed by the national press and many nurses throughout the country; within days the government had backed down and withdrawn the threat to remove the special duty payments.

▶ Clinical grading: clinical militancy enters stage left

But something else had been stewing during the winter months. It was not easily categorised or articulated but key themes were emerging. They were concerned with how nurses felt they had been treated and how they were perceived. Moreover, they saw this as being linked to how patients experienced care in the NHS and they saw staff shortages, managerial attitudes and the changing nature of the service, with its emphasis on shortening the patient's length of stay in hospital affecting their ability to nurse people in the way they had been trained to do. Until then, a significant number had been voting with their feet, leaving nursing altogether. Now they were talking about something completely different. This was reflected in contemporary statements to journalists, with nurses expressing, 'A feeling that something has to be done to stop patients suffering' (Pownall, 1988: p 18). They had seen 'the health service decline and services deteriorate over the past two years. In the past few weeks they have begun to react' (Sherman, 1988). The importance of pay within this cocktail was there for many nurses. After all, 40 per cent of them in 1987 were estimated to be earning below the Low Pay Unit's poverty threshold of £132.27p per week. There was also a relatively widespread understanding that the problems were due, at least in part, to government decisions about funding. A rapid decline had been seen during the decade, and the Social Services Committee estimated the accumulated underfunding was standing at £1.325 billion in 1986, rising by a further £1/2 billion in the next two years. It was this linkage to the concerns for patients and the actual care they, the nurses, were able to provide to them, that was the unique factor. One nurse preparing for industrial action was quoted as saying, 'The vote for strike action ... was absolutely unanimous. We want the full percentage pay rise we are asking for. We also want to ensure that there will be no more cuts affecting patients. Enough is enough' (Evening Standard, 20.2.1988). It was the fusing of the quiet revolution with something far noisier, creating a wholly incendiary combination.

The initial NUPE protest in January sparked off debate and actual calls for action in hospitals throughout the NHS. Nurses at the Maudsley Hospital, all members of COHSE, set the tone with a one day strike that created a whole new image for nurses taking industrial action. Being mental health nurses they were not wearing uniforms. But the Maudsley Hospital was not an old county asylum; it was a prestigious London teaching hospital with an international reputation, whose staff had already successfully staved off major cuts in 1986 in a highly publicised campaign. The nurses were supported not only by their ancillary and admin staff colleagues but, in a move that attracted enormous press attention, a number of doctors who briefly joined them 'on a picket line where grim messages of crisis failed to crush the carnival atmosphere and [car] horns tooting their support competed with the music and chanting, and cheering pensioners joined in' (Sherman, 1988). Next day, hospitals across the capital followed suit. The blaze of publicity from the Maudsley nurses' action guaranteed more of the same and the issue was now dominating the national political agenda.[3]

Behind the scenes, COHSE's General Secretary, Hector MacKenzie, was under intense pressure to bring his nurses into line with the TUC's official position, which was that the nurses were demonstrating rather than striking and there were protest rather than picket lines outside hospitals. The scars of 1979 ran deep and many NUPE full time officials, fearful of the Tory press dragging the Labour leadership into the dispute with demands that they condemn the nurses' action, argued behind closed doors for no further strikes. MacKenzie, a quiet, thoughtful Scot who had risen unobtrusively through his union's ranks, was not the obvious choice for a radical leader at this juncture but, whatever his private views, offered unequivocal public support for the nurses. Moreover, he gave a youthful and creative group of full time officials an unheard of opportunity to work in tandem with leading nurses in the campaign, warning of more problems to come if the government did not act, both on NHS funding and nurses' pay. He was right.

However, it did not come in the form of nationally co-ordinated action. With the TUC ambivalent at best, it was largely left to individual trade union branches although regions within COHSE's national structure did organise their own days of action.

One of the strengths of the way in which general management had been introduced to the NHS was that it was left up to individual health authorities to implement, within given parameters. This made it virtually impossible for its opponents, particularly the trade unions and the RCN, to organise effective opposition, given their First World War like chains of command and cumbersome decision making processes. The way in which the baton of leadership during this dispute was passed from hospital to hospital, however, had a similar effect on the government, who were the effective targets of the nurses' fury. They found it hard to counter the nurses' arguments. Even though newspapers supporting the Conservatives had run headlines such as 'Angels who nurse a death wish' (News of the World, 31.1.1988) and '490,000 nurses *will* be at work today' (Daily Mail, 3.2.1988), 79 per cent of voters polled declared their support for nurses taking industrial action – with even 67 per cent of Conservative voters holding that view. A TUC demonstration in March 1988 drew a crowd estimated at anywhere between 120,000 and 200,000.

---

[3] The strikes and issues around them garnered a great deal of international news coverage. It is interesting to note that by September 1989, similar concerns were being voiced by Californian nurses at the Oakland Children's Hospital, who went on strike for over two months in pursuit of special duty payments to accommodate the emotional demands made upon them by their patient group and because of staffing shortages which were pushing them to their physical and emotional limits (Smith, 1992: p 138).

In terms of actual action, there was still no cohesive line emerging, but there was growing dissent within the RCN, particularly when Trevor Clay was unwilling to call a special meeting for nurses to debate the issue of action from College nurses. There was also growing unease within the other trade unions that COHSE was letting its nurses run out of control.

The trade unions were uncomfortable with the heady mix of the clinical and the industrial. How would they take the campaign forward? How would anyone know when it should end and, vitally in such a climate, whether gains or losses had been made? For different reasons, the RCN were even more unhappy with the situation. If nurses had been 'rewarded' with the Pay Review Body for their 'good sense' by negotiating and ending their dispute in 1982, how much damage could be done by this current round of anti government campaigning? There was a considerable contest between the unions and the College – not just for hearts and minds, but also for members. The volatility of nurses was demonstrated to the nation when on 2 February, 'live' on Breakfast TV, Charge Nurse Paula Morrison from the Maudsley Hospital said she was leaving the College to join COHSE because of comments Trevor Clay had made on the programme about her striking colleagues. Nurses were both joining afresh or shifting from one union to the other in unprecedented numbers as a result of the respective organisation's stance on the issue that was dominating nursing: clinical militancy.

For the trade unions, the College and the political parties, there was a life raft in this sea of uncertainty, although it was heading on an uncharted course. It was called clinical grading. Barely prompting a mention in the press up until this point, it had actually been under discussion for nearly two years and was designed to extend the grading structure, respond to nurses' aspirations on pay and reward nurses for remaining in the clinical arena. Detailed consultation and working had been progressing well through the Nurses' and Midwives' Whitley Council until mid-1987. Despite a variety of problems, requiring hard nosed negotiation and compromise, agreement was finally reached on definitions for a nine point grading scale, from A to I, which was announced in March 1988. One key problem was to attach pay scales to the new grades, in the midst of the nurses' dispute. As was now common, both government and the staff side had put forward their evidence to the PRB about the merits of pay increases for nurses.

With this now allowing the unions to try to focus nurses' attention on pay, COHSE again did the unexpected and opened a second front against the government, by offering an alternative to the 2p in the pound tax cut the Tories had been trailing for several weeks prior to the March budget. The union argued that if this were abandoned and the money directed into the NHS, it would make up the £2 billion shortfall in funding that was at the heart of the current crisis.

Into the tumult, the PRB made its recommendations and, to some extent, the temperature was cooled when the government accepted these in full. Although every nurse in the UK had to have their post assessed before they would know which grade they would be assimilated onto, an immediate award of 4 per cent was made, with the remainder to follow as soon as the new structure was in place within their own workplace.

▶ Clinical grading: the aftermath – degraded and devalued

If this was an opportunity, finally, after forty years of the NHS for the work that nurses were doing to be valued and for nurses to feel their true worth was being recognised, it was one that was not taken. The task of allocating nurses to grades should have been relatively simple, the process having earlier been negotiated between the staff and management sides and guidance then being distributed to trade unions and managers throughout the NHS. A timetable had been agreed for each stage of the grading process, with 31 October 1988 the deadline for all nurses to be assimilated onto their new grades.

Given the backdrop to the implementation of such a radical development in the arena of nurses' pay, hindsight begs us to wonder at the naiveté of the key players. The track record of nurses' employers throughout history meant a smooth ride with such large sums of money should have been the last thing anyone expected. Equally, given the incendiary atmosphere in many hospitals, the government should have known that nurses' expectations were sky high and not meeting them would be costly indeed. Nurses had, after all, seen the grading criteria and virtually every nurse in the United Kingdom, being an expert in what they did in their own job, had decided for themselves what grade they should be on. By July 1988 it was clear that the process was going badly wrong in all kinds of ways. The sense of grievance and injustice grew.

An old problem within the NHS had been that the centre that is government or the Department of Health, would decide national policy, which would then be subverted, undermined or plain ignored in the regions or within the localities. This had been one of the factors that had led the government to want a general management system in place, where appointments were made from the centre and a direct line of managerial responsibility and accountability was drawn from the Department out to the most junior general manager. In a reversal of this historical circumstance, general management proved its worth as a means of delivering policy implementation as evidence emerged of collusion between the centre, the regions and those charged with actually carrying out the grading exercise. In some instances, it was more a case of coercion as nurse managers complained of undue pressure but it quickly became apparent that cash limits were secretly being imposed upon health authorities and that the management side at a national level was insisting that there could only be one 'G' grade per ward, regardless of the work being done by postholders. There were also claims they were manipulating the interpretation of 'supervision' in the clinical setting.

In practice, this meant two ward sisters who had been working alongside one another, doing the same work, managing the ward between them, would be graded differently, at 'F' and 'G' on the clinical grading scale, with the former getting a pay rise of 4 per cent while their former partner would be made the senior nurse and get an increase of 28 per cent. At the other end of the scale, untrained staff who had looked at the scale and expected a 'B' or 'C' grade according to the work they were doing found themselves anchored at the foot of the pay scale on an 'A' grade because of the way in which the crucial term 'supervision' was being interpreted, again receiving a meagre 4 per cent.

Ian Morton, the COHSE branch secretary at the Maudsley Hospital, summed up the situation: 'Nurses have learned over the past year that the way this government behaves is very much dependent on how it perceives what nurses are doing. They have massively misjudged the mood' (Brindle, 1988). As in February and March, the action was often spontaneous, unco-ordinated and lacked any national focus. Hector MacKenzie and the rest of COHSE's leadership was still strongly supportive of it, including an indefinite strike called at the Maudsley Hospital in September. This followed a walk out by the trade unions from national negotiations the previous month in protest at the Department's intransigence on the two major sticking points in the new criteria – continuing responsibility, which affected potential 'G' grades, and supervision, which had a bearing on 'A' and 'B' grades in particular.

The walk out had been led by national officers from COHSE and the RCN in the absence of Trevor Clay and Hector MacKenzie. Although the two general secretaries had fallen out publicly over tactics and the issue of nurses taking industrial action, any remnants of unity between the nursing unions rested on their relationship and the leadership they provided. Insiders reported that they had a genuine respect for one another, as well as understanding the constraints the other was facing. Both remained under pressure for different reasons. Senior figures from the other health unions, such as NUPE, and the TUC, as well as the Labour Party still wanted MacKenzie to 'control' his nurses and ensure there was no major fall out for the wider labour movement and, more particularly, the Labour Party leadership. Clay had been severely criticised by his own members, including senior, respected figures like Tom Bolger, for taking such a critical stance towards nurses taking or even supporting industrial action. There was also a significant, vocal minority within the College who wanted a rule change to allow them to join their colleagues in other unions on the picket line.

There were many senior RCN officials, however, who were arguing that the grading criteria were basically sound, the culmination of their demands on pay and professionalism and accusing COHSE of manipulating nurses' anger with a few militant branches creating the impression of more widespread dissatisfaction than there actually was. As she had in 1982, Margaret Thatcher endorsed this view, stating, 'These nurses would never have got this [pay] award but for the no-strike policy reaffirmed by the RCN' (Vousden, 1988). Although there was broad support for the principle of the grading structure within COHSE as well, both organisations had, in truth, been taken aback by the ferocity of nurses' reactions to it in the workplace.

Nurses' action took a new turn, attempting to force the government to meet the estimated shortfall to fully fund the new award, thus freeing up managers to, at least in the eyes of those involved, implement the new structure fairly. There were, by now, all kinds of allegations of 'fixing' being made. Mainly, these focused on regional cartels of senior nurse managers meeting to set grades together on a cash limited basis, receiving instructions from the DHSS on what numbers of grades could be afforded within a given region.

Kenneth Clarke had taken over as health secretary during the crisis. From the outset he was bullish, confrontational and apparently indifferent to whatever the nurses were doing, continuing the line that there was no extra money to fund the award. Until, in early October 1988, in time for the Conservative Party confer- ence, as if it had always been a part of the government's strategy, he declared that an extra £138 million was being made available. The following month, the NHS budget was increased by £1.8 billion, almost the exact figure by which COHSE had estimated the service was underfunded and for which it had so fiercely campaigned (Klein 1989: p 235).

That might have been that. Yet soon after, nurses were notified of their individ- ual grades and reacted with fury. Further walk outs followed. Nurses adapted their tactics to 'work to grade', carrying out tasks as close as possible to the criteria of their new grade and refusing to do anything which fell into the criteria of a higher grade. When frustrated managers pointed out that this meant they stopped doing nursing tasks and carrying out nursing care that had been part and parcel of their job before the grading exercise, they responded that this was entirely the point. Midwives, who had originally argued for a separate grading structure for their posts, had become more disillusioned than any other group. Their ballot about whether or not to abandon their 'no strike' policy was far closer than that of the RCN. One of the unnoticed fault lines in the grading structure emerged even more clearly with the allocation of their grades. Although touted as a *clinical* grading structure, the actual emphasis was very much on *managerial* responsibilities. Mid- wives' work demanded high levels of clinical autonomy and decision making, but little management. Consequently, they were being graded lower than those they viewed as, at best, their nursing equals. Forty-four midwives resigned their posts at the North Middlesex Hospital, whose Chief executive, David Hirst, said he was using lower grades to introduce a hierarchy, apparently oblivious that the midwives and nurses should have been graded according to the work they were doing in April 1988. Those like Kevin O'Brien, a COHSE branch secretary, took a more radical option. He led his members as they 'worked to grade' at Banstead and Horton Hospital, securing the upgrading of seventy night nurses without appeal. In other hospitals where similar approaches were adopted, its success was direct and swift. For others, it was to be a process that would be drawn out for years to come.

▶ Clinical grading: no appeal to reason

It's difficult to know who found the appeals process more difficult, the government, NHS managers or trade unions. By the mid-1990s clinical grading appeals had been heard at local, district, regional and then national appeal. A fast tracking system was eventually devised before the final appeal was heard, not far short of a decade after the new pay system was introduced. The damage had been immense.

A generation of nursing and NHS stewards were lost. They had led their nursing members in all kinds of campaigns, demonstrations and, in some cases, industrial action. They had attended local meetings, argued with intransigent managers, heard stirring speeches at their union conferences throughout 1988–89 and, in COHSE, roared with approval when their national leaders assured them every clinical grading appeal would be supported. Hardest to bear, however, was the attritional process of what was estimated for Radio 4's *Today* programme to be 120,000 appeals lodged in the aftermath of the grading exercise. They had sat through those appeals and represented individual nurses, often finding their evidence rejected and losing the cases, having to bear the brunt of nurses' anger – for nurses were furious that they had, in their view, been improperly graded in the first place and, in a system stacked against the appellant, still not achieved the point on the scale and, with it, the financial reward and status they believed was rightfully theirs. Rationally, unsuccessful appellants knew what had happened, how and why; they were grateful to the people who had, and still were, trying to help them. But on a more emotive level there was such pent up anger about the whole business and the stewards and union representatives were the people in the immediate firing line, who had that particular cross to bear, as nurses could find no way to vent their spleen directly at their managers. It became, even if only expressed in momentary dark, unforgiving looks, a case of 'the union that was to blame'. Even for those satisfied with their grade, or who won their appeal, there were mixed emotions and their view of their unions was undoubtedly affected.

Relationships within the national nursing organisations sank lower than was good for nursing, something that was reflected in a widening gap at local level. Trevor Clay continued to attack 'handfuls of nurses destroying the profession's image with silly banners', as well as their trade unions; Hector MacKenzie responded that it was time for Clay to decide 'whose side he was on, the nurses' or the government's'.

It would take years before midwifery recovered from the loss of status reflected in the grades they were awarded and for nurses in other spheres it was clear that more complex clinical work and innovative nursing brought no reward other than the satisfaction the practitioners derived for themselves and within their own team. Largely it came down to who and what the nurse managed, and how frequently, or how closely s/he was supervised – far removed from the original ethos of those involved in devising the structure. For instance, the difference between 'D' and 'E' grades was taking charge of a ward or equivalent on a regular basis – determined to be more than one shift per week.

Many managers faced a no win situation. Even if they had played no part in the grading process, they had to sit opposite highly aggrieved nurses and openly argue why they should not have a higher grade. Success won only the contempt of the nurses involved – and many of their colleagues – while losing an appeal would mean finding money from already stretched nursing budgets for the back pay. By the time of regional and national appeals that could be as much as £10,000 per person – if it was a successful group appeal involving several nurses, the financial consequences would be catastrophic for the local budget manager.

The – some might suggest 'rich' – irony was that, by many more objective indicators, the dispute about clinical grading had been a success. It had delivered an overall increase of 15.6 per cent. Most nurses were better off than they would ever have been. Moreover, it stopped in its tracks a triumphalist government re-elected for a third term, whose most radical and animated free marketeers were predicting a rapid end to the NHS. From a starting point of wanting to cut special duty payments, introduce local pay, limit the grading structure and hold the overall pay bill in check, the government had suffered reverses on all these points, not only having to implement the PRB's recommendations in full – for the first time in four years – but also make one of the biggest increases to the NHS budget in recent times. Even the main protagonists among the unions could point to financial success, given that COHSE reversed a five year decline in membership and gained an overall 4000 new members, while the RCN was even more successful, claiming it had gained 14,000.

Something far less tangible was lost, however. For those nurses who had not gained anything more than the basic 4 per cent, it was a bitter experience to see some others gain vastly more, especially where they could point to the fact that they had been working identically pre-grading. Concerns about staffing, patient care and the way in which people were nursed – the issues that had originally stirred nurses' imagination and spurred them into collective action – had been lost, never clearly articulated at a national level by the nurses' representatives. The unity nurses had found in campaigning together was replaced. Now the rebelliousness was something more private, taking place in an individualised world, characterised by even greater division and a system of nursing that was becoming even more hierarchical.[4]

---

[4] The appeals process, nonetheless, was undoubtedly a continuation of the same clinical militancy and unwillingness to accept any imposition of the management world view. Nurses of all grades who had never publicly disagreed with their managers, were now doing so in the most open and vivid manner, telling panels about their work, what they had done and why the manager and any witnesses they produced were incorrect. If a revolution truly needs a change in consciousness and the changed involvement of individuals, this was it. The importance and relevance of this aspect of the dispute was, perhaps understandably, lost in the melee and logistical nightmare of organising the people and the process and the nursing unions never made any attempt to harness it or make use of it in a collective way. Even as nursing became 'quiescent' in the 1990s, there was never any sense that there was a 'belief' in the new managerial doctrines that followed. The resistance had simply gone underground.

There were even more sinister consequences to come, that would have been almost impossible to foresee during those fateful months at the beginning of 1988. Interviewed in January of that year on BBC TV's, *Panorama*, Margaret Thatcher was facing intense questioning about NHS funding; it was almost a throwaway comment when she remarked, unscripted, that it was to be the subject of a ministerial review. The problems of nurses' pay had prompted the question and its answer was lost in the furore of the prolonged dispute. When that 'review' finally took place it was headed up by Kenneth Clarke, the new health minister who had made the financial and policy 'U turn'. It was a review that was to make the most far reaching changes the NHS had yet seen, in effect dismantling its national structure and framework. It was also part of the process that was to see the end of the era of modern nursing that had begun with the so-called Nightingale reforms.

▶ Conclusions

Too often, nursing histories have failed to get to the bottom of what has driven change or peered beneath the orthodox surface of events and the way in which they were related. It has, usually, been a 'top down' history written from the viewpoint of policy makers or those aligned with them, despite the honourable exceptions to this. Inevitably, there are any number of events, developments and issues that haven't featured in this account of forty years of the NHS. But, hopefully, it does connect policy with practice and politics in the clearest possible terms.

The histories of the NHS and nurses became inextricably entwined, although the fortunes of both have not necessarily followed one another as closely. Indeed, one could argue that nurses have sacrificed, for varying reasons, more than most for the 'good of the service'.

Nurses had already been placed at serious disadvantage, despite their numbers in the new organisation, by a combination of clever political footwork by the doctors, whose dominance prevailed within the healthcare system they favoured. Nurses had few real friends in the Department of Health, regional boards or local management committees and the trade unions and professional organisations were busy vying for power. The latter occupied the key positions on committees that would determine, within the constraints of the wider decision making process, what would happen within nursing – including how its needs would now be subordinated to those of the service, stuffed into an ill fitting, homogeneous straitjacket and not given any room to breathe any creativity into the new service. Despite a great sense of public and political hope, optimism and support for it – not least because of some significant achievements – the problems the NHS had inherited from its predecessors and issues of funding meant it faced increasing problems, had difficulty resolving them and found it even more problematic to change course. Its ambitions had to be scaled down and it was proving less effective at addressing inequalities and improving the nation's health in the way politicians had thought it would.

Wider social, political and economic change in the 1960s eventually found its way through to nurses. A long period of stability – or stasis – was followed by progressively rapid and radical change. Intricate rules and social mechanisms to keep individual anxieties had created dysfunctional institutions but, when changed without adequate support mechanisms, left nurses vulnerable to greater levels of anxiety and stress. Nurses went through a, largely unplanned, revolution. As well as positive benefits, this created more widespread dissatisfaction and grievances. The lack of mechanisms to resolve them at a local level became more apparent, particularly the main negotiating mechanisms, the centralised Whitley Councils. As the thread of consensus was pulled taut and finally snapped, the 1970s were convulsed with wave after wave of industrial action involving, at different times, virtually every sector and discipline. Some were enacting the class and social divisions institutionalised in the service – the struggle over private beds, for instance. Others reflected a wider conflict, with a trade union movement that had grown in size, confidence, influence and ambition pushing successive governments with their demands that culminated in a dispute too far. Like apparently invincible armies before them, the trade unions found themselves overextended and exposed to a cold winter of discontent in 1979. Yet both they and their opponent in that particular struggle – the Labour Party – were losers, the latter being ousted from government for 18 years.

As Thatcherism advanced, nursing continued on its twin paths. Clinical and training developments were taking place while pay and conditions were becoming even more of a pre-occupation. Thus the 1980s were marked by plans for Project 2000, primary nursing, the 1982 pay dispute and clinical grading. This period arguably represented some sort of high water mark – however brief – for nurses: many of them had been involved, to a lesser or greater extent, in steering through important changes in clinical practice and assumed more control over those aspects of their work. Moreover, their training had instilled in them a more reflective attitude. The new ways of working they were developing were further based on a more thoughtful, critical, questioning approach. These changes in turn brought nurses far closer to the people they nursed, allowing them the opportunity to develop a far more holistic relationship. Nurses also brought with them, and built upon, the confidence the greater economic freedom, social and intellectual independence had given their generation. Not least, they had become more demanding and better at articulating their demands. These factors were then clearly linked in nurses' minds and resulted in the clinical militancy demonstrated in 1988. The events leading up to, and including, clinical grading also represent as good a case study of nurses and politics as we are likely to get. All the essential ingredients are there. After that, nursing and nurses were to experience major change; that change impacted on the NHS and it would never be the same again. For the Thatcher Government had another agenda, of still greater commercialisation, a more disciplined, more business like, managerial culture. The gains that had been laboured over to make important and significant advances in nursing practice were rapidly eroded.

Clinical grading closed a circle opened in 1937 when a group of masked nurses marched through London's streets demanding better pay and conditions.[5] More than sixty years ago, nurses had been trying to mend the faultlines that ran through the discipline, largely caused by the problems that went back to the origins of modern nursing. These problems ran one off the other: how to find enough women to nurse the apparently ever expanding numbers of acutely and, particularly, chronic sick; how to maintain the funds to pay them; how to develop practice, education and standards, giving nurses greater status; how to exert the necessary control over such a large number of disparate, unwieldy groups, all labouring under the title of 'nurse', particularly when nursing has been subordinated both to the needs of the service and the medical profession as the dominant occupational group. The contradictions in that list are immediately apparent. They were to be made even worse by what was to come.

▶ Further reading

Ersser S and Tutton (eds) (1991) *Primary Nursing in Perspective*. London: Scutari.

Klein R (1989) *The Politics of the NHS*. 2nd edition. London: Heinemann: this gives a good overview of policy in and around the NHS, events and political analysis.

Menzies I (1970) *The Functioning of Social Systems as a Defence against Anxiety*. London: Tavistock: an essential read for anyone interested in understanding what nurses were experiencing during the period after the Second World War and the collective response of both them and those responsible for the organisation of nursing. In many respects, still relevant to contemporary nurses and their situation.

Morgan KO (1992) *The People's Peace, British History 1945–1990*. Oxford: Oxford University Press: this offers a good account of the political background to the changes affecting nursing during the period covered in this chapter.

Owens P and Glennerster H (1989) *Nursing in Conflict*. London: Macmillan: written just as clinical militancy was taking effect, this is based on a research study that focuses on the organisational repercussions of the Griffiths Report and its impact on nurses and nursing.

White R (1985) *The Effects of the NHS on the Nursing Profession 1948–1961*. London: King's Fund.

---

[5] It was one of the small coincidences of history that the key protest meeting held by nurses in February 1988, organised by London Health Emergency, was at the Camden Centre in central London. This was the same venue the masked nurses and their colleagues had attended that November evening, after their march and demonstration, just over fifty years previously.

4 Angels

Lost Angel of a ruined Paradise!
She knew not 'twas her own; as with no stain
She faded, like a cloud which had outwept its rain.

Adonais by Percy Bysshe Shelley

▶ Introduction

Angels are everywhere in nursing mythology. Nurses are angels. Everyone 'knows' this, because it's something we're constantly reminded of, in the media, by grateful patients and their relatives, in the portrayal of nurses in fictions, whether it be books, films or TV dramas. We even remind ourselves of it from time to time. Why? In some respects, the connection between angels and nurses might seem obvious and abundantly reasonable. It has existed so long that it is almost impossible to trace back to its origins. The earliest reference this author could find was a quote from Mr Macdonald, the man who arrived in the Crimea to administer the monies raised by readers of *The Times*, who said of Florence Nightingale, 'She is a ministering angel' (Bingham, 1979). Angels and nurses are apparently inextricably linked, yet the association is not as obvious as first appears and there is a subtext about its deeper meaning that is rarely explored in any nursing literature. If it has shaped, or symbolically represented, an image of nurses and told us something about nurses' relationships with the outside world, then we can be sure that something of the complexity of those relationships is to be found in the unravelling of the myths. Caring, nurturing, death, accepting hardship, suffering, subservience and subordination are all part of the myth. But, as with angels, there are two sides to the coin.

This chapter will explore the nature of angels and sources of information about them. Ministering to the sick and dying is only one aspect of the work of angels, but the nurses role in being with, and caring for, the dying was to be crucial in defining the characteristics of the earliest modern nurses and nursing. There is also a contemporary debate within nursing that mirrors that in philosophical circles about science and religion. For nurses, this reflects language and ideas but also sees a legacy in practice and education. As science and technology develop, what will be the implications for nurses? Will we truly witness, as is being predicted, the 'death of the soul'? As is discussed here, nurses understand and construct their work in very different ways. Nursing research and evidence based practice is akin to a new religion but can everything nurses do be measured and scientifically evaluated? Is there any credibility in the notion of faith and intuitive knowledge? Later in the chapter, the image of angels again arises, but this time illustrating the darker side of nursing, those who have transgressed or broken the rules of the discipline to which they belong. In its latter stages, there is an examination of why nursing is women's work, the images that are constructed to tell us about nurses and nursing and what factors might prompt change in nursing practice.

▶ Who are the angels?

Angels are common in many religions. In polytheistic religions the gap between humankind and their deities is far less pronounced and angelic functions are often performed by one of the gods through a human form. The angelic role is most fully elaborated in religions that emphasise a greater distance between man and God and are based on revelation. Judaism, Christianity and Islam are all examples of this. The greater distance means there is a requirement for intermediaries to bridge the gap and, as divine messengers, angels fulfil this role, amongst many others, but sit beneath humankind in the heavenly order.

Although little is really known about angels, as with nurses, they have been greatly mythologised. In recent times proponents of new age religions have appropriated the name and images of angels for their own ends. Concentrating on angels in Christian literature, which is those to whom they are most usually referenced, the obvious source of information about their origins is in the old and new testaments of the bible. Interestingly, however, much of the biblical image of angels is actually derived from apocryphal texts – themselves described as being mythological. The most influential of these is the apocryphal First Book of Enoch, which includes accounts of the actions of the four main angels, Michael, Gabriel, Uriel and Raphael.

The pages of the Bible contain few references to angels and even fewer that identify the angel(s) concerned, naming only Michael and Gabriel. Angels appear to pass on messages to Mary and Elizabeth about their respective births. It is angels that guide the shepherds to the manger. The book of Hebrews calls angels, 'Ministering spirits sent forth to serve, for the sake of those who are to obtain salvation' (Heb. 1:14).[1] It was an angel who brought Elijah bread and water while he was fleeing from Jezebel after his victory on Mt Carmel (1 Kings 19:5–6). A relatively modern phenomena – probably Victorian – is the concept of guardian angels which, presumably comes from verses when Jesus is described as having said,

---

[1] All biblical references are from The Bible (1952) Revised Standard Version. London: Collins.

'See that you do not despise one of these little ones; for I tell you that in heaven their angels always behold the face of my Father who is in heaven' (Matthew 18:10). Psalm 91:11 promises, 'For he will give his angels charge of you to guard you in all your ways.'

Angels were also on hand at crucial moments in biblical accounts as protectors or to encourage their mortal charges. When Paul and his shipmates were facing shipwreck, an angel appeared to him, assured him that not a life would be lost, and that he would live to stand trial before Caesar (Acts 27:23). Again, angels are described as being able to provide supernatural protection when, in Daniel 6:21–22, we are told of how an angel shuts the mouths of the lions when Daniel is thrown into their den.[2]

There are, however, two key incongruities in the association between angels and nurses. The first is one that is common to modern angel mythology as a whole, in that nurses have always been predominantly female – and were almost exclusively so when the tag was first applied. This corresponds with the romanticising, or sex-ualising, of the angels' image in songs, poetry and art. These associations are odd only because, of course, all the biblical angels actually given any identity were male. However, it's not just lascivious rock stars who accept such conventions: many depictions of angels within art are of females, perhaps attempting to convey the beauty inherent in the concept of the angelic being. Very few are male, with the remainder representing asexual creatures.

The second is that not all angels were 'helpful', nurturing and peaceful. Far from it. Even 'good' angels could bring death and destruction on a massive scale. It is an angel that appears, sword in hand, to Joshua, advising him how to bring about the destruction of Jericho (Joshua 6). Then there was Sodom. Although two angels come to remove Lot and his family from the oncoming carnage, they wreak their own havoc when necessary and presage the city's destruction (Genesis 19: 1–25). Michael is the senior of the archangels, traditionally regarded as the leader of the angelic armies and is mentioned in both New and Old Testaments. According to both the book of Revelation and the apocryphal book of Enoch, Michael led the heavenly armies against Satan and his followers, driving them from heaven. Perfectly reflecting the ambiguity of angels, Michael or Saint Michael is venerated as patron of the sick in East European countries while in the West he is held as the patron of soldiers.

And if there are 'good' angels, then there are certainly dark, or 'bad', angels. Although they were all created as holy angels, the bible tells us about one third rebelled against God and fell from their sinless position. Of course, Satan is the leader of these unholy angels and is described variously as a liar, a murderer and a

---

[2] For more information see, for instance, Sue Bohlin's 'Angel's' website or *www.probe.org/docs/angels.html*

thief. This angel hates God and passionately hates God's people. The Bible tells us that, 'The devil prowls around like a roaring lion, seeking some one to devour' (Peter 5:8). Satan and all his angelic followers are supernaturally brilliant, and Satan disguises himself as an angel of light (2 Cor. 11:14). God even gives Satan permission to strike Job with evil boils and an excoriating skin disorder, catastrophes, economic disasters and the death of his children. Ilan Kutz (2000) describes this story as one in which Job must struggle as a patient, with his various healers, with the process of loss and illness through adaptation and acceptance to being healed. It is only through the ultimate intervention of God – which has been interpreted as Job's own 'inner voice' – that he reaches this stage (Job 1–42).[3] Although Michael and his angelic army were able to defeat Satan, an angel is not someone you would want to meet when out alone on a dark night.

While the lyrics of many songs are not worth spending time on, latching on to popular imagery without thought or consideration, there are some that do explore something of the tension at the core of some angelic myths and concepts. Jimi Hendrix was a master of lyrical imagery and ambivalence. His 1967 composition (unreleased until 1970) 'Angel' tells us an 'Angel came down from heaven yesterday, She stayed with me just long enough to rescue me', and describes being taught to rise before affirming, 'Tomorrow I'm going to be by your side.' The song combines sexual and drug allusions with spiritual and romantic imagery almost reminiscent of William Blake. Mick Jagger's 1972 lyrics to 'Sweet Black Angel' are ambivalent in entirely another way. The song is about Angela Davis, a black activist, at the time awaiting trial on – what many considered manufactured – charges of conspiracy, kidnapping and murder. Jagger not only sings of her continued struggle and heroism while she awaits her trial but also hints that he 'is turned on by her heroism' (Weiner, 1995).

This ambiguity, these dark and disturbing undercurrents and different 'truths' – albeit in the context of a phenomenon many regard as mythical itself – can allow us to explore much more about the mythology, imaginings and realities of nursing.

Matters of life and death

Despite this, the common perception about angels and their visitations are that they are 'good' and will bring 'good outcomes'. Perhaps the most famous account of a visitation of angels is that from the First World War when, in August 1914,

---

[3] Kutz suggests that there is an important lesson in this for nurses and doctors. Only by confronting their own feelings of helplessness in the face of relentless deterioration of some patients, as well as empathising with the patient's own 'doubt, dissatisfaction, accusation or ingratitude', can the patient be helped into that stage of adaptation and accommodation of their circumstances (Kutz I, 2000). Job and his 'doctors': bedside wisdom in the book of Job. *British Medical Journal*, 23–30, December 2000, pp 1613–15.

British forces were fighting an apparently hopeless rearguard action against the Germans. Harold Begbie gave an account of how a British lieutenant reported watching three angels appear together for over forty-five minutes at around eight o' clock at night. He described a tall central angel flanked closely by two smaller spirits on either side. According to the account, the angels protected the officer and his battalion. The advancing German forces, which had appeared to be on the verge of capturing their position, recoiled in disorder. Begbie also claimed to have interviewed a German officer who verified the story. He reported that he, his men, and their horses were rendered powerless by the force of an apparition. And so, miraculously, these British troops survived. The story was given more authority because the British casualties elsewhere that night were horrendous. It received further confirmation – from a nurse who claimed to have heard the story from an injured soldier – and a number of other soldiers who survived the conflict. Although inevitably disputed by rational thinkers of the time it was written into folklore. One of the undoubted reasons the story did gain such wide currency and credibility in some circles at the time was that it captured the imaginations of those who wanted to believe that God was on Britain's side – indeed, that there might be a God in the midst of such awful carnage – and that their loved ones were not alone on the battlefield and in their time of death, important given that millions of young men would never return.

More modern, or new age, accounts of visitations from angels often centre on the sick, reflecting Psalms (91 : 11): 'He shall give His angels charge over thee, to keep thee in all their ways.' However, research into such 'visitations' has revealed a remarkable degree of consistency in the matter of so called near death experiences. Writing in the *Journal of Advanced Nursing*, Suzanne Simpson (2001) summarises the literature from nursing and medical journals of 'the personal experience reported by an individual after a perilous dance with death or temporary state of physical death' such as when someone has suffered a cardiac arrest and is being resuscitated. Estimates of how many of this group have undergone a 'near death experience' vary from between 35 per cent and 60 per cent. Some researchers think this an underestimate, due to people's reluctance to report such phenomena. All report a great feeling of peace and tranquillity during the episode but not all describe the latter stages, of an out of body experience and meeting with a spiritual being, including angels.

The way in which death takes people away, and the effect it has on those left behind, is something many nurses inevitably try to put to the back of their mind, given their proximity to it and the frequency with which it occurs. It is this aspect of being a nurse, however, that plays a part in linking the role to that of an angel in the public mind: a proximity to death – and, paradoxically, to life – and the bearing of witness to it. People rely on nurses to know something of death, about its nature and how to react to it. Whether or not this is a realistic or healthy expectation is not the issue.

In some respects, it is easy to see the link between the issues of life and death and nursing's religious origins – indeed, some early nurses who came directly from religious orders were as concerned about the state of the patient's soul at the time of death as they were about nursing the body through it. Yet, the legacy of nursing's quasi religious or spiritual role poses difficult questions for secular nurses working in the twenty-first century. Moreover, the underlying issues are even more complex, speaking of how the religious orders and ideas prevalent in Victorian England exerted an influence on the methods of working and the organisation of nursing.

Remedying the alleged filth and squalid conditions facing the wounded troops in the Crimea had been one of Florence Nightingale's earliest proclaimed victories. For her, sanitary hygiene was a matter of natural order and class. There was an order in nature which her class had understood and it was a matter of duty to pass that on to others involved in nursing and the care of the sick. Other leading nurses at the time of the Crimea, such as Mary Stanley and the Rev. Mother Bridgeman, who led an Irish group of nuns, saw these issues in an entirely religious context. In a difference of philosophy that was to assume great, but unspoken, importance for the very soul of nursing and its different approaches, Bridgeman and Stanley believed:

> ... the will of God was not to be found by personal revelation but through the teachings of his churches. Thus it was important that their patients saw their nurses not just as performers of a social duty but as performers of a *Christian* duty. And, of course, it was important to the nurses that their patients died in an appropriate state of grace [my emphasis] (Dingwall *et al.*, 1988: p 46).

In later years, this difference came to mean more than the pure, literal religious adherence to Protestantism or Catholicity; it took on a degree of political significance as it was also about the way in which nurses worked and were organised. The former was about an individualised relationship between nurses and nursing, that could only be understood because of the suitability of the woman to the vocation and adherence to a set of principles over which she could not exercise any control. It was a matter of individual submission to these principles and awaiting a personal revelation. The latter was based on notions of a collective approach whereby nurses taught one another, experienced nursing communally and moved towards an understanding of their role and their place in the world of nursing both through their own and others' efforts, all directed at caring for patients at all levels. This philosophy was expressed as recently as 1996, in *The Common Good and the Catholic Church's Social Teaching*, which stated that, 'The Church's social teaching can be summed up as the obligation of every individual to contribute to the good of society' and that it regarded it 'as no less important than fulfilling our religious duties' to show 'solidarity with people everywhere who are on low incomes, disabled, ill or infirm ... or who are otherwise vulnerable, powerless and at a disadvantage' (The Catholic Bishop's Conference of England and Wales, 1996).

There were other life and death issues, politically important to the evolution of nursing, that were shaped by events in the Crimea. These concerned those who were able to care for those facing death. Nightingale was able to lay claim to not only being able to organise the hospital, provide better nursing care and reduce the mortality rate of the wounded in the British army, but also that women from her background, social class and temperament were able to care for dying men in the most harrowing of circumstances – vital if the 'new' nurses were to gain any credibility. In reality, little had changed. This was largely still being done by male orderlies and soldiers' wives. Nightingale's ladies remained quite removed from the actuality of nursing the soldiers but their presence alone was one of the factors that paved the way for women of a higher social class to come into nursing (Summers, 1988).

▶ Science and religion

It can be seen then, that religion and religious thinking, as well as the 'religious' experience of being with patients as they were dying, were all important in the way that nursing developed. The significance of the relationship nurses have with death remains. The only people who have a closer acquaintance with it are undertakers; but this is only after the fact. Doctors experience the death of patients in an entirely different way and are rarely present at the moment it occurs. Even if they are, it is inevitably the nurses who are left to 'clean up' and perform the last offices – the moment when the body is washed, orifices filled to prevent bodily fluids leaking and wrapped in a shroud, all of which carries with it religious undertones. It is the nurses left with the relatives. Indeed, it is they who have to look those same relatives in the eye, and the patient, as the life begins to ebb away in cases of gradual death, knowing that the hope is fading with each glance. This observation and contact with death, people coming close to death or being nursed through critical illnesses or after near fatal injuries is something unknown to most people. As people move through later adulthood they will experience serious illness and the death of relatives, but this will still, generally, be an exceptional event in their lives. Yet most nurses will begin witnessing it within a short time of starting work in the clinical area, often at a relatively young age; for those who stay in adult nursing or who nurse older people, it will remain a fairly frequent occurrence. The first death is usually well remembered, with the experience the new nurse gets largely dependent on how it is 'managed' by the nursing team, and how s/he is helped through it.

There is evidence that supports the obvious observation that this is the most difficult aspect of nursing and that, however unconsciously, it can easily become one we wish to avoid, with any number of 'tasks' that apparently 'need' to be carried out to help us do so. A summary of the results of a survey based on continuous observation of fifty dying patients in medical and surgical wards in four large teaching hospitals revealed:

> The final period of hospitalisation ranged from six hours to 24 weeks. More than half of all patients retained consciousness until shortly before death. Basic interventions

to maintain patients' comfort were often not provided: oral hygiene was often poor, thirst remained unquenched and little assistance was given to encourage eating. By contrast, the patients' physical state was recorded regularly – the temperature and pulse of 84% of the patients and the blood pressure of 48% were recorded until death. Contact between nurses and the dying patients was minimal: distancing and isolation of patients by most medical and nursing staff were evident: this isolation increased as death approached (Buckley, 1998: pp 26–32).

For those nurses who distance and isolate themselves from the dying – in much the same way many nurses do from sex and the sexuality of their patients, for potency as much as death arouses primitive fears in us all – much of the difficulty is actually in 'being' with the person. It is not that relatively simple, or basic, nursing care is suddenly forgotten. Reasons might be given about workload, how busy the ward is, how the staff don't necessarily know the patient terribly well or don't want to intrude on visitors' grief as justification. But, essentially, what is difficult is allowing oneself to look at the grief of the living, the sense of loss of the dying patient and the life literally ebbing away, of trying to find the individual's understanding of their experience and the meaning they are able to attribute to their life and death, be that positive or negative. As Natalie Field, then a third year student, acknowledges, 'Through [observing the death of a baby and its effect on her parents] I learnt the difficulty of dealing with my own pain and emotions and coping with the fear and grief of others. I realised that to understand the importance of a nursing skill such as family support you have to experience the emotions and cherish each life as you would your own' (Field, 1998: p 28). There is little opportunity to talk about death in the work setting, few structures that facilitate any attempt to come to a shared understanding of it – even if it is only to conclude that, actually, people have very different ideas about death and the dying patient or experience death in very different ways.

Does the fact that nurses have lost contact with our religious roots change this experience? Most commentators – and, indeed, nurses – would agree, at least, that nurses have lost contact with their religious roots but, before considering whether or not that has actually changed their experience, we need to question that initial assumption.

Only a tiny number of nurses now come from religious orders. The number who would describe themselves as practising Christians has, presumably, declined along with the rest of the general population. There have long been non Christian nurses practising in Britain, but not in such significant numbers as to effect any major cultural change. With so many nurses now being actively recruited from overseas, with different religious beliefs, a different dimension is introduced but it is too early to assess the impact of this. However, as with many aspects of their experience, it will probably prove difficult to do anything other than subordinate it to the dominant culture of their workplace and peers, at least publicly.

Yet how much of the old language and practices of the religious orders has actually gone? How much of it remains, albeit being expressed and acted out in either a symbolic or secularised manner? There is still the language of vocation, as has been noted earlier, dressed up in terms of the 'needs of the service' or 'good of the patient', both implying that nurses need to subordinate their own needs to these higher ideals, and carrying with them connotations of sacrifice and duty. Poor wages and conditions are, again often in an implied way, justified by other rewards, those of acting altruistically and serving others. It is a commonly heard expression that 'nurses would not do the job if it were just for the money'. Ergo there is an assumption of something more rewarding, even if that is not necessarily defined or material. Moreover, the assumption is usually accompanied, in the public's mind, with one that there is something special enough about that work, that very few people are equipped with the necessary qualities to do it. Nurse training, with schools of nursing removed as they have been from the hospital setting and Project 2000 and its successors introduced, now carries less of the religious fervour for the vocation than was common in the older, apprenticeship based training. Nursing is undeniably different, without many of the initiation and socialisation rites and rituals of that older system. Some of these changes and differences, it has been argued, are responsible for the weakening of nursing as a discipline, resulting in a diminishing of the quality of nursing care provided to patients.

As efforts have been made to make education and practice more evidence based a new debate has emerged. It is sometimes characterised as science versus the art of nursing, sometimes almost caricatured as the embracing of new technology and a hi-tech approach to nursing at the expense of focusing on caring for the patient, an increasingly biological rather than psychosocial or holistic model. Proponents argue that nursing that accepts a more rigorous evidence base is more effective than a more intuitive approach based on experience and collective skills acquired through practice and with a knowledge base that is far more generalised in its development. Moreover, it is thought that evidence-based practice will be the element of nursing that will finally achieve that most cherished holy grail – status for nurses and the work they do. This dichotomy is given added currency as new technological developments are made. As is often the case, the internal debate within nursing reflects one engaging minds at all levels and is prompting ever more challenging statements – although these are sometimes most easily articulated by interested bystanders. For example, Tom Wolfe writes:

> Brain imaging was invented for medical diagnosis. But it's far greater importance is that it may very well confirm, in ways too precise to be disputed, certain theories about 'the mind', 'the self', 'the soul' and 'free will' that are already devoutly believed in by scholars in what is now the hottest field in the academic world, neuroscience.

Wolfe goes on to add:

> The notion of a self – a self who exercises self-discipline, postpones gratification, curbs the sexual appetite, stops short of criminal behaviour ... this old fashioned notion ... is slipping away ... (Wolfe, 1997: pp 6–10).

Rita Carter, a medical writer for *The Daily Telegraph* and magazines such as *New Scientist*, boldly states: 'The biological basis of mental illness, for example, is now demonstrable ... [and] ... it is now possible to locate and observe the mechanics of rage, violence and misperception, and even to detect the physical signs of complex qualities of mind like kindness, humour, heartlessness, gregariousness, altruism, mother-love and self-awareness.' However, she goes on to acknowledge that the 'mind mapping' work she describes 'does not settle the debate about existence', while critics of this approach can, for now at least, legitimately claim, 'A map of the brain can tell us no more about the mind than a terrestrial globe speaks of Heaven and Hell' (Carter, 1998). Advocates of an evidence based approach, or those who suggest that scientific advances which enable us to understand genetics and biology all the more clearly will offer us new mechanisms and techniques for better nursing (particularly so in mental health nursing), do so with almost a religious fervour bordering on zealotry. This is now embedded into official government policy as nursing research is only funded through the process of the research assessment exercise, where it is independently scrutinised, judging it against the same standards as all other disciplines, including engineering, physics and social sciences, all of which have long standing traditions of research and access to far greater funds to support it. Part of the debate is about whether or not nursing research should be separate, as there is about the respective merits of quantitative and qualitative research, with the former regarded as providing a stronger scientific base, with randomised controlled trials on all sorts of outcomes, but particularly identified nursing interventions, making the research applicable in different clinical settings. Supporters of research that does not simply look at how things are but seeks to change practice during that process, argue that this brings practice and academia necessarily closer together and, therefore, makes the research process far more apparent in its relevance to practice. So-called action research involves identifying a problem, selecting interventions, implementing change, reviewing the consequences and exploring the general findings, a model that bears obvious similarity to the nursing process (Gomm and Davies, 2000).

Those who question the evidence based, 'scientific', biological approach ask us to accept that there is more to the process of caring and healing than the eye can see or the tape can measure. Jane Salvage (1999: p 20) suggests, 'Faith has always been a crucial dimension of the healer's role, whether she was a village wise woman (or witch), a nurse or a doctor ... Anthropological studies in many cultures suggest that attributing special powers to healers assists cure ... Any practitioner can think of examples among patients ...' In effect the argument runs that we should have faith in our ability to care and accept that, in part, the efficacy of that care is based on precepts of faith, both for the patient and the practitioner. Attempts to gain understanding, through research, into the less tangible aspects of nursing care sometimes yield interesting results. 'An analysis of the nursing notes of 118 patients who had a cardiac arrest showed that in 41 per cent of cases nurses had been concerned about their patients in the hours leading up to the cardiac arrest. In a control sample of 132 patients who had not had a cardiac arrest, nurses expressed concern in only 9 per cent of cases.' However, while there were clear and consistent clinical indicators of the patient's deterioration, as one would expect, a key factor in any concern being expressed was the nurse's apparent 'credibility'. A view that came through was 'the perception that professional credibility could be damaged if nurse concern was poorly expressed to doctors' (Kenward and Hodgetts, 2002: pp 38–9).

Fergy (2001) further highlights the difficulties in unpicking all that a nurse does with a patient, evaluating its effectiveness in isolation from any of the other myriad interventions she is involved in, or analysing and articulating the process of cognition, decision making, use of experience, evidence based knowledge and practice or emotional labour. She ably describes the difficulty in the context of one nurse's care for 'a very ill, very frail and elderly patient ...' that involved, 'administering and evaluating analgesia, applying dressings, referring the patient to the medical, chiropody and physiotherapy staff, finding out why the patient wasn't drinking sufficient amounts of fluids, helping her to drink more, helping her to get to, and use, the toilet, talking to her about her anxieties about being put in a home, considering alternatives with her as well as giving space to speak with difficult relatives on the telephone'. Within these acts of, largely, physical care, there were a variety of emotional and psychological interactions. Fergy notes that 'giving the care did not pose insurmountable problems to the staff nurse ... [but] documenting the care did pose problems'. Fergy asks how such work can routinely be documented or simplistically summarised given that it is occurring on a variety of levels? Going on to argue that much of nursing is 'invisible, inarticulate and immeasurable', she puts forward the concept of 'innominate nursing' as a means of explaining why it is that so much about nursing and caring – women's work – remains elusive and so difficult to explain, let alone research (Fergy, 2001: pp 215–35).

Both sides in the debate have their own orthodoxy and beliefs, both have leaders and disciples, just as has always been the case in nursing. Thus, Kevin Gournay, Professor of Nursing at London's Institute of Psychiatry, could describe some of the advances made in DNA technology as well as those which mean, 'We are now able to study the structure of the brain', while arguing that contemporary research activity involving neuropsychological testing has important implications for mental health nursing. He suggests nursing interventions should be based on neuropsychological and detailed cognitive testing, with all mental health nurses requiring 'a basic understanding of neuroanatomy, molecular genetics and the various methods of brain imaging'. This, he writes, will benefits patients and their families but also 'put nurses on a more equitable footing with other mental health professionals'. In the same article, Professor Gournay cites the economic costs of treating schizophrenia, and, therefore, the economic benefits to be gained from adopting a particular type of nursing approach. Inevitably, given the 'rightness' of this cause, older, less scientific theories of nursing are heavily criticised, particularly those of Hidegard Peplau, something emphasised in numerous articles (Gournay, 1996: pp 7–12). Phil Barker, then Professor of Psychiatric Nursing at Newcastle University, with his colleague, Bill Reynolds, counters that Gournay's approach is 'potentially dehumanising' and that nurses should 'sharpen our focus on how all people differ from one another, and how these differences represent the distinguishing characteristics of the "person"'. Arguing that completing symptom checklists and working solely within biomedical constructs will further subordinate nursing to medicine, Barker and Reynolds suggest that viewing 'mental health in terms of human responses to the varied stressors associated with ill-health ... means that the primary role then becomes any response on the part of the nurse that assists the achievement of the most adaptive response possible to the traumatic life events that we call mental illness' (Barker and Reynolds, 1996: pp 75–80). Taking an even more direct view, Barker later wrote, 'Regrettably, many developments in psychiatry feign a knowledge of people by pretending that knowledge of the biological self – the brain – will help us understand the human self – the person.' He later continues, ' ... our behaviour, our interactions with the world of experience, the lessons we draw and all that life teaches us through our experience shape and mould the brain' (Barker, 1999).

It is, in some respects, a typical polemic. In fact, both Barker and Gournay hold complex views and, at the heart of their debate, was a very human concern about what might be the best way to care for people. It is also a debate that attempts to shape the very nature of nursing care, how nurses relate to the patient – from how we talk to people, what we talk about, how long we spend with them. The question arises, if we really are saying goodbye to our souls and that sense of self that has been inimical to human relationships is really slipping away, how do we relate to one another and how do we nurse each other?

In fact, the administration of 'simple' nursing care, the sort that it is argued should be carried out by untrained nurses because it is so simple and simply not cost effective to be carried out by registered nurses, has always had some aspects which are akin to religious sacraments. Feeding someone too infirm to do that most fundamental of actions, washing them, the laying on of hands, whether it be when bathing someone, treating pressure areas, applying dressings or moving their position, all have a direct, symbolic comparison in religious thinking and actions. And nurses continually ask patients and relatives to have faith, whether it is in the ability of the clinical team to discover what it is that is wrong in the first place, the treatment prescribed for them or their ability to withstand the distress, pain and uncertainty of their illness and 'get better'. And if Salvage is right, the efficacy of the *care* being given, rather than the treatment, is diminished as soon as either party, patient or nurse, loses faith. In those intimate moments when nurses are alone with the patient – or, at least as alone as two people can be in a hospital setting, although it is a far more profound experience when those acts of physical care are being carried out in someone's own home – they often hear an individual's most intimate thoughts and feelings expressed in an almost confessional way. This is at its most obvious when mental health nurses are deliberately probing in such areas but experienced wherever nurses have time to talk to patients. There is also a way in which the exchange between nurse and patient involves the working out of something like a penance on the road to recovery. In a mental health setting, this might involve the nurse and patient agreeing that the patient will confront something they have long avoided, possibly emotionally, possibly literally, often in both senses. In other settings, it might involve the patients making changes to their lifestyle, undertaking treatment they don't want or which is particularly difficult – for instance, chemotherapy. These are not, then, 'ordinary' interactions as the nurse cares for, and is with, the individual as they undergo that process.

In the moment of death, there is also an opportunity to see how nurses can bridge the gap between science, technology and the art of caring. 'Rosie is hooked up to balloon pump, ventilator, syringe drivers, dialysis machine, pacing box, defibrillator and mini jet syringes – a two nurse patient at the end of the road', writes Brian Belle-Fortune (1999: p 37). His account of how a decision is made to switch off this impressive array of machines at Rosie's family's request, how the nurses observe, on a monitor, her life fading away, the senior registrar staying to 'watch what we nurses do after a patient dies' and they all let Rosie go perfectly describes something that nurses so often think of as part of their job but which is far more. Joy Eden (1998: pp 32–3) writes an equally moving account of caring for Mr Nelson, a man who has had all his facial features either destroyed or disfigured by cancer. A combination of major surgery, radiotherapy, chemotherapy and comprehensive nursing care provides a quality of life that allows him an extended visit to his son in Australia and further time with his family. Nonetheless, all the treatment available cannot check the disease and it falls to a team of hospice nurses to care for him in his final days – still using supposedly hi-tech aids such as syringe drivers – but with the author able to come to an understanding of why she is so deeply affected by his death. There is a large body of evidence surrounding the grieving process, which is far from a concrete, easily measured and linear series of events, but rather a complex process composed of fluid phases that will be understood by individuals according to their own experience, all of which has contributed to the training and work of bereavement counsellors. Words like compassion, altruism, mercy and kindness might sound overly simplistic and sentimental to many in our postmodern era but, at times such as these, remain at the core of the process of nursing.

▶ Dark angels

Of course, those who transgress are also liable for excommunication – or, less prosaically, to be removed from the register. These are nursing's 'dark angels'. The news pages of the nursing press regularly features stories about nurses who have come before the NMC for some action or other and are facing removal from the register. Many hearings involve male nurses and sexual impropriety but over the years there have been a number of inquiries that have revealed that whole 'armies of angels' have lost faith and gone over to the other side, particularly in the old psychiatric institutions. At least, that is how it would seem. There can be no doubt that the litany of abuse and malpractice that emerged from twenty-four major public inquiries between 1968 and 1981 is not simply a case of a few rotten apples in a barrel that is basically pure. A whole range of issues, from petty pilfering, through minor acts of intimidation and gross acts of ill treatment to a series of suicides in one hospital and unexpected deaths in another were investigated. Yet the psychiatric unit, St Augustine's Hospital, was a good example of a dysfunctional institution that would not act upon concerns raised by two nurses until they eventually went to the press. The health authority then criticised the complainants, implying they were irresponsible. Even after a full and thorough investigation, which upheld most of the allegations (and during which the two nurses and many other staff members considering giving evidence in support of their allegations suffered harassment and intimidation by colleagues), no serious action was taken against the individuals concerned, virtually all of whom carried on in their posts with little sanction (Beardshaw, 1981: pp 84–9).

The reasons people come into nursing are complex and often hidden. Theories abound, of 'wounded healers' and can be traced at least as far back as Greek mythology. The notion runs that carers can carry their own vulnerability or a weakness that in some way reflects that of their patients. It is, in turn, reflected by the patient in his own capacity as a healer. Thus nurses, and other health workers, can be seeking to heal themselves in their act of caring (Barker et al., 1998). There is a large and important body of literature suggesting that there is no altruistic motivation for nurses or others providing healthcare. More, they argue, it is often a case going beyond the concept of the wounded healer and is about serving the helper's own needs, perhaps in controlling the patient or acting out a situation whereby attempts to control are frustrated. Nurses who are full of good intentions when they start their careers experience any number of influences that engender profound changes. Most of the nurses involved in the systematic abuses of the large institutions did not start off like that. Part of any understanding of nurses' behaviour, both in coming into the work and how they then respond to the experience of it, depends on adopting psychological, sociological and political theories but there is no doubt that the idea that people come into nursing simply because they are either 'good', want to 'help' others or purely out of a sense of altruistic compassion are to wholly underestimate human motivation and misunderstand how individuals are shaped by larger forces (Wilkinson and Miers, 1999). However, there is always hope that change is possible and Joy Bray (1998) highlights the fact that, perversely, in meeting their own needs, nurses can nonetheless still help their patients, particularly if they have some degree of self awareness and work to ensure that a degree of asymmetry, in favour of the patient, exists in the nurse–patient relationship, with the nurse working towards developing a truly collaborative partnership with the patient. However, as she points out, this can only really occur in a supportive environment (explored further in Chapter 6).

Without doubt, the most infamous case involving a nurse was that of Beverly Allitt, the 'Angel of Death', as more than one tabloid dubbed her. Allitt was found guilty of murdering four children and attempting to murder a further nine at Grantham and Kesteven General Hospital during an eight-week period in 1991.[4]

Speculation about the reasons behind this 'angel's' fall from grace has been covered elsewhere in detail. While not delving into those, it is worth asking whether or not the claim of Anne McDonald, director of quality at Manchester Children's Hospitals National Health Service (NHS) Trust and nurse member of the Clothier Inquiry team, was correct when she stated, 'The report of the Allitt Inquiry is not one that will gather dust on the top shelf' (McDonald, 1996). Or, perhaps, the question that needs to be asked is whether or not the recommendations made by the enquiry team were those necessary to remedy the actual problem. The report does address issues such as the responsibility and process of occupational health assessments and reference gathering, introducing more stringent health checks for new starters, targets for numbers of paediatric nurses on duty on a shift[5] and procedures for increasing the likelihood of identifying malpractice through incident reporting. But the political dimension to the events surrounding the Allitt murders were not

---

[4] There are numerous incidences of both nurses and doctors murdering patients. Robert Diaz, a Los Angeles nurse who liked to pretend he was a doctor, was sentenced to death in 1984 for the murder of twelve patients. Dr Sam Sheppard – immortalised in the TV series and film, 'The Fugitive' – was convicted of killing his wife in 1954. His mother and mother-in-law both died by apparent suicide and he was sued after two surgical deaths (Kinnell, 2000). Of course, many doctors and nurses also willingly participated in mass murder for the Nazi state in Germany while Britain's worst ever serial killer was Dr Harold Shipman.

[5] This was set at two RSCNs per shift but, in a subsequent DoH survey, only 50 per cent of units met this standard during daytime shifts and a paltry 20 per cent met the standard on night duty shifts (McDonald, 1996).

tackled, just as they were not in the inquiries into the malpractice, corruption and brutality of the old psychiatric institutions. Nick Davies, a journalist who closely covered the Allitt case, noting that the report made *recommendations* with national implications but no *criticism* that might have a national implication, summarised the context in which the murders took place thus: 'Nurse Allitt's success as a killer was the direct result of the government's failure as a manager of the NHS – she exploited a hospital that was underfunded, demoralised, and distorted by com-mercialisation' (Davies, 1994). One of the reasons the Clothier Inquiry Report probably is now stuck up on the top shelf, with most of the suicide and homicide inquiry reports that have been published since, is that they either fail to address the underlying problems and context or that managers believe they have neither the resources, will or authority to genuinely address them. Perhaps it is true that, in healthcare at least, we really do create our own heaven and hell on earth.

▶ Women's work

It would certainly be easier for politicians and policy makers if nursing was the work of 'angels', whose main reward was esoteric rather than material, who pos-sessed some supernatural qualities that would see them through the worst of the work and help them to keep coming back, regardless of how they were treated and the conditions they found themselves in. But, despite all of the above, this is not the reality. It is still assumed to be – and, in practice, still largely is – the work of women. This assumption is another that needs further examination and to be looked at anew. Perhaps the question should be put as: is nursing women's work or is women's work nursing?

In a sense, this shifts us back to the debate about care versus technological and biological innovation summarised earlier. But it also goes to the heart of the issues concerning the gender divide and division of labour in the healthcare systems of the nineteenth century. Orderlies working for the army were male. Attendants in insane asylums were predominantly male in the early years of those institutions. There were, historically, male carers or nurses from religious orders. Yet 'modern' nursing developed out of the work of the female religious orders, the female ser-vant class and the traditions of women 'healers' and nurses. It built upon the work of women in the home, not only in caring but also domestic management and housekeeping. Indeed, in nursing's early years, the men responsible for the organ-isation and structure of healthcare placed these skills above, and gave greater importance to, those handed down from healers and carers, who held a more inde-pendent position. Nursing the sick did not require the 'brute strength' that was seen as an asset for asylum attendants and, although male orderlies in the Crimea washed, fed and moved wounded or sick soldiers, as well as dressing their wounds, they were noted to lack the gentleness of the nurses brought out to the conflict – they certainly lacked the 'angelic' aspect that could be used to elicit public support.

In establishing nursing departments, the respective hospital committees, Boards of Governors and Guardians sought only women. Moreover, as we have seen, they sought women with particular characteristics. These were not just those that would lend themselves to a greater degree of compassion and care, or even an ability to learn new techniques and adapt to new situations quickly. Essential amongst these characteristics was a willingness to subordinate oneself to the 'greater good' and the needs of others, however these were defined and, most importantly of all, a male defined power structure and hierarchy, with doctors at its pinnacle. And it was doctors 'who defined femininity in terms of patriarchal feminine subordination to safeguard their own dominance' (Gamarnikov, 1991: p 111). Imagining how different nursing would have been if the work had been defined in such a way that would have allowed men to consider it as a useful and appropriate occupation and had actively been sought to take their place alongside the women recruited into the service may seem frivolous, particularly given the weight of history, we all know about how nursing has developed a notably feminine shape. Had men become nurses there would have been obvious and difficult issues of class difference but, immediately, we would have to re-consider the economic, social and political circumstances that ensured that nursing was the work of women and the gender relationships that developed between, particularly, doctors and nurses. Given that men *had* nursed historically, such a concept is not so fanciful. Nonetheless, it is perhaps apparent that, in such a patriarchal and rigid society as that of the mid-to-late nineteenth-century Victorians, nursing would always be a female occupation, particularly when it was being established as a means of addressing the healthcare needs and concerns of the wealthy. The emphasis on womanly qualities was important but there were also practical considerations. High profile leaders encouraged the entry of women of suitable status and background while, for lower middle and working class women it was an occupation where they could earn a living through an alternative to domestic service, shop or office work. Moreover, the exercise of power by men over women developed in relation to capitalism.

> The separation of the public (employment) and private (domestic) spheres under capitalism creates tensions for patriarchy which are resolved through men's dominance of families at the individual level, and of the institution of the family through the state and professions. This sustains general conditions for men to sustain power ... and masculinity, socially constructed maleness, is structured around the exercise of this power ... The situational logic of masculinity and the family can undermine men attempting other forms of action (Hugman, 1991).

The arrival of the male nurse into this predominantly female world, albeit one tightly regulated and controlled by men, was comparatively slow to come. The evolution of male nursing was very different. A very different type of man was sought for the asylums; nor had there been any particularly powerful attempts to initiate programmes of reform as there had been in general nursing. Indeed, the only significant changes that came to asylum nursing did so through female nurses, introduced, almost symbolically, to have a civilising effect, but practically to raise standards and bring the credibility they were gaining in the voluntary hospitals from which they were recruited. This often meant they were given preferential treatment when it came to promotion. The way into nurse training for men in London was barred during the latter part of the nineteenth century, as no training school would accept them. On the eve of the Second World War there were just over three hundred trained male nurses in general hospitals, with a further 120 in training (Pyne, 1982; White, 1985: p 11). After the war, male nurses formed their own association and aligned it with the professional associations. The vast majority of men were still working in mental hospitals and mental handicap institutions, with most being members of trade unions. The major breakthrough occurred in 1960 when, for the first time, the Royal College of Nursing (RCN) accepted men into membership. Following that, men were able to gain more senior positions, particularly in management, and nursing became a career with far greater potential. The balance of power slowly began to change, with men assuming more senior positions, proportionately, than their overall numbers would merit. As the influence of the matron declined, much of the practical leadership of nursing in the workplace was passing into the hands of men. The majority of men who still work in clinical posts, with care as part of their remit, are in a strange ideological netherworld, dominant in one sense but placed in a subservient, subordinated role because of the work they are doing and the fact that they have allied themselves with women to do it.

If this has distorted the gender divide within nursing, the relationship between nurses and doctors has always symbolised the male–female divide in a far more straightforward manner. A simple riddle illustrates the gender values and symbols involved quite well. A father is driving his son to school. Late for work, he drives too fast, hits another car and is killed in the crash. The boy, badly injured, is taken to the local A&E department where the consultant surgeon is called to see him. The surgeon recoils from the trolley in horror, gasping, 'That's my son!' How could this be? The surgeon, defying the expectations of many, is the boy's mother.

There are significant changes occurring in medicine, with vastly increased numbers of women being attracted into the profession. By 1991, 50 per cent of medical students were female. But doctors still represent a male view of the world; the socialisation process and culture for doctors remains male in its orientation. Medicine derives its authority from its scientific origins, with curing the sick as its aim. Certain characteristics are seen as being admirable if not essential for doctors: rational thinking, objectivity, decisiveness, assertiveness. Indeed, working within stereotypical gender frameworks, these characteristics become qualities. But the other side of those characteristics is being individualistic, aggressive, competitive, rash, aloof and unable to empathise. Although there has been some change in understanding and attitudes over the past two decades, as feminist thinking has been accepted into the mainstream, women would usually be described in negative terms whenever such characteristics were ascribed to them.

As has been discussed earlier, coupled to the very male world and attitude of the medical profession, the 'good' nurse was, by definition, caring, compassionate, supportive and nurturing and behaved in a dutiful manner during the period nurses and doctors were establishing their relationship in the country's hospitals. But it went a lot further than that. They were actually replicating the patriarchal Victorian society that shaped them, while aping that most important of Victorian institutions, the family. The doctor adopted the controlling, penetrative, dominating role of the father and it was the role, or 'duty' of the nurse to subordinate herself to, and support, him, nurture and care for the patient and manage the anxiety of the patient as well as that of the doctor and her own. The patient was placed in a wholly passive or helpless role, just as a child would be, awaiting the decisions and actions of the doctor to be effected upon him (Littlewood 1991: p 145; Carpenter, 1991: p 9). Arguably, it was easier for the patient to 'grow up' and change than for the nurses, who seemed perpetually trapped in this stultifying system. It is in this association with the oppressed mother, the sense that the nurse always has to 'be there', to care and tend to those in need, that defines the nurse's role. In the same way as occurred in the family, where father in a capitalistic society was defined by his work, so the doctor was defined by the clear parameters he placed around his work. Mother/nurse was expected to get on and do any and everything else.

▶ The past catches up with the present – what prompts change in the nurse's role?

That was then but this is now. How do those factors affect contemporary nurses in their everyday work? Even as the nursing role has expanded, it has led to even further role confusion and fits within that structure of doing the bits the patriarch – and others – doesn't want to, rather than defining the role through the work of caring, by helping patients adapt, cope or change through the way in which they work with them and placing all of this on nursing terms. Moreover, to an extent, this subordination to the needs of others was enshrined in the United Kingdom Central Council (UKCC) Code of Professional Conduct, when it stated that nurses must, 'act *always* in such a way as to promote and safeguard the interests and well being of patients and clients', as well as ensure that *nothing* a nurse does or omits to do harms patients and clients [my emphasis] (UKCC, 1992). As has been suggested by Steven Edwards, such moral standards are 'extraordinary' and could be said to be 'too high and unrealistic' (Edwards, 1996: pp 34–5). Yet we are not talking of principles enshrined in a code a century ago – this was written less than two decades ago. The code of conduct, therefore, still seems to point to a vocational ideal that many think not only outdated but actually long dead.

Legislation and policy pronouncements have apparently given nursing a cutting edge role in NHS and healthcare reform. Although nurse consultants and nurse practitioners have found a place in the hospital, where the nursing role has been expanded, the traditional hierarchies will always be slow to change. The medical consultant still sits atop the clinical and decision making tree. Indeed, it could be argued that nursing has taken several steps backwards. In primary care, one would expect to see positive effects of reform more clearly. Nurse practitioners are an obvious manifestation of this, as are the nurses working in Walk In Centres, answering calls at NHS Direct and taking their place as Board members on Primary Care Groups and Primary Care Trusts. In cases such as that of the Swanage Community Hospital, nurses combined running a minor injuries unit while taking on GPs' out of hours calls, using computer generated prompts for when taking a clinical history and fully worked out protocols to decide on what course of action to take or advice to provide. As a development it was described as an 'unqualified success' and cut GPs out of hours workload by an estimated 40–50 per cent , increased nurses' job satisfaction and improved an already good working relationship between the hospital and the GP practice (Legge, 1998). Yet a year later, the British Medical Association (BMA) GP negotiator was slamming the idea of Walk In Centres. This was only joining the chorus of doctors' disapproval that had greeted the extension of the nurse's role with nurse practitioners and followed NHS Direct like a rabid dog. At least some of the critics, such as consultant anaesthetist, David Wilkinson, were honest enough to admit they thought 'developments in nursing roles were "the thin end of the wedge" of nurses "doing doctors' roles"' (Cervi, 1996). There is early evidence to suggest that nurse-led Walk In Centres are, indeed, diverting patients from GP practices, with 33 per cent of patients treated at Walk In Centres saying they would have visited a GP had the Walk In Centre not been there (Clewes, 2000: pp 18–20).

GP's criticism focuses on the lack of an evidence base for new developments or expresses concerns about basic safety. It is never linked to money. But even before they came into office, the Labour Party had to create an 'escape hole to try to appease the then fundholding GPs, promising family doctors they would have their own budget for buying care. Given that according to *The Economist*, GPs were directly controlling £5.5 billion of NHS expenditure by 1997 and, during 1994–95, fundholders were able to keep 'savings' of £95 million from that overall budget, this is perhaps not surprising.

Although, when news of primary care reform came in 1998 it was broadly welcomed by the BMA, it met with 'little enthusiasm among GPs – and even outright opposition. One in ten of GPs surveyed threatened to refuse to join a PCG' (Brindle,1998). Two years on and GPs at the BMA's GP committee conference were still engaged in 'ritual denunciations of NHS Direct' and 'conveying the unmistakable impression of calamity' about the reforms, condemning the 'extra work, longer hours, too few resources and too much change too fast' (Health Service Journal, 23.3.2000). The government were listening – but, at the time of writing, change has shifted up a gear to breakneck speed as PCTs and personal medical services (PMS) are established, both of which are corralling GPs into the NHS in a way which has defied successive governments since 1948. It was, then, little surprise when the BMA decided to ballot all GPs to find out whether or not they were prepared to resign completely from the NHS because the government had not done enough to address their concerns about workload, administration overload and stress – with the result timed to coincide with the 2001 general election. Inevitably, it allowed them back to the negotiating table with ministers and civil servants. PCTs and PMS were top of the agenda.

If doctors are wary of changes affecting their relationship with nurses, particularly where this involves nurses eating into the edge of their role, some nurses view the apparent 'professional advancement' that comes from this as being no more than a means of disguising the fact that nurses are *having* to pick up the work junior doctors are necessarily jettisoning as their hours are reduced (Neenan, 1999). Many doctors have also been critical of the nurses who have qualified since the introduction of Project 2000, with complaints that 'something has gone catastrophically wrong' and that Project 2000 'doesn't fit in with the traditional role of tender loving care' (*sic*). Another criticism, articulated on behalf of his colleagues by Dr Nazim Mamode, then deputy chair of the BMA Junior Doctors' Committee, is that nurses are 'worried about the extra responsibility they may have to adopt', with the respect doctors have for nurses being 'subverted by problems and the issues of responsibility'. Moreover, there is a concern that nurses' theory based training means they are as ill equipped as newly qualified doctors for life on the wards (Robotham, 1999).

If the path to power for nurses has been made difficult by doctors, they have had to seek alternative routes. One of these has been the way in which nurses have subverted the hierarchy as defined by the medical profession in a feminine, non-confrontational way, for instance by suggesting a course of action in such a way that the doctor accepts it and is able to reframe it as his own (Gamarnikow 1991; Tellis-Nyak M, Tellis Nyak V, 1984: pp 1063–69). It has also been clear that both nurses and doctors have 'played' to their ascribed role in the family triangle referred to earlier (Gamarnikow, 1978). However, nurses have gradually asserted some degree of control over their own destiny and pulled away from that of the medical profession, through education and nurse training, registration and a code of conduct, developing models of nursing and a body of knowledge that has a distinct identity. After many false starts, was status to be achieved under New Labour with such initiatives as PCGs? Nurses serving on the board of these fledgling organisations, such as Jo Poole, describe how they initially felt intimidated as one of only two nurses on a board with seven GPs, either not asked for her opinion or having it discounted if it differed from that of her medical 'colleagues'. Her view that one of the main concerns of the GPs was for their own business, echoed that held by many nurses working in primary care. She points out that the move to PCTs, however, reduces the majority and consequent authority of the doctors on the board (Poole, 2000). While strongly advocating the position and involvement of nurses on PCG and PCT boards, Poole questions nurse attitudes to power and what they need to equip them in the role, yet does not acknowledge the inbuilt inequality, a factor that cannot be ignored. Nor can others such as the limited amount of time the nurse has to integrate herself into such a new body, the ability of her employer to provide adequate training and, ultimately, the weight of history that confronts every nurse in similar situations. Research has also shown that, on a wider level, nurses are rarely being consulted let alone included in decision making processes in PCGs and nurses wishing to become board members had to be subjected to rigorous interviews whereas GPs were simply voted on by their peers. Overall, the research showed 'disappointment and disillusionment among nurses', and the 'main finding was that "ordinary" nurses have been almost invisible in the PCG debate'. While nurses were initially pleased to be included in the process, GP groups lobbied hard and won concessions, increasing their power to the extent that other PCG stakeholder groups were effectively marginalised' (Smith *et al.*, 1999: pp 54–5).

The record of the medical profession as employer – largely in primary care, where practice nurses are employed by GPs – was declared to be one of 'injustice' by health secretary, Alan Milburn, at the RCN Congress in 2000. Despite a small minority described as excellent employers, too many fail to implement pay awards in full, hold nurses to worse conditions than their NHS counterparts and will not allow nurses sufficient time off for continuing education. Even when practice nurses were admitted to the NHS pension scheme, it took four years from the date it was agreed to actual implementation by their GP employers.

So, the question, 'Who wears the trousers?' asked by Jane Salvage and Richard Smith in a special joint edition of the *Nursing Times* and *British Medical Journal*, might seem to be missing the point by a long way. Maybe hedging their bets, the authors wrote, 'Everyone is confused' but then went on to make a crucial point:

> Celia Davies, professor of healthcare at the Open University, argues that the stranglehold of gender thinking must be loosened and the old doctor–nurse stereotypes must go. For decades we understood the professions as a conventional nuclear family, with doctor–father, nurse–mother and patient–child. But our hope for total wisdom and protection from father is forlorn, our wish for total comfort and protection from mother is unrealisable, and the patient has grown up. A new three way partnership should displace this vanishing family.

> Hastening its disappearance is a change happening in society at large. Just as women are occupying an increasing number of positions of power and authority, so too is the medical profession being progressively feminised. ... The easy equation of female sex with low status is no longer tenable (Salvage and Smith, 2000: p 24).

However, is it going to be enough to await the arrival of increasing numbers of women into the medical profession? Or, as they suggest later, that there be an open dialogue about professional training, regulation and rewards? These are obviously vital components in engineering change, and that change will only become a reality through a dialogue that changes the way its participants think, feel and behave. However, a report from the three royal colleges that, still, 'Women are being held back in the race to become senior hospital doctors because of the "working all hours" culture that remains in the NHS', does not bode well. The report noted that, in 1991, women made up half of medical graduates and could have been expected to account for a substantial proportion of doctors moving into senior positions. Yet, by 1999, only 17 per cent of consultants in medical specialities were female. The proportion in posts that combined academic and clinical roles was even lower (Meikle, 2001). Does this suggest that there is another dimension to the problem that will not be easily resolved through open dialogue?

▶ Reflections in a gilded mirror – or cage?

On the face of it, and despite all the difficulties, nurses have a positive image. There isn't another occupational group likened to angels. Comparative groups, such as the police, teachers, doctors and particularly, social workers are all viewed with more ambivalence than nurses. After Prime Minister Tony Blair launched one of his early attacks on public sector workers, the then health secretary, Frank Dobson, had to go to great lengths to assure anyone who would listen that Blair's criticism was not directed at nurses.

Even the case of Beverley Allitt, and others less serious but which might have concerned more widespread abuse or malpractice, don't appear to have dented nurses' popularity with the public. Another case that received widespread publicity but, again, didn't seem to rub off on nurses more widely, was that of the bizarre murder case in Saudi Arabia, after which Lucille Ferrie and Deborah Parry were convicted by a Saudi court but later released amidst a storm of controversy. The crimes of Dr Harold Shipman, the Manchester GP found guilty of fifteen murders but who is now believed to have murdered hundreds of his patients, seems to have resonated in the public consciousness in a way that Allitt did not. Admittedly, the sheer scale of his crime was far more horrific, as was the awareness that he could have got away with it for so long, with no apparent check from colleagues or anyone else. There was also the fact that his peers had some knowledge that his practice was, at best, dubious and he had abused drugs yet been allowed to continue practising. His trial coincided with other serious medical scandals breaking and, for many amongst the wider public, the old adage of, 'Trust me, I'm a doctor,' was becoming a sick joke.

The broad array of images generated around nursing only adds to the complexity of the bigger picture. When minor TV celebrity, Anthea Turner, was photographed in a specially shortened nurse's uniform at a publicity stunt for International Nurses' Day, she sparked a furious row with the RCN, whose spokesperson said, 'We are quite cross with Anthea's portayal' (Nursing Times, 20.5.98). The media has always loved nurses and they are regularly portrayed in literature, film and TV, readily recognisable to any casual observer, let alone nurses interested in seeing how they are portrayed. To an extent, these can be said to represent some images that had carefully been nurtured by the nursing elite. The self-sacrificing 'good woman', 'dutiful' and 'morally responsible'. The nurse as servant to the doctor, there to gaze adoringly into his eyes and mop his brow under the glare of the operating theatre lights. Inevitably, romance would creep into these latter scenarios, usually chaste and continuing to reflect the dominance of the male/doctor character. It wasn't just nursing stereotypes that were on show – female stereotypes were as much in evidence, from beautiful blondes, sophisticated brunettes, husband hunters, all white, Anglo Saxon, mostly middle class, well spoken and attractive. The few portrayals of working class nurses would show them as inferior: dizzier, less intelligent women, they would act as a foil to their more 'superior' colleagues and be almost as great a danger to the patients as the original conditions that brought them into hospital. Of course, the dragon like matron was always there, often so heavily caricatured as to be a source of some humour but also possessing great moral authority and integrity. Rarely were they portrayed as the source of unnecessary grief that many of their real life charges accused them of.

Nurses, doctors and hospitals provided rich material for a number of *Carry On* films, with Barbara Windsor and colleagues introducing seaside postcard sauciness as well as, in Hattie Jacques, probably the most memorable onscreen matron of them all. Again, despite Jacques apparent power, it was her job to be seen to yield to the dominant male, as it was every other nurse in the story, with the younger ones providing the *Carry On* style 'glamour' at the same time.

A darker side of nursing emerged by the 1970s, with Louise Fletcher's chilling portrait of Nurse Ratched in the 1976 film, *One Flew Over the Cuckoo's Nest*. An apparently maternal senior nurse, she is actually an authoritarian, repressed, malignant figure controlling and stifling the lives of her patients. Although one could argue that 'The Big Nurse', as she is referred to by the book's Native American narrator, is an obvious example of someone in a caring role for reasons very much of their own, these are not explored or given any space.[6] Rather, Ken Kesey's book actually uses the insane asylum and many of its characters as a metaphor for 1950s America, something the film did less successfully. Kesey wasn't alone in doing this, with a number of film makers and authors using the public's apparent familiarity with nursing images as a means of playing with audience expectations and creating a canvass onto which more subversive images and ideas can be painted. In the United States, writers have certainly taken that further than in England. Stephen King has an obviously disturbed nurse who finds an author with whom she has

---

[6] Nurse Ratched's vice like grip on her patients is only finally broken when JP McRandall, the book's anti hero and her constant foil, inadvertently rips open her blouse in the midst of a frantic struggle, revealing her full and womanly bosom.

long been obsessed, injured in a car crash. She nurses him back to health only so she can force him to write to order – her order – and brutally tortures him whenever he refuses.

John Irving goes a lot further. In his multi million selling, *The World According to Garp*, his nurse, Jenny Fields, has no wish to be saddled with a husband but does want a child. So she mounts one of her patients, a brain dead tail gunner from a Second World War bomber plane, while he lays dying on his hospital bed, and has sex with him to impregnate herself with the eponymous TS Garp. Jenny leaves nursing, writes about her life, sets up a home for distressed women and becomes an icon for feminists throughout the United States, who imitate her by wearing a copy of the white nurse's uniform she still clings to. Eventually assassinated by a right wing fanatic (male), her son is later murdered by a feminist fanatic – dressed as a 'Jenny Fields nurse'.

Although there are other themes being explored here, the relationship between nurses and women, gender roles, feminism, authority, caring and control is richly mined in all these stories. British fiction is altogether more prosaic, although it's inevitably moved on from programmes like *Emergency Ward Ten*. The nurses in *Angels*, from the 1970s, were more complex and the focus of the series was as much about them as young women trying to organise their personal lives in parallel with a career or student life as any of the clinical issues they faced on the wards. *Casualty* is now probably Britain's most popular hospital show – although it has to compete with a seemingly endless string of documentaries about hospitals, healthcare and nurses. A significant twist in this is that the role of 'matron' is given over to Charlie Fairhead, as played by Derek Thompson, the A&E Department's senior nurse – and probably the longest running nursing character on TV, as well as the most popular with nurses (Nursing Standard, 5.5.1999, p 5).[7] It is interesting to compare it with its American cousin, *ER*. Whereas Casualty is slower in pace, giving the nurses a lot of airtime – probably more than the doctors – and focuses on the 'human dramas' of the patients, *ER* is faster, glossier (with a far bigger budget, inevitably), more macho and follows the doctors as they heroically perform life saving procedures in between resolving personal crises that come as thick and fast as the gunshot victims.

ER is, in the widest sense, sexier than *Casualty*. And sex is never that far away from nurses, despite, or perhaps because of, the 'angelic' image. Nurses, or more precisely, women, in uniform, have long been used as a 'sex symbol', ranging from the apparently titillating to the overtly pornographic. The wider media like to exploit the sexual allure. One of the more salacious aspects of the case of Deborah

---

[7] Ironically, the model for Charlie Fairhead, the A&E head of clinical nursing at Bristol Royal Infirmary, Peter Salt, made relatively few headlines when he resigned his post because of 'intolerable pressures on services', saying, '"We find it increasingly frustrating to be unable to provide the kind of care we want to"' (Nursing Times, 98; 37, p 7).

Parry and Lucille Ferrie, quickly focused on by the tabloids, were allegations that, somewhere in the background to the crime, there had been an alleged lesbian tryst. Whether or not this threw any light on the crime itself, or possible motives, for many editors it added a sexual twist to an already intriguing story. Again, it has to be remembered that such images and representations of nurses echo ways in which women are portrayed and have a political as well as social and cultural context. On one level, Anthea Turner can claim her shortened dress is 'a bit of fun' while the RCN spokesperson, with the 'we are not amused' comment, sounds like Queen Victoria. On another, however, is the argument that she is playing to the gallery of the reactionary, male dominated culture that uses sexist – and, in some cases, pornographic – images to undermine women, particularly as they make strides towards greater economic, political and sexual independence. In looking at the 'sexiness', or lack of it, of nurses, there is no attempt to explore their sexuality. An old stereotype about male nurses was that they were 'all' homosexuals, as if this told us something about men who went into nursing, or made it easier to think about how men could care, show compassion, actually wash people and touch their bodily secretions. That there are gay and lesbian nurses seems of less interest to the public, just as questions about Florence Nightingale's possible lesbianism have not excited great curiosity in the media. It is now less of an impediment to career progress for nurses to be open about their sexuality and it is one area in which the unions have taken a progressive and significant role, with special interest groups for lesbian and gay members as well as advocating progressive policies for employers that are anti discriminatory.

Nurses do not seem able to project an accurate and coherent image of themselves as they really are (or, at least, think they are) and perhaps this is healthy, given the diversity and obvious differences that have become even more pronounced as the work has become broader in its nature. In fact, the public seems to have very clear ideas about nurses and issues pertaining to them. A MORI/RCN poll conducted in 2000, updating a *Nursing Times* survey from 1984, revealed few major changes in attitude in that period. However, the most significant of these were that 10 per cent more people polled thought nurses well educated and 42 per cent thought nurses did a lot to try and improve their pay and working conditions (up 19 per cent). Only 27 per cent , reduced from 42 per cent in 1984, saw nurses obeying doctor's orders without question and 13 per cent only thought nurses would be better at their job if they were women, a fall of 20 per cent (Payne, 2000). Maybe image isn't everything.

▶ An icon lives

Or maybe it is. The most powerful image in nursing, even now, even after all the changes, as modern nursing has been ushered into a postmodern age, is that of Florence Nightingale. Anyone who doubted that only had to look at the furore that was generated by an apparently innocuous motion that went before the Unison health conference in April 1999.

Unison's health conference had never before made the headlines. It had barely rated a few paragraphs in even the serious national press since the union's inception in 1993. Until Wendy Wheeler, a health visitor from Hackney, moved a motion that asked that International Nurses' Day not be held on Florence Nightingale's birthday, as the image and reality of Nightingale represented some of the most negative and backward thinking elements in nursing and had held the profession (sic) back for too long. That was it. In her speech, Ms Wheeler suggested Nightingale's reputation be re-evaluated, arguing that holding on to the image and myths surrounding her life, which had been appropriated by the nursing hierarchy and founders of the RCN, had left a legacy of subservience and subordination. Nothing particularly new in that argument. But the International Congress of Nurses was hardly likely to switch the day as a result.

So why the furore? For furore there was. 'Nurses abandon Florence', was the headline in the *Daily Mail*. with Emily Wilson writing, 'Nurses have voted to throw out Florence Nightingale in favour of more politically correct role models'. 'Nurses ditch Florence', was *The Times'* headline. *The Express* went further: 'Nurses snub St Florence', making her the first angel to be canonised in the process, while the *Guardian* joined in with a leader comment, no less, with a sub heading of, 'Florence was not such an angel after all'. The piece concluded, 'History shows that her motives were questionable, her science mistaken, and her results, to say the least of it, dubious' (The Guardian, 28.4.1999).

The debate, thankfully, went further than a broad condemnation of Wendy Wheeler and a dull attempt at attacking political correctness. Even in the more reactionary press, such as the *Daily Telegraph* and the *Mail*, space was given to some of the radical figures mentioned by Unison in its press statement following the intense interest expressed. Figures like Mary Seacole, Maud Gonne and the Rev. Mother Joanna Bridgeman were retrieved from nursing's secret history and held up to the light for re-examination.[8]

The news is not always about what is said. It is as important to attempt to examine what is not said. At that year's Unison conference there were far more important issues being discussed. Among them were delegates' fears that their own union was trying to dismantle its own health group and structure, the vitally important matter of the private finance initiative and the old perennial, pay. None

---

[8] In fact, the name and exploits of Mary Seacole, a truly remarkable woman who was a contemporary of Nightingale's in the Crimea, has in recent years justifiably been associated with a large number of projects, awards for nurses from black and minority ethnic backgrounds and, indeed, used as the name for a variety of health and social care premises. This followed a gradual uncovering of her history and exploits, led by her biographers, Alexander and Dewjee (1984). Until that point, Mrs Seacole was virtually unknown to any modern audience, despite having been the toast of Victorian high society and as famous as Nightingale in her day.

of these garnered any column inches, let alone headlines. Yet these were real issues, affecting not only the nurses and health workers who were involved in serious debates about them, but also the vast majority of the people reading about the validity or otherwise of Florence Nightingale as a contemporary role model.

Moreover, the debate – both at the conference and after it – about Nightingale, Mrs Seacole and the others was rarely about historical fact. It was largely focused on the myths. Much of it was revisionist. Current admirers of Mrs Seacole easily skated over the fact that she was happy to be feted by Victorian high society and enjoyed the company of the royal family. Nightingale is taken out of her Victorian context and judged by contemporary standards, while the legacy of those who appropriated her image is seen as hers alone. And within months the Reverend Mother Bridgeman and Maud Gonne had been tucked back under the veil of darkness from which they were briefly exhumed. Nightingale's position is, after all the 'fun', apparently unchanged.

This example of how a 'non story' can dominate the agenda to the exclusion of other issues that might actually be of more importance, however, can serve as a timely reminder that nurses today are the children of an imagined heritage as much as our real lineage. Myth and tradition are as potent now as they were more than a century ago. The images we see on the TV or cinema screen, that we read about in books, that we see in the news, are reflections not just of how we are but how we are imagined to be, how others want us to be seen, of how others want us to be. Just as Charles Dickens' Sarah Gamp and Betsey Prig were seized upon by mid-nineteenth century 'reformers', so the Unison debate was seized upon by conservatives and radicals alike, all mythologising and creating an imaginary historical landscape upon which to impress contemporary ideas or hold back discussion about issues that did not serve the interests of those in power, making decisions.

And yet ... like the weather, such issues have their own air currents and flows, moving at different speeds and in different directions. The Nightingale debate clearly reflected something about a changing political mood *within*, as well as about, nursing. Certainly, there has been no overt political change in nursing during that last four or five years, but perhaps this was something that registered at a deeper level. It seems to have been about how nurses felt about themselves and how they wanted to be perceived by others. Nurses did take part in the wider debate, whether by writing letters to the national papers or penning brief articles, for and against, in the nursing press. Once a story is kick started, there is no guarantee where it will lead.

▶ Conclusions: angels on fire

What has all this got to do with politics? Or nursing, for that matter? Angels, images, myths and inherited imagination. Of course, it is this that links angels to nurses. At least, for the purpose of this story. Angels have been mythologised and the term 'angelic' bastardised. The complexities of this celestial body have been ignored and sanitised for the purposes of popular consumption, just as nursing's popular history has been purged of anything that might disturb the myths and traditions or the political hegemony they shore up.

There were life and death issues for the early 'modern' nurses as they sought to establish themselves; the nursing of the living was an obvious one, but their care of the dying – or, at least, how that was perceived – was equally important. Inevitably, nurses never escaped that proximity to life and death, being played out in so many individual lives, and it has done much to shape the nursing experience and the perception of nurses by the wider public. Ironically, it is the way in which nurses care for people in death, as opposed to doctors, who have to relinquish their primary curative role at that time, that is one of the key, actual differences in their respective roles and offers nursing something that is wholly unique and different from the work of any others involved in healthcare. Once dominated by its religious origins, concepts and rituals, nursing has faced an increasing challenge from science and a more masculine approach, as evidence is sought, greater importance is attached to the biological, the visible and measurable. There has been a rearguard action in trying to promote the importance of the older precepts of faith and the role of caring but the theological divide has grown, as if the two sides of the debate cannot find any common ground – yet another example of the inability within nursing to adopt a more pluralist, inclusive approach.

Nursing's own dark angels continue to haunt the wider occupational group and, because of this, there remains the necessity to lay the blame at the feet of the individual, not at the door of the organisation or institution, or to suggest that there can be anything wrong with nurses, or for the deeper, less comfortable drives and feelings of nurses to be explored. But the 'bad' is not just out there, always. It is inside both institutions and individuals. It has to be acknowledged. Which involves being reflective and self critical without being persecutory and self blaming, if change is ever to be achieved and, paradoxically, if we are to understand the 'good' and this phenomenon that is nursing. It requires change within individual nurses but that can only be brought about by institutional and structural changes that facilitate the work of their staff through clinical supervision and better support.

Perhaps, in part, that has been difficult because the 'bad' has often been directed at nurses and projected into them because they are women, have low status and, like women in so many walks of life are expected to care and, in the process, are left holding the baby and having to clear up the mess. The division of labour established in Victorian Britain may have shifted slightly, but it has never been on nursing's terms. Old images, myths and straightforward political tactics are often employed, whether or not dressed up in new language or clothes, to maintain the balance of power. There will be no easy solutions, as can be seen by the way in which developments in primary care have taken shape and the battles that have taken place as a result. Moreover, beneath the 'veneration' of our 'angels' lies a more difficult ambivalence that is reflected in the ambiguity – or outright fear – of biblical angels, whom very few would ever want to actually see or meet. So it is with nurses, for contact with them in the context of their work will usually only occur in the worst circumstances.

Despite a complete change in the way in which the nursing media portrays nurses and their world of work, even today the national media and public perception remains resolutely close to the traditional archetype of the white, middle class hospital nurse. And, despite the continuing steps forward, nursing has yet to leave behind not only the images and ideas of dedication to a vocational ideal, forged from self sacrifice and sense of duty, subordinating themselves to the needs of the service and subservient to the medical profession, but also being kept in a subjugated position by those who have a vested interest in maintaining the status quo. The 'Nightingale debate' did eventually raise some genuine questions about the role and meaning of today's nurses and the names generated by the Conference debate itself, such as Mary Seacole, Elizabeth Fry, Joanna Bridgeman and Maud Gonne, as well as more recent, more radical nurses like Thora Craig (nee Silverthorne) and Avis Hutt, sparked a reappraisal of nursing history, albeit short-lived and superficial. This book will now attempt to take that debate further, but with a particular emphasis on the detail of what is happening 'now'.

▶ Further reading

Barker P and Reynolds B (1996) Rediscovering the proper focus of nursing: a critique of Gournay's position on nursing theory and models. *Journal of Psychiatric and Mental Health Nursing*, 3, pp 75–80.

Barker *et al*. (1998) The wounded healer and the myth of mental well-being: ethical issues concerning the mental health status of psychiatric nurses. In: Barker P and Davidson B (eds) *Psychiatric Nursing: Ethical Strife*. London: Arnold.

Bray J (1998) Psychiatric nursing and the myth of altruism. In: Barker P and Davidson B (eds) (1998) *Psychiatric Nursing: Ethical Strife*. London: Arnold.

Dingwall R, Rafferty AM and Webster C (1988) *An Introduction to the Social History of Nursing*. London: Routledge.

Edwards S (ed) (1998) *Philosophical Issues in Nursing*. Basingstoke: London.

Gamarnikow E (1978) Sexual division of labour, the case of nursing. In: Kuhn A, Wolpe A (eds) *Feminism and Materialism: Women and Modes of Production*. London: Routledge and Kegan Paul.

Gamarnikow E (1991) Nurse or woman: gender or professionalism in reformed nursing 1860–1923. In: Holden P and Littlewood J (eds) *Anthropology and Nursing*. London: Routledge.

Gomm R and Davies C (eds) (2000) *Using Evidence in Health and Social Care*. London: Sage/The Open University.

Smith P (1992) *The Emotional Labour of Nursing*. Basingstoke: Macmillan.

Summers A (1988) *Angels and Citizens: British Women as Military Nurses*. London: Routledge and Kegan Paul.

Useful websites

Temple of Angels *www.mts.net*

Kimbas Angels *www.kimbasangels.com*

5 Nurses and Nursing: A Common Good?

And thus I clothe my naked villainy,
With odd old ends stol'n forth of holy writ
And seem a saint when most I play the devil
                                Richard III, act 1, scene 3, 1. 336, by William Shakespeare

▶ Introduction

'The National Health Service, with the exception of recurring spasms about charges, is out of party politics.' That was the view of a former Conservative health minister, Iain Macleod – speaking in 1958 (Klein, 1989: p 32). By the new millennium it was one of the defining factors in the general election, having been pushed there by successive governments and their political opponents, by academics and trade unions as well as doctors and nurses. The key decade in that process was the 1980s. The first major re-organisations had taken place in the 1970s, as had the first round of significant public sector cuts. What differed in the 1980s was the ideological edge brought to the politics of the NHS (and much else in British life) by the Thatcher government.

The events leading up to and after the white paper, *Working for Patients*, are presented as a case study because it is a prime example of modern policy making. There was no extended period of consultation to study the conclusions of a committee with the intention of establishing a consensus about a process of incremental change in key areas. It could be understood using rational, organisational and political models of policy making (Lindblom 1959; Hogwood and Gunn 1984; Allison 1971; Ham and Hill 1984). It, therefore, tells us as much about the 'how' and 'why' as the 'what'. Similarly, the second of the case studies in the chapter, about National Health Service (NHS) funding, stands as much as an example of 'spin' and the manipulation of apparently objective facts as it does in explaining how much money is being spent on the NHS – and where the increased funding might actually go. In demonstrating the 'Gordon Brown accounting model' the reader should be aware that there is nothing new in this. It is a methodology familiar not only to all chancellors of the exchequer, but most politicians, civil servants and managers. Moreover, dealing with the original set of figures is only the beginning of such a story, while acting as a timely reminder, at this stage of the book, that virtually everything happening in nursing and to nurses occurs in an economic context. As such, it gives us a framework to think about how the proposed Foundation Hospitals might shape future service provision.

In the 1980s and 1990s, change was to run through the NHS like diarrhoea through an irritable bowel. Everything that nurses did was being overtly politicised and politics began to directly dictate much of what they did in the workplace, far more than had been the case when Macleod made his statement. Any political consensus was broken. The Conservative's political opponents made hay with the public perception of a government that wanted to privatise the NHS and its policies culminated in the reforms initiated through 1989's white paper, *Working for Patients*, which introduced the so-called internal market, local pay bargaining and the most profound ideological change the NHS had ever seen.

Such far reaching change cannot occur in a vacuum. There were key internal and external factors. Already, the system of management had been revised, with the introduction of general management. Noticeably, at that time, nurses had not been inclined to support their existing nurse managers, whose jobs and positions of relative power were threatened. Further change was brought about because the management and expenditure of the NHS – particularly in terms of how both could be controlled by central government – remained a major pre-occupation of Margaret Thatcher and her cabinet, just as it has been for successive governments since. An essential part of the process of change was to, yet again, re-define the 'common good' and the way nurses worked within it. A growing body of criticism had been used effectively to justify the radical overhaul.

So it is necessary to briefly outline the 'bigger picture' of these policy changes, to attempt an understanding of the academic and political criticisms being aimed at the NHS and the different perspectives on policy.[1] It is worth looking at what it is about NHS management, particularly in relation to nurses, that has proved so frustrating to ministers and, most fundamental to all policy initiatives, from ward to national level, money – the funding that comes in, how it is spent and what it means to the nurse at the clinical coalface and the patients she cares for. Within that, themes of power, decision making, pay and the nature of nurses' work come further into focus, as well as the way in which change initiated by nurses themselves is often marginalised. While these themes will also feature in Chapter 6, exploring these issues here will help us explore how the nurse's role was re-defined during this period.

▶ Market capitalism and nursing: the price nurses were to pay

Was it the intention of the Conservative Government to damage nursing in the way it did in the late 1980s and early 1990s? At the very least, nursing was an

---

[1] The importance of these reforms is that Tony Blair's government has increasingly struggled to shake off accusations that, despite its rhetoric and overall funding, it closely follows Thatcher's policies.

incidental casualty of major changes in healthcare policy. But for a government ideologically committed to the supremacy of the free market and reducing expenditure on public services, clinical grading had been a dispute too far. Although ministers may not consciously have taken the view, nurses had effectively priced themselves out of a job in wringing out all of that extra cash from the treasury in one year's pay rise. There was nothing of the careful, pre meditated planning that some writers argue precipitated the conflict with the miners in 1983–84. According to this view, the seeds of their defeat lay in the miners' victory over a former Tory government in 1972 (Marsh, 1992: pp 120–4). Nonetheless, the clinical militancy of 1987–89 had precipitated the second major nurses' dispute in little over five years and had cost far more than the government was prepared to pay in the long term. The need to resolve the problems and tensions involved in paying such a massive group of workers had been one of the prime motivators for having a nationalised health service. Now having to fund nurses' pay out of the public purse was one of the principle factors prompting the government to look to an alternative way of organising and funding the service, as well as determining how its staff would be paid.[2]

As had been the case with the Griffiths' Report, no nurses were involved, at any stage, in drawing up the plans that led to the NHS reforms. Nor were the plans fed through informal channels to obtain a nursing view while in their infancy. Change was happening *to* nurses via a top down agenda being delivered by civil servants on behalf of national government. The people charged with implementing it at local level, health authorities and hospital managers, were often relatively new to the NHS and had not been trained in, or 'grown up' steeped in its culture. Nursing, already weakened by the loss of positions at senior levels and being managerially accountable to non-nurses, was in no position to offer a coherent response.

One of the early characters portrayed by the comedian, Harry Enfield, was a Greek kebab shop owner called Stavros. In one of his weekly slots on the *Friday Night Live* show, Stavros summed up the view not only of the nation's nurses but the nation: 'The NHS is sadly bugger up. Is under-funded and under-peeped.' This was probably not the analysis that confirmed to the government it should act, but act it did. Its proposals were based on the work of an American economist, Alain Enthoven. The theory was that, despite re-organisation and changing the

---

[2] Chronic underfunding of the NHS during this period led to a pattern of bed closures each year. However, instructed by the then Health Secretary, Norman Fowler, *not* to close beds in the run up to the 1987 election, health authorities had 'saved' money by not paying bills to suppliers until the next financial year, 1987–88, which then made that year's cash crisis far worse. These bills had to be paid almost at the beginning of the new financial year, prompting more bed closures, even earlier, as well as making it more difficult for health authorities to fill nursing vacancies (Timmins, 1995: pp 11–13).

managerial system, the NHS faced a much deeper challenge. There were far too few incentives for staff to work efficiently. Moreover, competition was virtually non existent. Consumer choice could not be stimulated in any meaningful way. Because of these factors, it wasn't even possible to kick start greater efficiency. The net result was a funding 'black hole', which would swallow however much money government stumped up without delivering any great improvement in the service. This was exemplified by existing variations in performance, not just from region to region, but within districts and even hospitals.

The government had already utilised a welter of criticisms, often drawn from apparently contradictory sources, to justify its earlier attempts to make changes in the NHS. Perhaps the greatest irony was its use of critiques originally put forward by Marxist and other left wing thinkers.

Key policy themes had been subjected to a variety of perspectives. The social democratic perspective that had reached its apotheosis after the Second World War, sought consensus around creating a more just and equal society within a capitalist framework. It was distrustful of markets and favoured state intervention, particularly in welfare and health. Within the social democratic framework there was an emphasis on the redistribution of wealth and achieving change through a process of incremental reform. As the prevailing philosophy, it was the model most open to criticism. Marxist analysis of welfare provision was really developed in the 1970s, particularly by writers such as Gough (1973) and O'Connor (1975). They explored what was to be identified as accumulation theory and the inherent contradictions thrown up by the capitalist state as it relies on the provision of welfare provision as one of its tools of social control. Welfare is only one of a number of areas making demands on the government's economic resource. Within that category, health has to compete with social services and education, while the health budget has to be scrapped over by public health, acute hospitals, primary care, mental health and the like. Arguments that rising health expenditure damaged the wider economy disproportionate to the advantages it brought began to surface in the late 1950s but were developed by New right thinkers such as Friedman (1981) and Minford (1984) in the early 1980s.

Marxists had long argued that welfare provision and social policy were used by the capitalist state to ameliorate its worst excesses and mollify the working class. The State required a productive workforce. As such, the real priorities of the NHS were those of the State and not the patient. Welfare provision, in this way, was also used to legitimate the capitalist state and help maintain social harmony. This legitimacy was being questioned in the late 1970s and early 1980s, as evidence emerged that NHS users were feeling oppressed by, and alienated from, a service unable to meet their needs (Taylor Gooby, 1986). The argument ran that apathy, unresponsiveness and a decline in participation in resolving the problems facing it were leading to a collapse in support for the NHS as it was configured. This was linked to the state's perceived lack of democracy, mirrored in the health service, undermining people's confidence to direct their own lives (Held and Keane, 1983: pp 170–2). The paternalistic and overly bureaucratic nature of the service was criticised and, long before Enthovem, it was characterised by those on the Right as centralised, uncompetitive, inefficient, unresponsive and intrusive (Weale, 1987: p 151; Vaizey, 1984: p 102; The Adam Smith Institute, 1984).

As has been stated, one of the key planks of social democracy was the redistribution of wealth and it was always the intention of early governments that the NHS should 'redistribute welfare'. The recognition that the NHS had signally failed in this – as was argued to be the case in welfare provision more generally – became clear the longer the NHS was in existence. Essentially, this failure meant that those who least needed the NHS were getting the highest quality care and treatment (Le Grand, 1982; Doyal, 1979). This paradox was demonstrated by Tudor Hart (1971), who described it as the 'inverse care law', which showed that there was least expenditure on health in areas where there was greatest need. Moreover, feminist and cultural critics added their voice in the late 1970s and early 1980s, arguing that women, black and minority ethnic groups were even more poorly served despite having far greater need. These apparent problems were compounded by another of Mrs Thatcher's pet hates. The Grantham grocer's daughter saw, in the dominance of the professions, as much of an inhibition to her brand of politics as there was in the old major institutions, such as the BBC or universities. The medical profession, in ensuring the NHS had absorbed its prevailing model of illness and health, had secured its monopoly and, consequentially, maintained its dominance of the healthcare system (Navarro, 1987; Tonkin, 1988). Moreover, they were as much the architects of paternalism and culpable for the failure of redistribution as anyone else.

Within the broad headings of these criticisms, lay a range of other perspectives. For instance, radical anti racists claimed that not only was racism inherent in British society but a deliberate tool of the capitalist state and used to deflect criticism of the state and its systems. Broader explanations tried to tease out issues such as direct and indirect racism, institutional and intentional racism and how the adoption of a 'universal' approach to healthcare provision meant the needs of minority groups were inevitably ignored. The wider body of feminist critics also contained a wide range of sub-groupings. The ambivalence towards, or contradictions in, healthcare provision does not make it any easier to develop coherent policies within any political framework. Women can gain from healthcare as individuals yet still experience the state provided service as oppressive (Doyal, 1985). Socialist feminists also argued that broader welfare policy perpetuates the male breadwinner model of the family and subordinates women within both the domestic and public spheres. More radical feminists put the case that separate women's services, provided by women, are necessary as all women are oppressed by men and the welfare state inevitably perpetuates this, with the source of this oppression being biological and 'directly related to [women's] sexual relationships with men in the domestic sphere' (Bradshaw, 1997: pp 9–19).

In the 1980s, the Conservatives were able to argue that these issues were not just the finer points of academia but had changed voting patterns and paved the way for their electoral victory (Rose, 1986: p 162). However, after several years in power, and despite the changes they had already made, the problems remained. Politically, they also had to deal with the widespread perception – in this case, actually based on reality – that 'for the first time "real" spending on the NHS went down' under their stewardship (Charmley, 1996: pp 209–10).

It is overly simplistic to suggest that the solution of the New Right was to privatise all aspects of welfare provision – although advisors such as Patrick Minford did urge such a course of action – and they adopted that approach with utilities such as water, gas, electricity and British Telecom. However, as the New Right dominated the intellectual agenda, they prosecuted the argument with great vigour that increasing individual choice and freedom through the market and reducing the level of state provision would provide the answer to the problems of the economy and the health service. Politically, these were difficult courses to chart, particularly reducing the level of state provision. But the reforms were seen as the ideal vehicle to match a practical solution with the government's ideological agenda.

▶ General management and nursing: appropriating the language and culture

With this debate as the backdrop, innovations and research into new nursing practice methods were still occurring, generally continuing to be driven by those nurses most directly involved in patient care. The pace of clinical change had slowed slightly from the 1980s as the altered managerial and organisational arrangements took effect and tighter fiscal controls were introduced. The loss of a nursing voice at higher decision making levels also meant such initiatives were often met with a sceptical response. There was a reliance on the quality of relatively new relationships between nurses and their managers in decisions about how cuts or organisational changes would affect clinical practice. Inevitably, these were highly variable. Two examples of this can be taken from contemporaneous research in Oxford, where nurses responded to the researchers' questions about working in the NHS and being under the authority of new general managers:

'I am not "the manager" of my ward, but merely the supervisor. I have only partial control over my environment and cannot change most things';

'Feeling undervalued by managers, is reinforced by attitudes of doctors and even patients as they don't seem to understand the constraints [nurses] work under. This ward is a popular ward, there is a queue of students for jobs here. But with higher pressures to push patients out, more complicated surgery, and complex treatments for terminal conditions, greater skill and patience is required of the nurse to meet individual needs of patients, and it requires an increasing amount of effort to do the same job. Most of our staff nurses only stay six to nine months' (Owens and Glennerster, 1990: pp 146–7).

What nurses valued was not necessarily valued by medical or managerial colleagues and old alliances sometimes took their toll. Cuts were becoming more widespread and even innovative units, such as Beeson Ward, of the Oxford Development Unit, which had housed a variety of nursing and organisational developments – including the introduction of nursing beds, where nurses made decisions about patients being admitted and discharged – were not exempt. In this case the reason given for closing it was ostensibly one of cash shortages facing the health authority but followed severe pressure from doctors, with whom the unit had been unpopular.

The most significant change for nursing during this period was the implementation of Project 2000, the long awaited new training system. Even that was not impervious to other policy initiatives, as schools of nursing were taken into higher education. Almost inevitably for the period, cost cutting was part of the process. Tutors began to face redundancy just as the new system was about to come online, further changing the culture of nurse education. If innovation and new practices could be either lost or stifled among the welter of policy, managerial and organisational initiatives, it could also be appropriated if managers saw advantages to systems they might otherwise have been unenthusiastic towards. An example is the nursing process and primary nursing which, as we have seen, were used to create a system that strongly emphasised the role of individual nurses.

Another thing that was appropriated in the new NHS of the late 1980s and early 1990s was language. Patients became clients or users, reductions in services, closures of wards or even hospitals became the rationalisation of services. Objectives, human resources, performance management, change management, budget management, cost effectiveness, cross charging, deficit levels, virements, rationalisation and downsizing were all buzz words in the new, business-like NHS. Some of them were fairly obvious and straightforward in their meaning. Others were far less so and obfuscated more complex and, sometimes sinister policies. For example, often what was deemed 'cost effective', i.e. delivered the best level of service efficiently within a given cost banding, was in fact simply cheaper. Nurses were given the responsibility of managing ward budgets but no authority to do so and no control over the extraneous events that might make that task so much harder. Much of it was actually linked. Terms like 'clients' were designed to signal a new relationship between nurse and patient. On the one hand, this seemed to fit with a progressive agenda many nurses were willing to sign up to, wanting to facilitate a shift in the power relationship between service providers and users. But there was another message incorporated in this changed language, implying a more business-like relationship, even one with a financial component.[3]

Some of the language of the nursing process could also be used in interesting ways. Nurses were now individually accountable for their practice, pressed home through

---

[3] While many nurses are anxious about terminology in this area, as noted in the introduction, research has shown that people who come into contact with health workers still prefer the moniker of 'patient' (see Introduction).

the United Kingdom Central Council (UKCC) code of conduct (1983), and re-inforced by educational institutions and employers. The trade unions and professional organisations inevitably picked up on this, producing advisory notes and briefings. But what were nurses individually accountable for? Little, if anything, was advertised about the employers' responsibilities towards its employees, their welfare, health and safety. Information about a collective form of legal responsibility, vicarious liability, was not produced or spoken about in any such depth. Yet vicarious liability meant that employing organisations were legally responsible for the actions of employees.

The meaning and the language used in describing these issues was used to communicate an associated relationship and meaning, both of which were far less welcome as the years rolled on. Nurses found themselves accumulating much more responsibility, with no status or the authority to allow them to manage it properly, and accountable for things over which they had little actual control. For instance, a nurse in charge of a ward would be told she was accountable for all its patients, even if additional patients were admitted against her advice when the ward was short staffed, leaving it much less manageable and its nurses unable to provide the necessary levels of care to all its patients. The UKCC's code of conduct requires her to inform her manager of her professional opinion that the ward is unsafe and patients are at risk. In reality, few nurses would do that very often. Besides, it's unlikely to cut a lot of ice in the middle of a winter bed crisis. A community mental health nurse working with a caseload of thirty plus when she knows it should be closer to twenty is often in much the same position. A 'D' grade community nurse covering the absence of a 'G' grade district nursing supervisor without being paid acting up pay or receiving any extra support faces a similar dilemma.

In situations like this responsibility brought higher levels of anxiety but little – if any – reward. The idea that the nurse was then accountable for anything and everything that might happen was highly oppressive, and far from the increased status expected from autonomous and accountable practice. It did, however, provide a far greater ideological framework for controlling the nature of nurses' work and played a part in progressively isolating them one from the other, individualising not only their practice but thinking. Moreover, it placed the nurses' accountability to senior nurses and managers above that to her patients and even her own professional body, though that was one of the original precepts of the code of conduct. At the same time, the institution and higher management were absolved of their responsibility to ensure there were sufficient beds, adequate staffing levels, support and an infrastructure that would facilitate not only safe but good clinical practice.

Primary nursing, which had been advocated as a means not only of improving patient care but also flattening hierarchies and democratising clinical practice, could be inverted into creating a more elite group of qualified nurses prescribing care that would then be carried out by more junior, often untrained, nurses. Thus the separation through hierarchy is increased and a new division of labour created. All of these factors were now contributing significantly to a shift away from collective responsibility, collective practices and that 'catholic' aspiration of nurses achieving progress through their own and other's efforts. One other factor that was highly significant in this period would also play a huge part in the process: the shift in resources – and most particularly nurses – from hospital to community.

▶ Case study 2: The internal market – working for patients?

Having a legitimate body of criticism, both from the political left and right, the government had, in some senses, an open goal at which to kick its new policy initiative, *Working for Patients*. Their plan was to retain the principal of funding the service through taxation and universal access for all at the point of need. But the problems of efficiency, variations in service, inadequate financial control and, above all, the lack of competition would be addressed through establishing an internal market in healthcare. One of the cornerstones of the white paper was consumer choice. Obviously, this made it far easier to sell to the electorate. It was claimed it would break the stranglehold exercised by the medical profession which the government saw as a major obstacle to change. Moreover, the white paper stated explicitly that massive funding increases were not the answer; it was a matter of how that money was managed, and the best place for that to happen was at a local level, well away from the remote hand of central government. A 'review of funding' had made an enormous leap of faith and become a blueprint for the largest re-organisation the NHS had faced since 1948.

The key trick Health Secretary, Kenneth Clarke, was keeping up his sleeve was that he wanted to achieve increased local responsibility for things such as service provision, pay and funding arrangements but even more accountability to the centre – and thus control – than had been achieved thus far.

Hospitals were to become self-governing trusts, GPs were to take control of their own budgets as fundholders, management was to be restructured at every level and, most importantly, the commissioning of services – or purchasing, as it quickly became – was to become a separate function to that of providing them, carried out by completely different bodies. It was expected that patients would receive an improved, more equitable service overall. With bureaucratic and administrative barriers removed, patients would be able to travel to the NHS hospital of their choice. Waiting lists would be reduced and rigorous auditing would deliver best practice and, that ubiquitous term of the period, value for money.[4] Nursing practice was virtually invisible as far as the document was concerned.

---

[4] Compare this list of expected achievements for self governing trusts with Alan Milburn's claims made for Foundation Hospitals in 2002 and the far reaching influence of Thatcherite ideas and philosophy on New Labour and its health policy is only emphasised, despite the fact they were almost wholly discredited in the intervening years.

There were a few problems with the concept of an internal market, as it was being defined by the government, but these did not seem to trouble the ebullient Mr Clarke. Its system of capitation funding, or funding provided per head of population, hit inner cities and deprived areas hardest, where additional cash was needed to meet greater levels of need. Trusts had to pay what were, in effect, interest charges on all hospital buildings and premises, designed to encourage more efficiency by using fewer buildings but which also had the biggest impact on inner cities. Moreover, all the country's major teaching hospitals – again, usually situated in inner cities – had to bear the increased costs of their teaching and educational functions, as the local health authority purchasers would not.

Yet even this, the most radically Conservative government since the war, had not gone as far as it could. It had stopped significantly short of introducing a true market in healthcare. The local NHS was still, to all extent and purposes, the monopoly supplier of healthcare. Their function was still heavily regulated by government. Nor was there the homogeneity of 'product' to allow a market to function efficiently. Fundamental to any effective working was information. Trying to introduce an effective market without adequate information systems was like trying to fly a plane without a navigation system but this was the situation most managers found themselves in, with inadequate accounting, manpower and ordering systems. Even more important in market terms was the information required by consumers to assist them in making choices. Having a hip operation was not like buying a new car. Models couldn't be test driven, the patient couldn't sit in the operating theatre and watch the surgical team at work. The district nursing service in Northampton might be better than in Brighton but it would be unlikely that someone would make the journey there to have his or her ulcers dressed. A health consumer magazine couldn't effectively do a survey of operating techniques or measure district nurses' performance in monitoring diabetes and administering insulin throughout the country and give out meaningful star ratings, while Commission for Health Improvement visits might offer a rough guide but could not take into account the many variables and complexities required to compare one service against another. Indeed, GPs and the new purchasing authorities didn't have sufficient information to bypass a reliance on local providers or allow them to make informed decisions about strategic services (Le Grand and Robinson, 1984: pp 38–9). The only way to challenge that was to make decisions based on inadequate information or notional costings, quickly put together by managers with no experience or training in doing that, but which purchasers began to do more frequently nonetheless.

Any analysis of market forces has to deal with supply and demand. Demand on the NHS had, to that point, increased year upon year, with politicians making bolder claims for the service, usually spurred on by the medical profession's confidence in its ability to cure illness and disease, all of which fuelled the growing expectations of society at large. More people were being treated but waiting lists were still growing. In a true market, increased demand would give the supplier or provider increased power. The other factor in this would be the price, which would rise and fall as demand fluctuated. Health, however, produces a situation of inelastic demand. More people do not fall ill or get well quicker according to changes in the market. The only way to change demand was through a change in the purchaser's capacity or willingness to buy services from a particular trust and little, if anything, to do with the incidence of ill health in the local population.

Achieving greater efficiency was, therefore, associated with 'increased throughput' – another use of language which was supposed to sound better than acknowledging that more patients were being admitted because others were being discharged earlier or, even more significantly, sending them home before they were ready for discharge – rather than increasing capacity. Although advances in operating techniques, increased use of technology and better use of more community health provision, had all enabled clinicians to properly discharge patients earlier, 'increased throughput' was often simply synonymous with lower quality care.

An inelastic demand side was met with an equally inelastic supply side. Just as news about clinical grading wrongly inspired the hope that nurses would be paid more according to their qualification and the clinical work they did, some nurses at least thought that if they worked in an efficient hospital and were providing a good quality service, at last that service would have the opportunity to grow through improved funding. There was also a hope that, just as in business, hospitals would be able raise cash for service investment and development. Again, such hopes proved unfounded. The overall NHS budget remained fixed. The entire premise of the internal market was undermined. Moreover, the speed with which implementation was begun generated its own inefficiencies, while the 10–15 per cent additional funding needed to kick start the system was never provided by the government (Barr, Glennerster and Le Grand, 1989). Nor was the new system helped by the financial situation within the NHS at that time. Cumulative underfunding of pay review board (PRB) awards since 1984 had reached £193 millions, which health authorities had had to find out of their own budgets. And each annual NHS funding award failed to meet the cost of inflation. For example, the Retail Price Index stood at 7.7 per cent in 1990 but health authorities were allocated only 4.5 per cent. Nurses were already working in difficult conditions when the internal market was introduced. Janet McCabe, the then theatre manager at St George's Hospital in Tooting, was warning that unless she could increase her nursing levels, theatre lists would have to be cut. She was running six theatres with a nursing establishment designed for four and nurses working on their days off to provide cover. But with her health authority facing debts of £3 million, there was little chance of any improvement (Gaze, 1990: p 19).

For nurses there was something else about the new white paper. It didn't grab the headlines in the early days. Bubbling on the edge of the nursing agenda for a few years, it had largely remained an internal debate within COHSE. Local bargaining was necessary if the government was to deliver on its promise to devolve all policy making to a local level. It meant that effective consultation and negotiating machinery had to be in place within each NHS trust, with a completely re-defined relationship between local unions and employers, national unions and government. For nurses, it also threw the future of the PRB into doubt.

Just as with general management, privatisation, trade union legislation and almost every other government policy to which they had been opposed, the unions campaigned. The shape and form of the campaigns was difficult to design and co-ordinate because, initially, there was only a concept and no one was sure how that would develop into practice. Again, there were lots of local variations – as was the very point of the policy. Privatisation and trade union legislation had only had a very indirect affect on the BMA and RCN. In fact, the latter had been able to make major advances while its main nursing rival, COHSE, was embroiled in unsuccessfully defending its members and its political position against a determined government. Yet it hadn't all been plain sailing for the College. Griffiths had delivered a major blow against its senior nurse members. The failure of that campaign was made all the worse because its own members, in more junior positions, essentially ignored their union's call to action.

The unions were unable to co-ordinate their opposition in any unified way and each pursued its own agenda. But the opposition was widespread. 'Polls revealed upwards of 90 per cent of health workers opposed to opting out.[5] British Medical Association (BMA) ballots of consultants in twenty-eight opting out hospitals found an overall 69 per cent against, with clear 'no' votes in twenty-one (Timmins, 1995b). Sixty per cent of nurses surveyed believed the reforms would not improve patient care (Snell and Gaze, 1991). The BMA mounted one of its biggest campaigns ever, personally attacking Clarke after he had refused to give ground in negotiations. As a government, the Conservatives had immediately looked favourably on the doctors. One of their first initiatives had been a relaxation of NHS consultants' contracts to enable them to further develop their practice privately, even though this eventually led to an inevitable conflict with their work within the NHS. Doctors had also received far bigger pay rises than nurses and other health workers, while their system of merit awards was not challenged, despite the enormous cost and concern that they were awarded without any assessment of a contribution to improved health (Mohan, 1995). Almost as important, their

---

[5] 'Opting out' was the term given to those hospitals and NHS service providers who were choosing to depart from direct NHS control, via their health authority, and adopt the status of a self governing Trust. Opponents argued that this meant leaving the NHS completely. The government, supporters of the reforms and those NHS managers who felt trapped between the proverbial rock and hard place and saw opting out as the only avenue open to them, explained that they were remaining within the NHS and would still be bound by its policies, ethos and practice while having more independence.

clinical authority had been left untouched, even after an attempt had been made to draw them into the managerial fold with Griffiths.

The medical profession's serious concerns about *Working for Patients* were appeased after protracted negotiations with Clarke ensured it retained its position as one side of the policy making triangle at the centre of the NHS, with the civil servants and politicians. The unions, despite their overwhelming opposition to the policy, resisted calls for industrial action. Trevor Clay, the Royal College of Nursing's (RCN) general secretary, again emphasised his organisation's position on delivering on the government agenda rather than supporting nurses' views: 'I believe we will only win if our focus is on making the health service work for the patients and clients, and not making the rights of those who work in it our only priority' (Clay, 1989: p 16). The College strategy suggested amendments to the white paper but was as unsuccessful as the trade unions.

One of the RCN's leading lay members, Sally Gooch, perhaps summed up the confusion and antipathy of many nurses at the time: 'The NHS white paper is such a preposterous set of proposals that without the experience of ten years of Thatcherism it would be impossible to believe that the government means to implement it in the face of almost unanimous opposition, natural justice and common sense. While the principles behind it are inhumane, most of the content is simply unworkable' (Gooch, 1989: p 42).

▶ The 'common good' is re-defined

It was obvious that Kenneth Clarke, with steel toecaps under his trademark Hush Puppies, was determined to see the new system introduced. When Gooch recommended that nurses be 'subversive', she was perhaps unconsciously recalling the principles of an earlier, more feminine type of opposition. Yet, in the face of a policy that Confederation of Health Service Employe (COHSE) had warned put the future of the NHS at stake, the nurses' organisations were left wrong footed again and again, unable to organise any coherent opposition. Perhaps it was because of the scale of change and the unlikely nature of it, as it was perceived at the time. There was also an increasing expectation that, after more than a decade of Conservative government, Labour might be able to snatch victory at the next election. The nurses who had been so radical a few years earlier were relatively quiescent. With far more emphasis on hospital admissions and discharges, waiting lists and finished consultant episodes (note the inherent superiority of the medical profession within that term), 'cure' was again assuming more importance than 'care', with the consequence that nursing was being cast even further out of the decision making loop. The government moved its agenda forward so quickly that even the managers charged with local implementation struggled to keep up.

In the midst of all this, the general election came and went. John Major had succeeded Margaret Thatcher as leader of the Conservative Party and thus prime minister in 1990, following her unceremonious dumping in the wake of the poll tax fiasco, as well as growing tension about Europe and the running of the economy within Tory ranks. He was probably one of the few people in the country not surprised when he walked back through the black door of 10 Downing Street after the poll in 1992 but was then relatively quick to act on the health service. Despite the introduction of the market, the government had actually been anxious about major unrest in the NHS prior to the election; now it let the market move into another gear. The profound changes and the speed with which they were brought in caused major problems across the country but especially in London. Apart from the problems outlined above, purchasers in the Home Counties switched contracts away from the high cost teaching hospitals. If the market would work anywhere, it would be in a city like London, with a large number of hospitals sitting cheek by jowl. But was the government really prepared for the consequences of major hospitals, in one of the largest capital cities in the world, being closed due to the decisions of a handful of relatively uninformed and inexperienced managers in brand new purchasing authorities? There was now a real possibility it could happen.

Its solution was another inquiry, actually initiated in the autumn of 1991 but not published, as the *Tomlinson Report* (1992), until after the election. As far back as 1979, the Tory Government had drawn up plans for the closure of 6000 of London's 50,000 beds over a ten-year period. The closures actually accelerated at double the planned rate. Nonetheless, Tomlinson thought there was scope for far more, especially if primary care was given a significant boost. Accepting this proposition, the government's own proposals, *Making London Better*, enlarged even upon Tomlinson's estimates about potential closures, taking the capital's health services to the brink of chaos (DoH, 1993). Now it wasn't just hospital beds but entire hospitals that were facing closure. It looked as if the government was prepared to take a political step no other had yet dared. But while this part of the drama was unfolding, a parallel policy development was about to impact. The market was taking its course alongside planned and carefully managed change – with both resulting in reductions in levels of service not just in London but most of the cities where there were a number of hospitals in relatively close proximity to one another.

For the first time since the beginning of the Second World War and before the inception of the NHS, nurses were facing redundancy in large numbers as the new self-governing trusts desperately tried to balance their books. Despite accepted nursing shortages throughout the country, trade union officials, particularly in central London hospitals like University College Hospital, the Royal London Hospital and Barts, found themselves trying to save hundreds of nursing posts. As outlined in *Making London Better*, it looked bland enough: 'The changes we are setting in hand have significant implications for staff. It is vital that their skills and commitment are retained in the NHS wherever possible ... Redundancies may, unfortunately, be necessary as a last resort. Staff will, of course, be entitled to their statutory rights ... ' (DoH, 1993: p 17–18). This process was begun in late 1992 – early 1993 but did not stop there. By 1996 hospitals were still engaged in a process that was not just sapping skills and commitment from the service, but its ability to function properly. Trusts like Croydon's Mayday Hospital were reduced to asking all patients coming in through the A&E Department whether or not they had private insurance. Far worse, with redundancies still occurring on an annual basis, the Trust issued, 'A warning that staff who are left behind must expect a tough new policy of non replacement for colleagues who leave, are sick, on maternity leave or on holiday. The action will be about saving money not necessarily in a fair way.' This was all in the context of the hospital spending 'A massive £811,000 on redundancies and early retirements: more than was spent buying medical equipment for patients' (Brook, 1997). Moreover, spurred on by the government, necessarily looking for ways to both increase efficiency at the same time as cutting staffing costs, trusts moved towards negotiating local terms and conditions. To all intents and purposes, the NHS was dead. The needs of the service, the common good, was very clearly re-defined. Now, it was to work within budget.[6]

▷ Everything must change

The importance of *Working for Patients* was that, through the internal market, GP fundholding and introducing local pay bargaining, it changed everything. None of its parts could be said to have been a complete success in policy terms and, in their own ways, all came to a sticky end. However, this was genuinely a case of the sum being far greater than its parts. One of the key elements in this was that the culture of the NHS was altered in a way that general managers had not been able to achieve. The imposition of financial controls was no longer an abstract proposition but a reality. They were dictated by another new phenomenon, that of the service level agreement (SLA). These were agreed by managers from the purchasing authority and provider unit that is NHS trust, with targets being agreed to be met by the provider against a sum of money that would be paid over by the purchaser. This might be for a specific number of operations or a 'block contract' to provide, for

---

[6] Has the definition of the common good changed under New Labour? In July 2001, the South London & Maudsley NHS Trust had patients with serious mental illness sleeping in armchairs, on mattresses on floors and in corridors, which involved nurses in practice that lies outside virtually every clause in the UKCC Code of Conduct. 'Staff are feeling the strain, with sickness rates and stress levels soaring on the worst affected wards' (Unison Eyes, No. 9, July 2001). The reason? The trust, with its health authority, had agreed it would no longer overspend on purchasing private beds for those people who could not be accommodated within the trust's existing number of beds, despite knowing that, given the demand within its catchment area, that number was insufficient.

instance, midwifery services. The problem was that, once that money was gone, there was no more to come in. Therefore if a trust completed its quota of operations nine months into the financial year, surgeons might be left with no work to do, despite waiting lists. Wards would be temporarily closed, as happened quite frequently in the early days of the market. More likely, there simply wasn't enough money in the SLA to allow the provider to undertake its work properly and pay staff throughout the financial year. These agreements were often negotiated and agreed without a lot of medical input and certainly none from nursing staff, unless it was by a nurse in a very senior position and with no clinical contact.

But managers were quoting these contracts and waving budgets in front of clinicians. For nurses, it meant that the expectation of working within budget was even greater – even though they hadn't agreed to it and it meant not having nurses to cover absent colleagues, losing places on training courses or finding themselves unable to order what was deemed essential equipment. Having their own budgets and having it drilled into them that they were limited, they took it upon themselves to limit their involvement with anyone or anything that could adversely affect their spending position. At its worst, this would lead to ward sisters trying to 'cross charge' one another for nurses who had worked on a different ward for a few hours. Always hoping that there would be advantage to be gained from performing effectively and within budget, previous levels of co-operation often broke down. 'Efforts to modernise pathology services in the East Kent region, of which the cervical screening service at Kent and Canterbury Hospital was a part, were paralysed by "turf wars" between several newly "freestanding" hospitals for nearly four years. While ambitious entrepreneurial schemes were being promoted, the women of the region were meantime getting an inept service officially condemned ... as "an appalling series of events which should never have been allowed to happen" and which led to five deaths and many more women being damaged by cervical cancer' (Lashmar, 1997). At the time of the report's publication in 1997, Professor David Hunter of the Nuffield Institute of Health, commented that this was not a unique problem but 'a good example of a national problem. I think we can say that the internal market has not worked'.

Strategic planning was now seen not only as less important but actually inefficient and harmful to the functioning of the new system, which had serious consequences for planning the annual intake of nurses into training, as well as specialist services across the regions and the country. Keeping track of bed closures across the regions was impossible.

Bureaucracy became a byword of the new service. Teams of new managerial posts were necessary to administer the SLAs, chase money, monitor performance and monitor the monitors. This change in numbers and emphasis of the work gave 'the men in suits' (for these posts were dominated by men and, with them, a masculine culture to rival that of the medical profession) far more influence. Nurses were given more administrative work than ever before. Much of this was gathering statistics, which had to be compiled on a regular basis, generally about patient activity and staffing issues. Different forms had to be completed with demographic information and patient details for the purposes of admissions. There were massive attempts at information gathering, even down to the numbers of chairs and cupboards, in the initial preparation for capital charging. And nursing documentation was becoming increasingly bureaucratic and inclusive at the same time. It all took nurses further away from their patients.

Two things happened that affected the relationship between the public and their healthcare services. Inevitably, the whole promise of consumer choice proved hollow. Not only did patients not have the opportunity to pick and choose where they wished to be treated but, because their local health authority might have ceased contracting with specialist hospitals, the option of accessing services that would have been available prior to the market (which was usually made on their behalf by their GP or another referring doctor) was lost. However, expectations were raised by the way in which the government sold its new policy, with the constant emphasis on increased choice and improved standards. It meant there was an implicit encouragement to come to the health service with every possible ailment, including social ills as social services became increasingly under-resourced and criticised.

There were counter-prevailing voices, saying that, if anything, explicit rationing was going to be necessary rather than the implicit and underhand rationing that was occurring. This would require a very frank public debate and, although MPs, clinicians and academics were willing to enter into it, neither the government or Labour's shadow cabinet would touch it – even when some health authorities made it clear that there were some specialist referrals they deemed to be not cost effective and would not fund, no matter how desperate the individual patient's circumstances. Equally, although the medical profession was holding up its collective arms in despair as the workload increased and resources failed to keep up, sections of it were quite willing to maintain the façade that virtually every ailment was curable or should fall within their ambit, while some GPs who had led the march towards fundholding were embracing the market along with the increased power and finances it gave them.

The respective fates of two London hospitals revealed the prevailing political reality of the time as the government responded to the working of the market and the apparently more rational and planned policy making implicit within the Tomlinson Report. Camden and Islington Health Authority publicly consulted on proposals to remove its contracts with one of its main service providers, University College London Hospitals (UCLH), incorporating the University College and Middlesex Hospitals. Given that Camden and Islington was the 'host' purchaser, i.e. the local and main purchaser, it was clear that this course of action would effectively close two of the biggest NHS hospitals in the country. The health authority argued they could purchase the same services from other local hospitals more cheaply and were following government policy to its logical conclusion.

Quality of care, patient choice and the strategic hole that would be left in specialist services and London's A&E provision were immaterial. Unison members within the new trust balloted for industrial action, and with nurses taking a leading role, led a major Unison campaign to save the hospitals, mounting the most high profile strike action since 1988. With the internal market firmly at the top of the political agenda, Secretary of State, Virginia Bottomley, intervened and the proposals were withdrawn. However, having survived, UCLH was forced into radical action in terms of cutting costs – initiating massive redundancy programmes in the process – and, in finally bringing the supermarket philosophy to the NHS, found itself being accused of starting a 'price war' by announcing 'reduced prices' for 1994–95 (Cresswell, 1993: p 4).

Only COHSE and London Health Emergency had taken a wholly critical stance against Tomlinson. Even the RCN had given lukewarm support, despite the impact there was to be on its members. Almost everyone assumed the report had a strong intellectual rigour underlining its recommendations and consequently concurred that London's health services needed 'a shake up' (Reid, 1993: pp 41–5). Despite ensuring UCLH's survival with the promise of additional funding to help it through its 'short term difficulties', Bottomley confirmed that, post Tomlinson, St Bartholomew's and the Royal London Hospitals were to merge and Barts A&E Department would close. A massive public campaign followed, but one which did not engage the nursing staff, who remained inactive throughout, despite significant attempts by Unison to rouse them. The A&E department closed, with a minor injuries unit opening and a shift of significant services to the Royal London.

▶ New Labour's first two years in power – what was the difference?

New Labour had already committed itself to the Tory's spending plans in the run up to the 1997 election, a substantial problem given that the wily Ken Clarke, now chancellor, would inevitably hand them a poisoned chalice were they to be elected. Following on from eighteen years of Tory underfunding, by Labour's own account, the new government was then tied to perpetuating that for a further two years. Clarke's legacy quickly became apparent. NHS Trusts and health authorities were carrying a collective deficit of £300 million from 1996–97, with a further £1 million debt being added *each day*. Tory promises to increase spending on patient care services by £1.6 billion or 2.9 per cent in real terms hid the fact that most of the increase would come from cuts elsewhere in the health budget, with projected NHS investment slashed in real terms by 10 per cent in 1997–98. Only £470 million of new money was allocated to the NHS in what became the first year of New Labour's government, on top of zero growth planned for the previous year. The spending increase of a miserly 0.3 per cent in real terms, once inflation was taken into account, over a three year period to 1999 was wholly inadequate, given that the

NHS had struggled with what had averaged at a 3 per cent annual rise in the previous two decades (Caldwell *et al.*, 1998). Writing in early 1999, Will Hutton observed:

> 90 out of 100 health authorities are in the throes of major closures and cuts, and almost every local authority is scaling back community care. The NHS is no longer governed principally by considerations of public health, clinical need and patient care. Its overriding values are cost reduction, operational efficiency and the need to reproduce the managerial culture of a privately owned PLC. Patients' interests have become secondary to those of ideological public accounting principles and the enthronement of market values in public provision. A policy begun by the Conservatives, which the nation voted to change, has been continued largely uninterrupted by New Labour (Hutton, 1999).

As events were to show, the re-definition of the common good had, indeed, survived a change of government.

The warnings had been accumulating throughout the decade for Tony Blair and his party. In 1995, 13.5 million people attended the nation's A&E departments, a rise of 25 per cent since 1989, but the number of departments fell by one-third, to 200, during the same period. The Audit Commission found that 25 per cent more senior house officers and 43 percent more Registrars would be needed even to meet government targets (NHS Federation, 1996). Tales of increasing waiting times, patients being stacked up on trolleys in corridors, were almost so common as to lose their news value. Almost every local Trust was struggling, many having to take similar steps to those of Croydon's Mayday Hospital. There, twenty posts had to be lost and nurses were asked if they wanted to accept redundancy to make savings of £700,000 as the management announced it was developing 'a new marketing team to win back business from fundholding GPs', having lost contracts worth £200,000 as those GPs moved their patients to other hospitals (Croydon Advertiser, 25.10.1996). Virtually all clinical areas were pleading for more money, with warnings of crisis coming from Trusts up and down the country.

In London alone, an estimated 15 per cent of beds had been closed post Tomlinson, even though emergency admission rates were increasing at 2 per cent per year, with the length of stay decreasing by an average 4–5 days. A further 125 staffed homes were required to meet the Conservative Government's own planning targets for accommodating mental health patients requiring twenty four hour nursed care, with an accompanying 875 qualified nurses, all at a cost of £70 million plus (Unison Greater London Region, 1997).

There was also another part of the Tories' new agenda for health that its New Labour successor took into its policy nest uncritically: the Private Finance Initiative (PFI). The predictions were equally dire. 'More than £5 billions of taxpayers money is to be handed over to construction consortiums over the next 30 years to build, own and run the first PFI hospitals recently approved by Labour. Waves of redundancies, bed shortages and cuts in patient care will signal [their] arrival' (Leigh *et al.*, 1997).

Despite New Labour's stated concern for nurses and nursing, as well as its grand policy design, which was becoming apparent through its legislative programme, without the cash to support it or a serious initiative to redesign the power structures within the NHS, these too often were claimed to be hollow noises. 'The decision by Swindon and Marlborough NHS Trust to slash its nursing budget as part of a £4 million savings package is yet further proof that, for many trusts, the NHS white paper is hardly worth the paper it is written on. What happened to those worthy intentions that nursing would be at the cutting edge of the health service of the future?' (Nursing Times, 10.6.1998: p 3). The stories of poor care in filthy surroundings continued as they had under the previous government. '[The renal ward at Guy's Hospital] was filthy beyond belief. You couldn't walk with your bare feet on the floor and there were mice running about at night. All around us was degradation and dirt. The ward had blocked sinks full of stagnant water, no clean bedding, and inedible food. I have never witnessed such callous treatment. Animals are usually treated with more respect than my mother was' (Revill, 1998). Cash crises continued to cause cuts. With a £1.3 million overspend within the financial year begun in April 1999, The Royal London Hospital, closed twenty children's beds seen as essential and which it had promised would be safeguarded following the closure of the Queen Elizabeth Hospital in Hackney the year before. Geoff Martin, director of pressure group, London Health Emergency, branded the closures 'a complete betrayal' of those assurances. Nigel Crisp, then director of London's NHS region and later to become Chief Executive of the NHS, said, 'The closures were an example of "prudent housekeeping"' (Revill, 1999 b).

The cumulative effect of these financial pressures obviously had a direct impact on patients' care and treatment. Eastbourne NHS Trust had to admit that the care of a woman who bled to death after a routine operation was compromised by nursing shortages. Following a colleague ringing in sick, the only trained nurse on a surgical ward with thirty five patients had reduced the frequency with which the woman's observations were to be carried out, to once every four hours from every thirty minutes, after an HCA had informed her they were 'ok' (Gould, 1999: p 8). When an independent review of skill mix and staffing levels at the Eastbourne Hospitals NHS Trust was carried out by the National Health Service Executive South East, it found that ward sisters and charge nurses were often working as the only trained nurse in a team, that healthcare assistants were assessing and planning care, were responsible for patients following major surgery and undertaking one-to-one nursing requiring 'a high degree of nursing knowledge and competency'. Students were being placed in 'highly stressful situations on grossly understaffed wards'. Nurses 'did not feel valued' and had 'lost faith' in management, finding their managers 'unwilling to listen, complacent and autocratic'. Having previously denied there was a shortage of nurses, the Trust's chief executive and chair both resigned, the latter blaming financial shortages for the problems outlined in the report (Coombes, 1999a: p 7).

The devastation was continuing and widespread, affecting all areas of the health service. Of course, not all of the ills of the NHS were due to funding problems, as ministers and civil servants are quick to point out. Nonetheless, research conducted at Ninewells Hospital, Dundee, between 1992 and 1995, suggests that workload plays a significant part in treatment and care outcomes. The research team involved found that patient mortality increased by more than 100 per cent when the workload was high for doctors and nurses in the hospital's Intensive Care Unit (ICU). Workload measures included the proportion of occupied beds, the average nursing requirements of patients and the ratio of occupied to appropriately staffed beds. Designated as full when its six beds were occupied, it frequently admitted a further two patients, bringing the total to eight and a further two ICU patients could be cared for by the unit's staff in a high dependency area elsewhere in the hospital.

▶ Case study 3: NHS funding

Yet the money, according to the government, was piling in. An extra £1.2 billion was pledged in 1997 as new chancellor, Gordon Brown was forced to break free of Tory spending proposals as the scale of the problem became apparent. It represented an increase of 2.25 per cent for 1998–99 and his first budget also pledged a new hospital building programme, albeit under the PFI scheme. Most commentators observed, however, that it was unlikely to match demand. By 1999, new initiatives were being announced outside the annual budget increases, such as a £100 million single increase, comprising a £20 million boost for primary care, with the remaining £80 million going to the acute sector. Amongst other things, the money was to be used to improve buildings and working environments and providing nurse practitioners in A&E departments. By 2000, a total of £4.17 billion was being pledged, representing real term growth of 7.9 per cent, with the promise of 6.3 per cent average real terms increases over a four-year period. Any government throwing this sort of cash into public services might feel they had earned the right to a bit of gratitude. It wasn't forthcoming. The reason for this is complex but worth exploring. It also goes some of the way to answering the question asked by so many nurses. Why is it, if so much extra money is coming into the service, they seem to be working harder than ever and don't see the benefit of it?

▶ NHS funding: the chancellor was in his counting house counting all our money ...

On the positive side, millions of pounds was being directed into capital schemes – building projects which were either to refurbish existing but seriously dilapidated NHS buildings or for new hospital departments, health centres and premises. These are 'one off' projects but which generally swallow up huge amounts of funds.

Less positively, New Labour continually announced 'new' spending initiatives, only for it to be later discovered that the money had already been allocated to the NHS in a previous announcement. In early 1998, Gordon Brown announced the NHS would receive an extra £21 billion between the financial years 1998–99 and 2001–02, of which £3 billion was earmarked for new hospital buildings as part of the widely publicised modernisation fund. This left £18 billion. It was to be allocated over the three years as outlined in Table 5.1.

The obvious question is, how does this add up to £18 billion? Where is the missing £9 billion? If the increases are added in a different way, it can be found. There is a £3 billion increase in the first year. Add that to the next financial year's increase and you have a total of £6 billion. If the original £3 billion is counted for Year 1 and then again for Year 2, along with the actual second year increase of £3 billion, that adds up to £9 billion. For the third financial year, count the original £3 billion *three* times, the second year increase twice and the final year's £3 billion once and you have a grand total of £18 billion by 2001. As can be seen, this is not just double counting, but treble counting. Nurses may be familiar with it as an accounting system, for it was one New Labour learned from the Tories, when it was often used to suggest that nurses had received, e.g., an 18 per cent pay rise in the previous three years when they thought they had only received 3 per cent each year (see Table 5.2).

Table 5.1   Increase in NHS funding, 1997–2001

	NHS budget (£ billions)	Increase from previous year (£ billions)
Base Year	36.00	N/A
Year 1	39.00	3.00
Year 2	42.00	3.00
Year 3	45.00	3.00
Total increase		£9.00 billion

Table 5.2   Increase in NHS funding, 1997–2001 according to the 'Brown formula'

	NHS budget (£ billions)	Increase (£ billions) in year	'Brown formula'	Brown Increase (£ billions)
Base Year	36.00	N/A	—	—
Year 1	39.00	3.00	+ 3.00	3.00
Year 2	42.00	3.00	+ 3.00 + 3.00 = 6.00	6.00
Year 3	45.00	3.00	+ 3.00 + 6.00 = 9.00	9.00
Total increase		£9.00 billion	3.00 + 6.00 + 9.00 = 18.00	18.00

The problems do not end there. To the average person in the street or working nurse, the difference in buying power between £9 and £18 billion pounds is almost impossible to imagine, with both sounding like incredibly large sums. However, £18 billion is barely enough. Using the 'Brown formula', if inflation during that period runs at an average of 2.5 per cent, which it has to the time of writing, that will account for approximately £6 billion of it. With nurses' pay settlements just edging over the rate of inflation, even though non-PRB staff have been less generously treated, the pay bill will swallow up a further £3 billion. Demographic and technological change is likely to require an additional £7 billion during the period, given that the NHS is treating an increasingly ageing population, as well as continually broadening its treatment base and using new techniques and equipment. This leaves £2 billion of 'new money' to cover the cost of increased recruitment and all the other initiatives the government are showering upon us.

All in all, it adds up to vastly raised expectations followed by a profound sense of disappointment, like receiving a letter informing you you've won a vast amount of money only to be confronted with nothing more than a time share salesman when you go to collect the cash prize. Put another way, spending 3 per cent more than inflation on the NHS, year on year, was not enough to ease the pressure on hospital and health authority budgets and one reason why the Tories were perceived to have failed as a government. 'More money is needed to take Britain closer to the share of the nation's income that other advanced countries spend on healthcare, and behind which, on current plans, we shall continue to lag behind by a significant margin' (Kellner, 1999). As the debate continued, a specially commissioned report for the Treasury on NHS funding, *Securing our Future: Taking a Long-term View* (*www.hm-treasury.gov.uk*, 2002), known as the *Wanless Report*, concluded the UK had achieved less in terms of healthcare than other developed nations because it had 'spent very much less and not spent it well'. It was estimated that NHS spending would have to increase from £68 billion to £184 billion by 2022.[7,8]

---

[7] In nursing terms, these vast sums of money can be further broken down. As Brown continued to invest more in the NHS, with promised rises from a base of £65.4 billion in 2002–3 to £105.6 billion in 2007–8, the *Nursing Times* decided to announce a Nurses' Plan, stating what it thought nurses should be getting from the NHS Plan. These included pay modernisation, education reform, computer training, flexible working, clinical supervision and leadership skills, with an estimated first year cost of £1.5 billion (Munro, 2002 a pp 10–13). This is probably a conservative amount and certainly wouldn't meet the costs of placing student nurses back on salaries, equal pay for work of equal value, regular study/research time for nurses as doctors currently get or establishing staffing levels matched to the clinical and service demands facing nurses.

[8] Scotland had a variation of the Wanless Report in *Fair Shares for All: The Report of the National Review of Resource Allocation for the NHS in Scotland* (1999), also

▶ New nursing initiatives – what influences spending in the NHS

When times are hard and there is not lot of cash to go around, it is inevitable that everyone is going to be fighting that little bit harder for their share – as well as anyone else's they can lay their hands on. Despite the hard accounting that is detailed earlier, more money has come into primary care and nursing initiatives under New Labour. Nonetheless, the acute hospital sector still gets the lion's share of funding, clearly reflecting the continuing dominance of the medical profession and its model of illness and health remains strong under the new government. Looking at other areas of the health service shows how the battle is fought out for the scraps that fall off the hospital table.

Launched on three pilot sites in early 1998, NHS Direct quickly expanded and was allotted £50 million of funding – but with the expectation that it would both take pressure off A&E departments and GPs, as well as save substantial amounts in the long term. This is one of the reasons for the twenty-four-hour health advice line's popularity amongst ministers. It was intensely unpopular with the medical profession, with the BMA initially branding it as dangerous and misguided.

With the service two years old, a further £1 million for mental health leads on each NHS Direct site was made available, as well as the introduction of its first nurse consultant's post. Opposition mellowed in some quarters, partly because of its success in minimising the impact of the 'flu epidemic in late 1999–early 2000 and the way it was being embraced by larger numbers of GPs, especially in out-of-hours services and GP co-ops, with whom it was working increasingly closely. But not completely. Professor Robert Winston put the criticisms in their bluntest, most politically obvious form. The prominent Labour peer and fertility pioneer quoted two instances when nurses had not picked up on a serious condition when dealing with callers and argued strongly that NHS Direct was unsafe. Nurses, he stated, would always be inadequate because they don't have a medical training. When he argued, however, that the money would be better spent on better GP cover, he got closer to an issue that many medical critics had strenuously avoided. The serious flaw to his case was that the problems were not about nurses' experience and training but that they were performing a service 'blind', i.e. at the end of a telephone. Moreover, he did not consider the number of cases where GPs and A&E doctors have misdiagnosed with the patient in front of them. This was rather similar to the scare

---

contd.
known as the 'Arbuthnott Review'. This was originally established in 1997 under the chairmanship of Professor Sir John Arbuthnott, Principal and Vice Chancellor of Strathclyde University. It reviewed the methods used to allocate funds for the NHS in Scotland and was re-convened by then minister for health, Susan Deacon in 1999 (for further information see *www.scotland.gov.uk*).

stories which emerged after *Health Which?* (2000) had reported that in two cases when its researchers had rung up NHS Direct feigning a heart problem, they had only been given 'adequate' advice. This was seized upon by the opponents of NHS Direct and, yet again, the nurses providing the service throughout the country were branded as putting lives at risk because of their lack of training and experience. Of course, no comparative research was done in A&E departments or GP surgeries.

There is a far deeper issue at the heart of the medical profession's rearguard action. If all calls that would go to GP out of hours' services are routed through NHS Direct, doctors will lose their twenty-four-hour, seven day a week, responsibility for patients, which will undermine their contractual status with the NHS and, ultimately, their pay, an attractive option to government.[9]

Nurse prescribing has been another key initiative in extending the role of the nurse. First piloted in 1994, a formulary for nurse prescribing was designed containing eleven items but the pilot process was dogged by problems. The RCN demanded that this be scrapped, allowing nurses to administer any drug or dressing within their competence. The BMA offered cautious support but the UKCC did not take a formal stance and Unison urged the legal position be resolved and seemed to be vindicated when an occupational health nurse was cautioned by the UKCC for the unauthorised ordering and supplying of prescription-only medicines. The union, which represented the nurse, called for the ambiguities to be ended, saying that the Department of Health's existing guidelines for nurses administering medication needed clarification as they conflicted with the Medicines Act, which had failed to keep up with the development of nursing practice (Mahoney, 1998). It wasn't until early 1999 that the consultation process for two tier prescribing powers was unveiled. These were to allow independent and dependent nurse prescribing, according to experience and training, but only from a range of medicines restricted to their own specialist area. The RCN was critical, having been lobbying for the proposals to get onto the statute books quickly. Unison remained cautious. The issue remained, however, about what was driving this policy. Was it about improving the service to patients or saving money? Nurses were as split as their unions on the issue until, eventually, the government announced in November 2000 that it was now willing to allocate £10 million to train up to 10,000 nurses and give them new prescribing powers – with the stated aim of improving patient access to drugs and breaking down professional boundaries. What had changed? In 1996, there were serious doubts that the Treasury

---

[9] By 2002 NHS Direct was receiving 120,000 calls per week and been listed as one of the modern innovations that had changed the way people lived. Caller satisfaction with the service has consistently been audited at more than 90 per cent and an Audit Commission study has shown the service to be as safe as any other in the NHS (Munro, 2002b: pp 10–11).

thought an investment in nurse prescribing would be cost effective (Nursing Times, 1996: p 3). Those financial considerations laid to rest, it was now deemed to be in the patients' best interests, or in the common good, for the policy to proceed.[10]

▶ With all this going on, who wants to be a nurse?

Retaining nurses in the climate stimulated by the internal market, never easy, as we have seen, was not going to be any easier for New Labour. This was a task exacerbated by the Tories' failure to implement PRB awards in full in successive years leading up to their election defeat. But the cost of replacing each nurse who left a post within a Trust was estimated at £5000, including absence cover, advertising the vacancy and training replacements. With an average of 300 nurses leaving each trust every year, the costs for 1997 were estimated at £1.5 million by The Audit Commission and Institute of Employment Studies, who submitted a special report to the Department of Health (Audit Commission, 1997). Given that this was money 'lost' to the organisation, it only compounded the problem.

A Unison survey, 'Cause for concern' (1998a), found that 65 per cent of nurses reported frequent staff shortages due to sickness, while 53 per cent complained of shortages due to staff having left and not been replaced. Yet the work still has to be done. Who makes up for absent colleagues? Usually those nurses 'left behind'. Obviously, nurses would want to be paid overtime but this is almost unknown in the NHS for nurses. Wherever possible, it used to be done on a 'time owing' basis but, as the shortages worsened, it was recognised that there would have to be some financial inducement and nurse 'banks' were set up. This allowed nurses to work additional shifts or hours through the Trust, as well as those who were not employed by the Trust but wanted to work on a part time, ad hoc or temporary basis. The bonus for employers – and it was a big one – was that bank rates were not only significantly lower than overtime but, because they were usually paid at a

---

[10] Although the government is carefully guarding the results of initial research into the work of the Walk In Centres, there are indications that they are not achieving their objective of diverting patients away from GP surgeries, despite attendances rising steadily and far exceeding the already ambitious targets set by government. Moreover, a number of clear tensions about the role of the nurses, their preparation, training and experience for working in the Walk In Centres were surfacing. Both recruitment and retention were as much of a problem as anywhere else although, to an extent, initiatives like the new Centres and NHS Direct were asset-stripping places like A&E departments in terms of experienced and skilled nurses. As the problems became more obvious, the Department of Health appeared to be cooling, moving key personnel onto other projects and not planning to establish new Centres.

'basic' rate, often a 'D' or 'E' grade, even cheaper than paying an experienced nurse at their own grade for the extra hours. It also allowed Trusts to 'fill' vacancies with bank staff who might be paid at a lower rate than the substantive grade they were covering while, until recent EU directives, bank employees were ineligible for sick pay, holiday pay or many other employment rights.

It is inevitable that nurses would be deeply unhappy with this, realising that they were being exploited. As in so many instances, the resistance was not overt or confrontative. It does, however, further compound the original problem when nurses either leave the NHS only to continue working through an agency or opt to work their extra hours through the same route. In this case, not only are they earning more but, with the commission fee paid to the agency, adds to the trust bill. Under the Tories, agency numbers – and costs – peaked with the introduction of the internal market in 1991–92, when costs were £120.8 million. They then crept back to this level by 1995–96.[11] The percentage of the nursing workforce employed through a bank system had, almost trebled to 4.25 per cent. Patient care is undoubtedly affected as continuity breaks down, agency nurses have no time to build-up relationships with people, there is a lack of familiarity with local procedures and nurses who are, effectively, self-employed will always have difficulty keeping up to date with changes in practice when there is not only the matter of paying course fees but losing money for the duration of the course. With a pretty poor press, agency nurses are rarely looked upon favourably by their permanent co-workers (although this often changes when they are employed in an area 'on a line', over a longer period of time) and nurses working in areas reliant on agency staff often complain of low morale and increased stress levels.

The reasons for nurses exiting the NHS vary enormously. Remarkably, given the real nurse shortages and reliance on temporary cover, there are still some areas where nurses are leaving because of the frustration of being unable to get promotion. For example, Angela Hughes and Fiona Kelleher were both highly experienced, had undergone post-graduate education but were unable to move out of their respective 'E' and 'D' grade posts (Gulland, 1999 a).

For other groups, the reasons are more about staff shortages and working conditions. School nurses saw major cuts in their services under the Tories and those remaining found the work increasingly pressured and difficult. Inevitably, it became more difficult to either fill vacancies or those posts which were re-opened when the effects of the shortages became apparent. Mental health nurses working on acute wards faced increasing levels of violence, racial and sexual harassment, with larger numbers of disturbed patients staying for shorter periods. With inner city hospitals having had bed numbers slashed, occupancy rates of 130 per cent were common – with the 'record', held by a London Trust, standing at a staggering

---

[11] As we shall see in Chapter 8, spending on temporary staff under New Labour was to leave these sums way behind.

230 per cent (Lister, 1999). Agency and bank staff made up a third of ward based nurses, but for those on duty there was a chance of being assaulted, on average, every three days. With acute psychiatric units reportedly close to collapse, the main focus had become 'bed management', or admitting, discharging and transferring people around an increasingly fragmented system, leaving nurses little time for real contact with patients (Department of Health, 1999 a). This has led to them finding themselves de-skilled and without adequate training for the work expected of them. Indeed, The Mental Health Act Commission (1999) had identified that one consequence of this was that 25 per cent of patients would have virtually no interaction with nursing staff during their time in hospital.

A 1999 survey of London based health visitors carried out by the Community Practitioners and Health Visitors Association (CPHVA) revealed that 33 per cent did not have time to carry out essential duties. Only 6 per cent had mobile phones, although they were considered important for staff safety, while 35 per cent of their managers had one. Fifty-five per cent did not think their professional judgement was valued by managers. Caseloads had all risen and one of the ways in which managers were trying to manage this was by being more prescriptive about what health visitors could and could not do, rather than letting them make their own judgements based on clinical need.

These illustrations only reflect the problems nurses face in almost every clinical arena in which they work. The pernicious cycle of low staffing levels is one which shall be explored in later chapters, but has run like a virus through every part of nursing and through every era. Limited career opportunities are linked to the loss of senior posts and higher graded posts disappearing due to budgetary cuts. It then becomes inevitable that patient care suffers, patient demand increases, as does workload for those still in the service, morale sinks as stress rises and many nurses would concur with the views of those London health visitors surveyed, when 37 per cent said they would leave their jobs immediately if they could.[12]

► Out of the ruins, hope can rise

There seems to be no hope. But is there? Sometimes, out of adversity comes opportunity. The closure of A&E departments meant a small number of nurses were able to establish themselves in nurse-led minor injuries units and an increase in numbers of emergency nurse practitioners within A&E units. The chaos that ensued in mental health following the Conservative's catastrophic bed closure programme in the 1980s, when thousands of beds were closed in little over a decade, meant that

---

[12] 60 per cent of nurses reported in a separate survey they had considered leaving their posts in the previous twelve months, with 71 per cent of those citing the fact that they felt undervalued (Unison, Cause for concern, London, 1999).

nurses had to develop innovative ways of working with people with severe and enduring mental illness in the community. Nurses started providing case management, assertive outreach, a new range of psychological and psychosocial interventions and sophisticated assessments, as well as new techniques and services for helping patients in crisis, including home treatment teams. Many of these services operate in a genuinely multi-disciplinary way, with doctors, nurses, occupational therapists and psychologists working alongside one another clinically, undertaking training programmes together, and making decisions in a far more collective way than once would have been the case. Although integration with social services is a slow and painful business in most instances, it is still inching forward, breaking down old barriers to joint working and shared care. Nurses, particularly, have adopted techniques and work that once would have been the province of most of the other disciplines and are much the richer for it. Moreover, many mental health Trusts developed genuinely close partnerships with user groups during the same period.

With greater difficulty discharging chronically ill people and the elderly from hospital and acute beds being 'blocked', new ways of working have had to be developed. Some of the successful initiatives from mental health have been replicated in community nursing, with 'hospital at home teams' and short-term acute services providing intensive nursing input to help people remain in their own homes rather than be admitted to hospital. Nurses are also involved in services such as housing medical teams, which try to resolve people's health-related housing problems. The growing numbers of asylum seekers and refugees have also sparked new and innovative services, often nurse led or with nurses forming the hub of the service, while it was nurses in the vanguard of using assertive outreach techniques for providing care for rough sleepers, as homelessness went beyond crisis point to becoming a chronic problem.

Those nurses involved in innovative projects almost always describe them as rewarding and claim to benefit from the additional training that is usually part and parcel of the service. Perhaps the most striking aspect of the comments nurses make in such posts, however, is about having the opportunity to be creative, make their own decisions and work differently, in such a way that they are able to make a palpable difference to their patients' lives. Often, this entails stepping outside of the traditional nursing role, whichever area of nursing, assuming greater autonomy and authority in the process. These themes recur when nurses are involved in highly functioning teams or projects which take what might be termed routine practice to new heights. Midwifery is a service that has gone through even more turmoil than almost any branch of nursing since clinical grading. Despite falling numbers, enormous steps forward have been made in clinical practice, with midwives becoming even more autonomous and now, in some areas, guiding women through their pregnancy, birth and post-natal care exclusively. As a discipline, it has almost certainly been strengthened by distancing itself from nursing and retaining a link with its historical roots, something which has been easier as direct entry training has become more established.

Renal nursing and haematology are examples of where nurses' autonomy has grown. Service changes elsewhere have partly shaped their extended role but, collectively, they have grabbed the opportunity. At the other end of the technological scale, nurses have been instrumental in movements that have taken the care of the elderly into new realms. The innovative work of those like Ian Morton and Christine Bleathman in the care of elderly people with dementia has overlapped with that of psychologists and psychiatrists while holding onto many of the virtues which stem from their nursing backgrounds (Morton, 1999).

The need to cut both costs and things like waiting lists will always offer nurses opportunities as well as posing a threat or serious problem. Examples of this are nurse led rheumatology clinics, which were used not only to slash waiting lists but improve the service at the Bristol Royal Infirmary. Nurse specialist posts were introduced for people with suspected colorectal, breast, lung and gastrointestinal cancers at the Blackburn Royal Infirmary while, elsewhere, nurses were taking on the work of preparing patients for surgery. Again, the more holistic and biosocial approach of nurses means that patients often get a far more comprehensive service than that offered by surgeons and anaesthetists (Shamash and Gallagher, 2002: pp 20–3).

There are other elements that crop up time and again when reading about innovative nursing practice. Although they are going to feature in far more detail in subsequent chapters, it is worth linking them with what has gone before, because they are factors that have, in some respects, survived *despite* the changes that have been heaped onto nursing in the last couple of decades – and we have not even come to the plethora of policy that has piled out of New Labour's first term of office yet. Working together, a strong team identity, a clear focus, commitment to shared ideals, creativity, resilience, interdependence, reflective practice and radical thinking, sharing decisions in an open, involving way, combining theory with practice, all suggest a collective tradition that was almost destroyed by the internal market, the onslaught of general management and clinical grading. These were not long standing traditions in nursing; in fact, they really only developed in a way that would be recognisable to contemporary nurses in the late 1970s and early 1980s. They came together from different strands of nursing, combining factors that, decades earlier, had been alien to one another. When they did, however, they were regarded as radical and dangerous: a threat to the 'common good'. In these relatively recent traditions, which are still alive in pockets of nursing, there is something important in helping us think about where nursing might go in the future, away from practice that is driven by economic and ideological factors or inter-disciplinary power struggles beyond its control. Maintaining a clinical radicalism, as opposed to clinical militancy, they balance the tension between what is good for nurses and what is good for nursing with the needs of the patient, but recognise those tensions are not irreconcilable.

▶ Conclusions: nursing taken to the brink

The white paper, *Working for Patients* and subsequent legislation, made no specific mention of nurses. Nonetheless, as policy was put into practice, the consequences were terrible indeed. The degree of commercialisation begun by the privatisation of ancillary services crept further into the heart of the NHS, not least because clinical services were being taken into the private sector in a variety of ways: in the massive, poorly regulated growth of care homes for the elderly, the increased use of private beds for mental health patients who couldn't be accommodated on NHS wards, the relaxation of consultants' contracts, enabling them to spend more time in private practice (in the process giving them less time in which to see NHS patients or perform duties in the NHS) and, most pertinent for nursing, the increase in the use of agency and bank nurses.

The NHS had been under intense scrutiny, and subject to criticism from both left and right, and the Conservatives could argue that they had used a rational model of policy development in responding to those criticisms, applying their own diagnosis to the problems afflicting it and the way in which they introduced their solution. The internal market may not have been a true market in the economic sense but it was used to establish a whole new set of relationships, such as those between purchasers and providers, and to devolve some aspects of decision making as far away from central government as possible while tightening the grip on finances far more successfully than any previous government had managed. Strategic and long term planning were banished as the new self-governing trusts and purchasing authorities were left to get on with the task of managing change – primarily through setting short-term targets and negotiating year long SLAs. The cultural revolution begun with Griffiths was almost complete. But the problem with constant change was that it brought a degree of chaos that was making the service almost unmanageable.

With nursing posts being made redundant on an unprecedented scale, the workload was increasing beyond the already high levels of the 1980s. Stress went up and morale plummeted. Accountability and responsibility were, in many cases, a burden and threat rather than a liberating route to improved status. With pathways to promotion diminishing, nurses and nursing had nowhere to go. Their work was being more and more individualised and traditions of collectivity broken down. With 'gagging' clauses used in the most authoritarian manner, trade unions weakened and split, a workforce that had raised itself to new heights under the banner of clinical militancy was broken. Perhaps most disturbingly of all, the change that nurses – and, indeed, a substantial part of the country – thought it had voted for in May 1997 didn't come. New Labour accepted the Tories' financial strategy for its first two years in government and, far more decisively, its overall policy thrust, leaving in place a system where patients' interests had become secondary to those of ideological accounting principles and the enthronement of market values in public provision.

With the gulf between nurses and managers having steadily widened and with the loss of any meaningful leadership, nursing innovations were often left hanging in the financial wind. Judged by criteria in which clinical effectiveness or advancing practice were not high up the scale, they were as likely to founder as survive. Project 2000 was an initiative that had government support but such radical change would always have been a struggle to implement successfully, let alone in the climate created by the market. Doctors, on the other hand, may have been critical and resistive to change, but always used their power to consolidate their place at the negotiating table and in the policy making process. They supported nurse led initiatives when they eased the medical workload but, when those changes posed a more serious threat to the status quo or doctors' earning power, their position was far more strident and oppositional, such as with NHS Direct.

And yet. Through it all, pockets of excellence have flourished. Nurses, albeit in small groups, resisted the doom and gloom that appeared to pervade the NHS, finding new ways to work effectively together, to create and develop new services. And the vast majority got on with the job of caring for their patients as best they could. Under New Labour, money did flow into the NHS – although nowhere near as much as they wanted the public to believe – and they promoted major changes to nurses' roles in particular areas. However, there had been no real difference in the way that policy was usually made without the active involvement of nurses. The definition of the common good, which actually determined how the broad thrust of nursing was shaped, hadn't changed.

▶ Further reading

Barr N, Glennerster H and Le Grand J (1989) Working for Patients? The Right Approach? *Social Policy and Administration*, 23 : 2.

Coxall B and Robins L (1994) *Contemporary British Politics*. 2nd edition. Basingstoke: Macmillan.

Doyal L (1979) *The Political Economy of Health*. London: Pluto Press.

Ham C (1992) *Health Policy in Britain*. 3rd edition. Basingstoke: Macmillan.

Navarro V (1979) *Class Struggle, The State and Medicine*. London: Martin Robertson.

North N and Bradshaw Y (eds) (1997) *Perspectives in Healthcare*. Basingstoke: Macmillan.

6 Power, Decision Making and Leadership

My answer to this is that a powerful prince will always be able to overcome all such difficulties, inspiring his subjects now with the hope that the ills they are enduring will not last long, now with fear of the enemy's cruelty, and taking effective measures against those who are too outspoken ... So the subjects will identify themselves even more with their prince, since now that their houses have already been burned and their lands pillaged in his defence they will consider that there is an obligation on his part. The nature of man is such that people consider themselves put under an obligation as much by the benefits they confer as by those they receive.

The Prince by Niccolo Machiavelli

▶ Introduction

Were this an episode of the TV series, *The X Files*, this would be the point in the narrative at which Mulder would turn to his ever sceptical partner, Scully, and whisper, 'Do you think there's something going on here we're not being told about?' Scully would scowl, responding earnestly, as if to a precocious but wilfully recalcitrant child – and without taking a breath: 'Are you suggesting that the fact that nurses are still poorly paid, working in a low status occupation, unable to resolve any of the long term problems and grievances that have affected both their work and their relationships within their workplace while their core role, to care for their patients, is at once exalted into an almost unachievable goal and, at the same time, hopelessly undermined is a *conspiracy*? That would be crazy! Why would successive governments and people in positions of power and authority want to do that? Governments need nurses to perform their jobs well. They do all they can to make that possible. And even if you didn't accept that, it makes no sense that they would deliberately undermine the position of such a potentially powerful group of staff:' Mulder grins wryly, raising an eyebrow. He says, 'Explain it to me, then.'[1]

---

[1] For the uninitiated, or anyone reading a copy of this book lost in someone's loft for several years, *The X Files* was a very popular television series in the 1990s featuring FBI agents, Mulder and Scully, investigating paranormal events. Almost everything they encountered was part of one conspiracy or another. Or was it?

Politics matters. Many nurses might like to think that they breathe a purer, apolitical, air, or haven't the time to think about anything as base and boring as politics. This is, in itself, perfectly understandable and mirrors attitudes outside nursing. But it misses the point. As nurses, we live politics. Or, more precisely, we work with the consequences of political decision making each day when we turn up for duty. To not think about the political dimension of an issue but decide upon an apparently rational response, is to implicitly submit oneself to the political and ideological agenda of those in power.

In this chapter, the policy process will be further explored, particularly at a local level. As has been the case in previous chapters, the overall emphasis will be to tease out how and why particular decisions are made. This is taken to be of more value than simply recounting events or listing out so-called facts. The decisions actually looked at are regarded as important in themselves but also as representative of a process that needs to be understood, just as with the earlier case studies. Walk In Centres, Primary Care Trusts, innovations in critical care nursing or NHS Direct are only of fleeting historical importance. But the way in which governments, policy makers and managers impose political and ideological agendas will remain much the same.

Since New Labour came to power in May 1997, it has been striving to make the NHS 'modern and dependable', introduce the national service frameworks, the *NHS Plan, Making A Difference, Improving Working Lives, Shifting the Balance of Power* and much more.[2] If these policies are successful, New Labour will rightly be able to proclaim itself one of the great reforming governments. The NHS will be more responsive and patient centred. Staff will be empowered at all levels. Having established PCGs, these were transformed into PCTs, which will have the role of running the NHS and improving health in their areas in a reformed service. Key targets, such as the reduction of waiting lists will have been met, suicide rates will have been reduced by 20 per cent, the maximum waiting time in A&E departments will have been reduced to four hours by 2004, patients will be seen by GPs within 48 hours at most, 25,000 lives a year will be saved from coronary heart disease by 2008.

Having signed up to the European Union's social chapter, legislation followed that changed working conditions, the environment and more. Some of these policies impacted upon one another, occasionally in contradictory ways. The overall thrust and effectiveness of New Labour policy will best be picked over by historians but, towards the latter half of this chapter, it may be possible to discern some clear trends, particularly about how any government might set such ambitious performance targets while devolving decision making and empowering staff at the same time.

This chapter will also seek to tease out just who makes the decisions that affect the working lives of nurses, the structures in which those decisions are made and, perhaps most important of all, the factors that influence them, whether it be within a ward or community team, at trust level, within the Department of Health or

---

[2] See the Department of Health website for more details: *www.doh.gov.uk*

government itself. A framework for thinking about this is featured, with reference to issues networks and the so-called 'iron triangle' of decision making that occurs between the medical profession, civil servants and government. Power is an obvious influence in these processes but how is it used and what, exactly, is it? Importantly, why are some policies championed while others are left to go stale in the policy cupboard? Its focus goes beyond the political dimension that currently shapes nursing and into the world of our own workplace. What do we do, as nurses? What shapes those decisions, actions and, again, non-actions? Importantly, it will seek to contrast the external world to the internal, the way in which nurses perceive themselves, with the ensuing consequences. What the main political parties say – and, wherever possible – how that correlates with what they do is a good starting point. Again, a model for understanding power is discussed, with examples from nursing experience.

Managers often come in for harsh criticism and, for many nurses, are a soft target. Yet, in most cases, there are not actually 'good' or 'bad' managers, just people responding in the context of a particular system. There is strong evidence that NHS managers increasingly perceive themselves as having to respond to an agenda that is not theirs, that even chief executives have difficulty in stamping their own personality and direction on their trust as they respond to an ever tighter central, government-driven agenda. As this chapter will demonstrate, the job of being a manager is not a lot easier than that of being a nurse. It will be seen that the vast majority of managers are no better or worse then the organisational structures in which they find themselves allow them to be; the notion of the 'bad' manager is almost as much a social construct as the 'bad' nurse. Focus on the relationship between managers and managed, between nurses and the people to whom they are expected to answer, thus becomes all the more important. It is inevitably a complex issue but it is one where change has to be exercised if nursing is to take the position that the government says it wants it to within the NHS. Indeed, it is virtually impossible for the government to transform the NHS into something that is 'modern and dependable' – or anything else – unless nurses lead that process on their behalf. This was a point made by the RCN when faced with proposals for widespread change in Northern Ireland as part of the process of devolved decision making following the establishment of the Northern Ireland Assembly. This chapter also includes a further two case studies. The first provides a relatively brief account of devolution and the effects it has had on nurses in Scotland, Wales and Northern Ireland. It is a subject worthy of a book in itself but, given space, can only be looked at in the context of the broader development of policy, practice and politics as they affect nurses and nursing. Indeed, devolution offers perhaps some of the most profound evidence of the power of politics when it is seen how it can transform the nursing landscape, especially in Scotland. The second uses the example of the government's objective to reduce waiting lists to illustrate how an apparently 'good' policy can actually create at least as many problems as it is designed to solve while obscuring far more important issues.

▶ Promises, promises, politics, politics

Of course, talk comes cheap. Nurses do not. This has always complicated politics and nursing for government ministers. In 1997, Simon Hughes, then Liberal Democrat spokesperson for health, was promising £200 million each year, ring fenced (set aside) for recruitment and retention alone. That was in addition to an extra £550 million for the NHS, a single pay spine for *all* healthworkers, doctors and senior managers included, and three-year service level agreements, as opposed to the single year the Tories had used for the internal market. Labour's Chris Smith was more circumspect, undoubtedly aware his Party were likely to have to make good their election pledges. These included, considering a loyalty bonus for 'D' and 'E' grades, piloting a nurse retainer scheme, discouraging the use of agency or bank staff, a national minimum wage and, of course, matching but not exceeding Conservative spending plans. The then Secretary of State for Health, Stephen Dorrell, spoke of increasing the number of nurses qualifying each year by 2500 within five years, increasing spending, making further efficiency savings (sic) and continuing local pay bargaining The Liberals were circumspect on the internal market but wanted to increase public participation at trust board level, while one of Labour's few firm commitments was that it would scrap the market, with nurses and GPs leading on locality commissioning. They were also promising an independent review of the NHS funding formula. The Conservatives wanted to use GP fundholding as a means to achieving 'a primary care led NHS'.

Within a year of New Labour's spectacular romp past the winning post, 'ecstasy had changed to cynicism'; nurses had received the lowest of all the public sector pay awards and New Labour had staged it, just as the Tories had before. Waiting lists had risen to 1.3 million, the much vaunted funding review was looking at things like introducing 'hotel charges' for hospital patients and means tested prescriptions for people over sixty. Asked to comment on its performance in that first year, it is interesting to note that practising nurses took a far more measured and critical view than union leaders such as Christine Hancock of the RCN (Gould, 1998a: pp 32–3). Members of the public, polled by ICM, shared the nurses' view. Only 12 per cent thought the NHS had improved under New Labour, with 42 per cent thinking it was worse (ICM state of the nation poll, The Guardian, 8.10.1997).

By 2000, further promises were being made in preparation for the election that would follow in the next year. Labour was pointing to its record of having implemented the Pay Review Body (PRB) recommendations in full for the last two pay awards, claiming to have increased nurses' pay by 15 per cent in three years. The Liberal Democrats were now a little more timid, limiting their promise to 'going further than Labour in putting the case for more nurses who enjoy better conditions'. The Conservatives had decided to 'decide on pay when we come to office'. However, then leader, William Hague was promising tax cuts as well as matching 'Labour penny for penny on the NHS and sweeping away Labour's dogmatic opposition to private provision' – which only suggests that Hague's maths were as confused as his understanding of government policy towards the private finance initiative (PFI) and a range of other policies involving partnership with the private sector.

In fact, the cripplingly low standing of Hague and his party with the electorate, was having a debilitating impact on the political process, just as had occurred due to Labour's unelectability in the 1980s. One commentator was moved to write, 'The only explanation I can make for William Hague's disastrous leadership is that he is secretly working for the other side' (O'Farrell, 2000). The arrant nonsense being put forward by Dr Liam Fox, the Conservative Party Shadow Secretary of State for Health, who described himself as a GP, did not help. In a speech to the Society of Apothecaries on 20 February, 2001, providing 'an authoritative guide' to Conservative health policy, Dr Fox pledged to 'reform nurse training' yet again and 'look at new ways to organise nursing rotas so that ... more medically trained nurses are available in the winter months when they are most needed, while surgically trained nurses are available in greater numbers in summer when surgical activity is at its peak'. The logistics of this might be workable with a non- or semi-skilled workforce in areas of high unemployment but, in nursing, do not bear thinking about. Fox was also for 're-establishing matron's values' with matron's posts to provide 'a clear chain of command throughout the hospital so that there is someone personally responsible for overseeing and supporting the nursing staff (Fox, 2001).[3] This was said almost as if the Tory engineered Griffith's revolution and internal market never happened. Such intellectual and political weakness meant that it was almost impossible to mount any serious opposition to Labour's failure to make good on many of its election pledges and difficulties on health from within the House of Commons.

▶ Political pressures on policy and practice

To paraphrase Roy Griffiths, were Florence Nightingale's ghost seeking to haunt those 'in charge' in the twenty-first century, she wouldn't come anywhere near the NHS. It had become so highly politicised – and centralised – since the 1980s that more and more decisions were being made outside of its corridors, in another building altogether. The Treasury, of course, is one of the places where the most important decisions are made about the NHS. As was the case with Margaret Thatcher, Tony Blair has at times completely surprised his ministers with off

---

[3] This represented a big shift in attitude from first taking up post, when Fox apparently had 'little time for nurse consultants, matron and PCGs' (O'Dowd, 1998a). Alan Milburn and his New Labour colleagues were apparently impressed enough with re-introducing matron's values as this was a policy they quickly adopted, with 'new matrons' being introduced to hospitals in the same year.

the cuff announcements that have effectively set policy – if not in detail then certainly in its direction and overall shape. This happened when he announced the introduction of nurse consultants but, more importantly, when he stated that it was his intention to match the percentage of Britain's gross domestic product (GDP) spent on health to the EU average. These are obviously the exceptions; but the national service frameworks developed by New Labour, structures to set and maintain national standards through mechanisms such as the Audit Commission and the Commission for Health Improvement (CHI) have all extended government's reach far into the decision making corridors of the NHS.

As was the case with these latter examples, most national policy does evolve through more appropriate channels; acts of parliament are passed and policy documents come out of the Department of Health as civil servants translate government decisions and aspirations into hard policy. New Labour's approach was thus a significant departure from its Tory predecessors, who were less inclined to churn out and enforce policy in the same way, having introduced the internal market and worked hard to devolve policy – although it retained its power by controlling that framework, finances and, particularly, ruling on what *could not* happen. For New Labour, a number of factors influence their policy making. Most significant of all are its election commitments from both 1997 and 2001. With a relatively successful economy, unemployment and inflation consistently low, health moved sharply up the agenda to take pole position in the nation's expressed concerns.[4] In 2001, having been judged poorly on their record in managing the health service during their first term of office, Tony Blair and his party staked their credibility on overseeing major improvements in the National Health Service (NHS). The obvious human concern to see people receive the most effective healthcare possible is a factor while, financially, there has always been enormous concern about pouring money into the infamous funding black hole that some critics saw as the NHS. Maintaining a healthy and economically productive workforce remains a key policy driver.

Politics and government is, however, far more complex than a relationship between the party that wins the election and the people who directly elected them. Tony Blair made clear his belief from the moment he was elected leader of New Labour: winning power was the only goal a political party should seek. Once attained, the goal shifts to keeping it. What many of his supporters didn't understand was that, for Blair, this involves balancing any number of competing interests, forces and influences through a delicate process of compromise and

---

[4] Although a number of political commentators point out that, while people tell pollsters they would be willing to pay more taxes for better public services, every government elected since the 1980s has pledged not to raise direct taxes. Many within the labour movement thought the tax plans of John Smith, then Shadow Chancellor to Neil Kinnock's Labour leader, cost the Party the election in 1992.

negotiation. One way of understanding this is to view the party of government as only one of a number of competing groups, which includes their elected political opponents, the civil service, judiciary, industry and business, the church, trade unions, media and electorate. The net spreads even wider in the modern age, incorporating European politics and legislation, multi national companies, the International Monetary Fund and World Bank. Government attempts to maintain control and its hegemony, or general and intellectual dominance, can thus be seen as a complex process requiring the building and dissolving of different alliances, some of which may look strange indeed if viewed in isolation (Gramsci, 1971; Wilkinson and Miers, 1999).

These external factors can influence the work of government far more directly than any parliamentary debate, especially when it has an unbeatable Commons majority. Government should abide by legal rulings and draws serious criticism when it doesn't. It can be vulnerable to media reports and campaigns, moves by groups like the Confederation of British Industry (CBI) and trade unions. Many would assume that civil servants are doing the work of their political masters, impartially enabling legislation and smoothing the policy process. Few ministers talk openly about the issue while in power – an indication of the power of the civil servants, perhaps – although many recorded frustration at their inability to get their political wishes enacted by reluctant officials within the Whitehall bureaucracy once out of office. Under New Labour, civil servants began to complain about the way their work was being politicised and the difficulties they were having with special advisors brought in by ministers and working directly to them, with a wholly political brief, which eventually blew up into a major political row in early 2000.

Globalisation has been propelled by economic mechanisms that enable multi nationals to transfer money, manufacturing and employment to the place that they believe offers them the biggest market returns, allowing huge corporations to exert far greater pressure on national governments with the threat of withdrawing investment and jobs, seeking favourable conditions if they are to base their work in any one place. So it is that events in Germany, the United States or Singapore can have a significant impact on Britain's economy – and thus its politics.

▶ Case study 4: Waiting lists: just why are patients waiting ?

A criticism thrown at New Labour's attitude towards the health service has been its propensity for attempting short-term political fixes in the face of what are actually complex and long-term problems. Attempts to reduce waiting lists is one example. New Labour attacked the ever lengthening lists under the then Tory Government and made reducing them one of its key manifesto promises. As such, it was relatively simple to measure, rolled off the tongue easily and, above all, shorter waiting lists were desirable. Weren't they?

Yet reducing waiting times for *all* operations meant shifting resources to ensure that operations can take place more quickly when particular lists – such as hip replacements – are lengthening. However, should waits for relatively minor operations have equal priority with life-saving surgery? Should political prerogatives override clinical judgement? Nor does such a policy actually resolve the problem of why some hospitals are unable to provide surgery, or why waiting lists are so long, nor how needs can be prioritised. Nursing shortages that affect a hospital's ability to carry out operations go unrecognised. Moreover, a long waiting list does not, in itself, necessarily signify a problem. It does not always follow that a long waiting list means people are waiting a long time (Hamblin *et al.*, 1998: pp 28–31). Such considerations were, however, ruled out in favour of a populist political position which could be sold to voters and enable ministers to trot out favourable statistics. Other aspects of government policy or elements completely beyond the scope of NHS nurses or managers can also impact on targets. The reduction of waiting times for hospital operations, as well as outpatient appointments and A&E waiting times, was central to the NHS Plan (Department of Health, 2000). Yet, with 13,000 nursing and residential care home beds closing in 2001, an increase in a growing trend that brought the total to 63,000 beds closed in a six-year period, this task was inevitably made far more difficult (Akid, 2002a: p 4). It can, therefore, be seen that setting the target of reducing waiting lists is erroneous. Moreover, it prevents other questions being asked, which might actually be to the advantage to nurses, such as why are there shortages of nurses in particular areas or clinical fields? Thus, as seen in the previous chapter, such problems might create opportunities for a few specialist nurses but do little, if anything, to benefit the majority. Moreover, it creates an impression that the NHS is failing when as Revill (2002a) points out, patients are 'more likely to be given the correct medication, more likely to survive on the operating table. Childhood mortality is at an all time low, women dying in childbirth is now a rarity'. The annual winter crisis has been addressed and largely effective measures put in place. Revill argues persuasively that both nurses and doctors are working more effectively – even if she does not address the problems resulting from nursing shortages.

In fact, the concentration on waiting lists proved not only a policy mistake but also something of a political disaster for New Labour, with any positive announcements about reduced waiting lists being countered by opposition claims that the figures were being 'fiddled', that the government had ordered trusts to devise 'unofficial' waiting lists for patients to get onto official waiting lists, ironically, something the Tories had been accused of when they were in office. Worst of all, the government had to publicly admit throughout the lifetime of its first term that, in fact, the lists were actually getting longer, with an increase of 18,000 from the previous year recorded in 2002, bringing the total to 1.05 million (Revill, *op. cit.*). A further blow to this whole initiative came in late 2001, when the Audit Commission discovered that a number of NHS Trusts, including Barts and the

Royal London, had indeed been publishing inaccurate statistics in order to make it look as if they were making better progress in reducing their own waiting lists. When, long after this furore had died down, there were yet more sordid revelations, one might have expected public outrage. Ian Perkin, finance director at St George's Hospital, Tooting, the tenth largest NHS trust in the country, 'was fired after revealing his hospital's financial problems... and alleged waiting list fiddle' and then 'lifted the lid on what he claims is the culture of deception now endemic in the NHS', claiming 'the pressure from Ministers on managers to meet government targets was making it impossible to openly talk about problems in the NHS' (Revill 2003: p 4). That there wasn't perhaps spoke to the perception that people had come to accept that the massaging of waiting lists and government statistics was part and parcel of the political life of the NHS.

▶ The politics before policy

Policy taken through the legislative process involves parliamentary debates taking place, a green paper being issued for wider consultation, then debated again in the House of Commons before moving on to the House of Lords. Any legislation needs to be voted upon, with the majority vote carrying it through. New Labour's enormous parliamentary majority makes this a relative formality: in effect it is able to operate an 'electoral dictatorship' similar to that of the Thatcher Governments of 1983 and 1987. The Lords can 'send a bill back' to the Commons if they disapprove of it in total, or parts of it, suggesting amendments where appropriate, but the bill can still be passed by special legislation on a subsequent reading in the Commons designed to stop the Tory controlled House of Lords effectively stymieing Labour or Liberal governments.

Government is also scrutinised and called to account by Select Committees, made up of MPs of all parties, with a remit to examine policy and issues in a given area, such as health. These committees hear evidence from experts and contribute to the policy process via their reports, inquiries and response to government. Their real power rests in their ability to embarrass government with critical reports. Ultimately, however, it depends on public perception of how serious the issue and how serious it regards the criticism. A small majority, such as that of John Major's in 1992–97, does change the political landscape as backbenchers can combine with the opposition to pressure the government into making serious concessions or even changing policy. Otherwise, it is essentially the power of persuasion versus naked power.

The political process can nonetheless never be discounted. The key drivers in reforming mental health practice in the 1990s, notably with the introduction of the Care Programme Approach (Department of Health, 1995), but also with the decision to concentrate the efforts of community mental health teams on people with severe and enduring mental illness, were serious incidents that attracted massive press coverage, including several homicides by people with mental illness.

Frank Dobson announced that 'care in the community had failed patients and the public' and the government wanted to look again at the option of compulsory treatment in the community. They also paved the way for the National Service Framework on Mental Health in 1999. On one level, this was perfectly reasonable and rational. However, the furore being stoked up in the national press did not match the reality. A study based on Home Office figures had shown that the number of murders by mentally disordered offenders had actually halved in less than twenty years. Four hundred and eighty people were convicted of murder in 1979, with 121 of those having a mental disorder, reducing to sixty people with a mental disorder being convicted of murder in 1995 out of a total of 522 (Radcliffe and Munro, 1999: p 10). The backdrop to the policy change was a sustained campaign mounted by understandably aggrieved relatives and groups such as SANE, which received highly favourable coverage in the media and, almost inevitably, raised concerns with which most people could empathise, as opposed to the plight of thousands of people with mental health problems who were being poorly cared for in unsuitable conditions or not even receiving treatment and care, living in dreadful circumstances.

In January 1999, a high-level inquiry team recommended the closure of Ashworth Hospital, a top security institution in Merseyside, 'at the earliest opportunity'. Frank Dobson rejected this, instead drafting in a former Royal Navy admiral to develop an action plan to 'turn the hospital around'. The inquiry team had found evidence of 'financial irregularities, drug abuse, pornography and poor quality of care' and 'a child being brought in to be groomed for paedophile purposes'. The inquiry chairman wrote that, 'We have no confidence in the ability of Ashworth Hospital to flourish under any management.' Dobson retorted that he though the ex admiral would 'bring to this task the leadership and management skills he demonstrated in the Royal Navy'. He made no mention of sinking ships. Instead, he stated that 'there is no practical alternative in the short term' – by which we can assume he meant affordable alternative (Department of Health, 1999b; *The Guardian*, 13.1.1999). In this case, there would be no public sympathy with the patients of Ashworth and, given that they were locked up, out of sight and not posing a danger to the public, they were clearly politically expedient.

The use of publicity and news in the media can often be used to pave the way for politicians to push through policies that might otherwise have been unpopular, or to put a populist aspect of the policy forward, or create a more favourable context for the policy to appear in. This is widely known as 'spin'. All parties have done it, even though 'spin' is a relatively new term, and the opposition parties' attacks on New Labour's success in using it in opposition, as well as during its first term in office, often appear to be driven more by jealousy than genuine moral outrage. However, New Labour's success backfired, becoming a story in itself and reaching its zenith when Jo Moore, special advisor to Stephen Byers, the government's then transport minister, was revealed to have emailed colleagues to suggest that there was a good opportunity to 'bury' unpopular government announcements. It was

11 September 2001, and her email was sent immediately after the terrorist attacks that sent passenger planes ploughing into the World Trade Centre in New York.

▶ Putting policy into practice

Policy that passes through the legislative process and onto the statute books to be enacted is then sent out to the appropriate NHS bodies (now including organisations in both the voluntary and private sectors), which are then expected to enact them. Although the NHS has been subjected to such frequent changes it is impossible to indicate how services will be organised for any length of time, the common model is one of a board structure, made up of a chairperson, chief executive and members who occupy both executive and non executive positions (see Figure 6.1 for the configuration adopted in 2000).

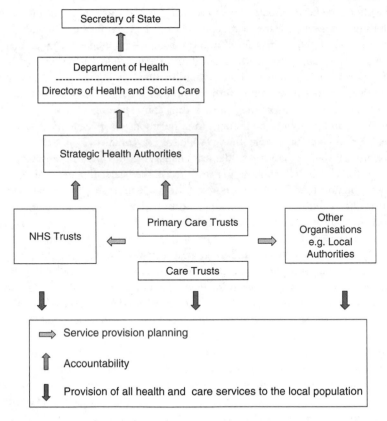

Figure 6.1 The new NHS in England (2000 model)

Source: Department of Health website: *www.doh.gov.uk/about/newnhs.htm*

There are no elected representatives on boards and the chain of command is even more tightly controlled with PCTs and the new strategic health authorities. Non-executive, or 'lay,' members have limited input into the trust but are expected to provide some degree of scrutiny on the work of the executives, who occupy managerial positions within the organisation. The board oversees all matters pertaining to the work of the organisation. Executive teams will have direct operational control of key areas, such as nursing and medical services, finance, planning and support services. The medical director will be an automatic member of the executive team; the nursing position might afford this level of seniority but could equally be a non-executive post.

One of Frank Dobson's earliest moves when he became Health Secretary was to 'purge ... Tory placemen on NHS [Trusts]', with hundreds of directors appointed under the old government being told they would not have their contracts renewed as they would not meet the new criteria he was introducing. Ostensibly, this was about ensuring non-executive directors lived locally to the trust and could demonstrate a commitment to the NHS. It still served its wider, political purpose (McSmith, 1997).

Directorates cover a specific clinical speciality, such as surgery, headed up by a directorate manager. In mental health and community trusts the directorates are more likely to be based on geographical localities, with specialist directorates, such as forensic psychiatry or children's services, running across the whole trust. However, it is the medical director who invariably 'manages' the medical staff throughout the organisation rather than any specific, non-medical, director or service managers.

Senior nursing staff within a trust these days will have a variety of titles. These might include ward sister or charge nurse, ward manager, team leader, nurse practitioner, senior practitioner, clinical or professional supervisor. These are, as can be seen, inconsistent and not that senior, given the hierarchy within the NHS. All will report to a general manager, who in turn will report to a more senior general manager, who will be likely then to be reporting to someone at board level. Nurses no longer have a direct managerial reporting mechanism through to board level, which means that, even if there is a nursing directorate within a trust, the nurses are not line managed through that but by operational managers. In some respects, it could be argued that this allows nurses to address nursing issues within their specific hierarchy without the conflict of interest that might arise were their line managers fellow nurses who also had to balance 'professional' development and financial issues. In practice, however, most nursing directorates have very few direct opportunities to address the day to day nursing concerns of the nursing staff and are occupied with much the same 'top down' agenda as other senior staff within the organisation.

The position of nurses within PCGs has already been discussed in Chapter 4, but it is worth noting that the culture, values and direction of the PCG or PCT board is largely shaped and influenced by the doctors, their experience, background and needs from the outset, while lack of time prevents nurse board members either canvassing colleagues' opinions or consulting with them.[5]

If the board of an NHS trust is its 'governing body', it is the senior managers operating inside the system who wield a particular type of power. It is they who will actually decide on how policy is implemented and begin the process of interpretation that will continue all the way to 'shop floor level'. Vast sums of public money can thus be committed to projects following decisions made either behind closed doors or when the real discussion, examination of options and sharing of information has taken place. For example, even with something as significant as purchasing decisions to be taken by local health authorities at the heart of the Tory Government's reforms, local consultation was 'more about communication of the inevitable to the public than about participatory purchasing, let alone higher level planning (Paton *et al.*, 1997: pp 24–7) Budget setting for ward sisters, charge nurses and team leaders rarely reflects the important role of the nurse, but usually involves little more than being given a pre-agreed financial framework that allows senior managers to demand that the nurse keeps the nursing team within the 'agreed' budget, whether or not that is actually within her and her colleagues' control.

Similarly, most hospitals or community teams would have regular meetings for senior nurses to discuss their service, developments and ongoing managerial issues. However, few would get sufficient information in advance of the meetings to enable them to make genuinely informed decisions. Moreover, often they are not setting their own agenda and would not usually be in a position to make any decisions that went outside a relatively small policy area; certainly not anything that would seriously affect the organisation of non-nursing services. In these circumstances, senior nurses from teams often end up relaying what is seen as important information from their own workplace to their managers but get little response as managerial time is taken up with its own 'top down' agenda, often already passed on by their own superiors in order for specific tasks or objectives to be delegated. When a team of nurses have expectations that their issues will be addressed,

---

[5] The lurch towards a 'primary care led NHS' was actually an unplanned consequence of the 1991 NHS reforms, which introduced GP fundholding and new initiatives involving community services. The emphasis towards primary care provision has then been continued by the Primary Care Act 1997, PCGs and PCTs. However, this has been in 'the absence of good quality evidence of the effectiveness and cost-effectiveness of shifts in the balance of provision towards the primary care sector (Robinson *et al.*, 1997: pp 26–9) Indeed, there was evidence that any gains made from this policy were only realised 'at significant cost', that they failed to address public health issues, the problem of inequality and access to services and failed to resolve the problem of weak primary care services in some deprived areas, while further fragmenting, weakening and dividing the 'NHS family' as a whole (McCullough and Ashburner, 1997: pp 22–3).

however, and their nurse in charge returns with yet more work or demands that are expected of them, the whole process can easily become discredited, and the participants disaffected.

▶ Case study 5: Politics in policy: devolution and nursing

Devolution has, perhaps represented New Labour's greatest reform, and is in stark contrast to many of its other policies, which have been deeply centralist. Not going as far as its nationalist critics would have wanted but far further than the Conservatives would ever have wanted (and, in Northern Ireland, the so called loyalist parties and paramilitaries), the government has established a Scottish Parliament and Assemblies in Wales and Northern Ireland, this latter as part of a delicate, lengthy and, at times, torturous peace process. Within the devolution programme, there have been clear differences: Members of the Scottish Parliament (MSPs) have far greater authority and decision making powers than Assembly members in either Wales or Northern Ireland, including the ability to raise taxes and enact primary legislation. In part, the decision about the level of local autonomy was determined by referenda carried out early after New Labour was elected, when the people of Scotland decided they wanted devolution in the face of a strong campaign by the Scottish Nationalist Party for full independence, strongly supported by a number of well known Scots such as the actor, Sean Connery. There were more overtly political concerns about Northern Ireland, which saw its Assembly suspended twice by the Westminster government due to internal disputes between the different political parties and problems within the peace process.

Early appraisal of the effects of devolution showed that Scotland was spending more on health and social services per capita than any other UK country, at £1,271, compared with a United Kingdom average of £1,072 and spending in England pegged at £1,041. The three devolved countries also had more available hospital beds than England. The private sector had made far less inroads into service provision in all three countries compared to England. Although some of the 'inherited policy factors' from the United Kingdom, such as the 'Barnett formula', used to determine funding in Scotland, Northern Ireland and Wales, were still clearly in place and dominant. However, some differences were quickly emerging in relation to style. Anna Daley from the Community Practitioners and Health Visitors Association (CPHVA) was confident that transparency in decision making had improved in Scotland, with the Scottish Executive committed to developing the role of the nurse, saying, 'I think some of the other countries are envious of our public health policy.' Dave Galligan, Unison's head of health in Wales, was one of the critics of the Welsh Assembly's lack of power, arguing that its role was limited, in some ways, to that of, 'Moving a pot of money around and ... having the appearance of a super county council.' It should have, he argued, been seeking greater powers although, like his Scottish counterparts, he was finding devolution brought with it greater democratic accountability and transparency. Despite policy changes in Northern Ireland, it was, according to RCN acting regional Maureen Scott, still 'lagging behind', with greater spending on health and social services than was the case in England not having sufficient impact. Nor was the apparent head start of having integrated health and social services, although devolution did offer access to a minister with direct responsibility for issues such as the downgrading of particular hospitals (Dinsdale, 2002: p 12).

While devolution signals different approaches to policy making – and, indeed, as it has taken root, differing policies altogether – nurses already had some experience of devolved bodies, not only in their own national health networks but also in the national boards that had been established in the 1980s alongside the UKCC. England and Wales had retained the closest relationship in policy making and structural terms, although there were still notable cultural differences. As such, devolution only emphasised those differences. The early implementation of *The NHS Plan* (2000) is a case in point. Perhaps summing up the views of a large number of nurses, midwives and health visitors in England, Beverley Clarke, an inner London health visitor stated it would be no more than 'words on the page' or 'simple ideology' unless recruitment and retention of staff were central to government policy. Pointing to the difficulties in delivering a public health agenda in England, Ms Clarke went on: '[Health visitors] used to be linked into nurseries and nursery schools, but now the resources aren't there. The community needs to be involved so we can develop services that would reduce inequalities in health and improve access to health.' Her view was that this led logically to decentralisation of decision making (Clarke *et al.*, 2001: pp 246–50). This was certainly something nurses in Scotland, Wales and Northern Ireland all felt they had going for them, as their host nations all fashioned their own versions of the policy. In that sense, devolution signalled, if not the death of the NHS then the birth of four semi-autonomous national health services, with the other three having an advantage over England in that decentralisation and greater ownership of the policy agenda could exist at local level within a firm national framework.

▶ Devolution: Scotland

As Scotland was seen to be leading the way in developing transparent decision making, so some practitioners viewed its public health commitment as having the edge over the rest of the United Kingdom, with the existing local health focus becoming even sharper. Contact with parliamentary representatives was greater than pre-devolution and the Scottish NHS Plan was seen by many as taking a major step forward to creating a new national health service that was finally divorced in its entirety from England. Unified health boards assumed responsibility from the existing NHS trusts and health boards. In a major change to health policy in England, staff could elect representatives onto these boards and take part in accountability reviews of boards' performance.

The devolved Scottish government, known as the Scottish Executive, assumed its powers on 1 July 1999, the same date the Wales Office came into being, with the powers of the old Welsh Office being handed over to the National Assembly for Wales. It was established as 'a policy system of incomplete responsibilities, focusing on the delivery of non-cash social services to individuals' (Parry, 2002). Scottish devolution was dealt a body blow with the tragic and untimely death of its principal architect and inaugural First Minister, Donald Dewar, a giant not just in his home country but on the British political scene as a whole. Undoubtedly, this affected Labour's confidence, especially as his successor, Henry McLeish, had to resign amid a financial scandal. And, in the Scottish National Party (SNP), Labour also had an effective opposition capable of making significant electoral gains and snapping at its heels, e.g., prepared to make capital of claims that ministers had presided over a decline in staffing levels, problems over infection control or 'a massive rise in hospital bureaucracy' (MacDonell, 2003). It was also ready to offer nurses in key specialities enhanced pay packages, SNP leader, John Swinney, saying the party would encourage Scottish hospitals to use their authority to pay higher rates and give them a competitive edge in the recruitment and retention of staff.

In part, some of the notable differences in policy since devolution had been the result of a changed voting system for devolved government, based on proportional representation rather than the 'first past the post' arrangement used in English local elections and the general election for the Westminster parliament. This produced an electoral coalition of Labour and the Liberal Democrats. For example, tuition fees for university students were abolished in a move led by the Liberal Democrats, opposed by the Labour majority but supported by the SNP. Similarly, Labour was forced to accept that the personal care for older people in long-term accommodation should be free.

As noted above, Scotland had a long tradition of independent action in health. Administration of the health service largely fits within this independent or devolved model. There continues to be an interface with Westminster in some areas, such as the ending of the mechanisms for the internal market (although, interestingly, while the principles of the market could be argued to have survived in England and Wales, having already arrived later in Scotland, it was also more clearly eradicated). The greatest change could still be to come. The political control of the Executive has some policy areas where it is in complete or partial alignment with government in Westminster. But a change of political majority, with the SNP breaking the Labour – Liberal consensus would almost certainly signal a period of direct opposition between Holyrood and Westminster (Parry, 2002: pp 315–24).

Its independent tradition had, in fact, protected the health service in Scotland from some of the effects of the internal market for a number of years. With a much smaller population than that even of London, its decision makers will have grown up together. A stronger sense of shared identity between ministers within the new Executive, MSPs, civil servants, trade union officials and, in some cases, NHS managers, provides an opportunity for a more cohesive vision of how politics can shape the policy agenda and a consensus approach to service delivery, as shall be seen below.[6]

As the *Scottish NHS Plan* (2000) noted, 'Scotland's health, compared to that of other European nations, is poor and our life expectancy is shorter ... For too long, health policy and health services have focused on the treatment of ill health rather than on its prevention. We are now working to shift that emphasis' (p 13). Part of that was to be an ambitious target of securing greater public and patient participation than was ever envisaged in England, with an implicit recognition that patient need would be the most important factor in developing services. While the English plan created the scope for even greater involvement from the private sector, the Scots decided to use revenue raised from the tobacco tax for the Health Improvement fund. A range of initiatives were used to deliver on this expectation, including working in partnership with staff. With staff shortages nowhere near as acute as in England, the news that 10,000 more students than originally planned were due to qualify in the period leading up to 2005 was a major boost while 120 specialist nurse posts were funded to help manage winter pressures (p 82). However, NHS Scotland has a shared legacy with its English counterpart, facing the retirement of 14,000 nurses between 2002 and 2012. With much of its increased investment being directed at staffing costs, Malcolm Chisolm, health minister declared this was 'central to investing in reform', in contrast to his English counterpart. Chisolm was able to put this in the context of a 1.5 per cent increase in nurses and midwives in the year ending September 2001 while announcing a £1.75 million boost to skills training for nurses, while the RCN were able to state that the Scottish Executive had met almost all the action points the College set in its Value Nurses campaign, including bursary increases, free return to practice courses and time off for post registration training. Reform was progressed in primary care, fuelled by significant shifts in resource (Making the Connections, 2002: *www.scotland.gov.uk*).

Yet there is still room for criticism. Audit Scotland released a report revealing 'up to 40 per cent of wards were staffed below recommended levels, with 'two trusts singled out as having "Dickensian" practice for failing to provide any cover for nurses on holiday or sick leave' (O'Dowd, 2002a: p 4). Partly as a result of trying to meet shortfalls in staffing, agency costs for NHS Scotland rose sharply, as they did

---

[6] The strength of the Scottish national identity has even been demonstrated to reduce the number of emergency psychiatric presentations to hospital during and after successive World Cup football competitions! (Masterton and Mander, 1990: pp 475–8).

elsewhere in the United Kingdom, increasing from £19 million in 2000–01 to £24.5 million in 2001–02. The creation of new posts was a contributory factor, as well as actual vacancies and the Scottish health service was on track to begin a recruitment drive of overseas nurses in a bid to find a temporary solution to its staffing problems, alongside a £5million recruitment drive. The Executive's declared aim of making inroads in the battle against health inequalities and to establish a serious public health agenda was helped by the introduction of free personal and nursing care, which was actually introduced in July 2002. It could also point to minimal success with its waiting lists but significant problems remained.

Caring for Scotland: the strategy for nursing and midwifery in Scotland (NHS Scotland, 2002), recognised the importance of the role of nurses and midwives in improving health and delivering health services, looking at a wide range of initiatives, from introducing effective support and supervision for newly qualified nurses and support workers to linking leadership with broader education and training programmes. The language and targets are similar to policy documents in the same vein issued from the Department of Health. A range of other policies are referred to emphasising the Executive's 'joined up thinking' and recognition of other areas of social and economic policy on health. Yet there is a significant difference i.e. part cultural, part ideological, part political. Leading figures like First Minister, Jack McConnell and Bill Speirs, General Secretary of the Scottish Trades Union Congress (STUC), 'grew up' politically with many of those now involved in making key decisions affecting domestic policy, including health. There is, to a large degree, a shared understanding of the issues and a different type of approach, partly forged not only out of long opposition to the Tories in Scotland (when the Conservatives had barely any parliamentary seats north of the border but absolute power due to their majority in Westminster), but also a more positive image of how their country could be shaped for the future. Bill Speirs and his small group of staff at the STUC attended approximately fifty ministerial meetings in the first year of the Scottish parliament – more than double the amount the STUC were invited to in eighteen years of Tory government. Indeed, the problem for the highly regarded Speirs and his team now is actually keeping up with the vast number of committees and official bodies in which they are expected to participate (Hassan and Warhurst, 2002).

These relationships also translate into action. One Hundred and Four community psychiatric nurses working for Lanarkshire Primary Care NHS Trust, engaged in a difficult three-year battle to get themselves upgraded from 'E' to 'G' grade. However, Unison officials involved in supporting the claim went on to suggest that up to 20 per cent of nurses throughout the United Kingdom could be under-graded. Bridget Hunter, Unison Scotland's lead officer for nursing and Jim Devine, its head of health, developed a resource pack to help nurses with similar grading claims and were 'flooded with enquiries from all over the UK'. Almost immediately, Scottish health minister, Malcolm Chisolm, committed the government to considering a wholesale review of nurses' grades (O'Dowd, 2002b: p 5).

With Unison members taking on a number of trusts and private contractors in the NHS in battles over low pay, Jim Devine was able to negotiate above average deals for admin and clerical workers and an astonishing 16 per cent extra for 14,500 ancillary staff, whose hourly rate would rise from £4.62 to more than £5.00. 'A' grade nurses were to see the bottom three points of their salary scale removed, increasing their salary as a consequence. Yet, while Devine could praise his own members and view this as 'the beginning of the end of the scandal of low pay in the NHS', he was able to acknowledge that 'the Scottish Executive and, in particular, the health minister Malcolm Chisolm ... worked with us to do something about it' (Unison News, 20.1.03: *www.unison.org*). In fact, insiders within the Scottish political scene were surprised to find officials from both Unison's London head office and the Department of Health attempting to exert pressure to have this latter deal at least delayed for fear it might undermine *Agenda for Change*, which was not going to deliver anything so lucrative. Such was the power of devolution. Indeed, given the views of some Unison national officials about how the health group in Scotland can conduct its affairs and arguments that have come from some of the RCN's regional offices (*sic*) about the College not paying sufficient regard to the devolved nations, it may well be that the unions have at least as much trouble – if not more – than the Westminster government coming to terms with devolution.

▶ Devolution: Wales

Before the Welsh Assembly, there were those who complained of a planning vacuum in the principality. Having had to overcome the not insignificant problems of massive debt – the NHS in Wales had an accumulated deficit of £25 million for 1997–98 – the Assembly had its work cut out in shaping a clear identity for the Welsh NHS (Clarke *et al.*, 2001). Although policy decisions for the NHS were always regarded as taking effect for England and Wales, these were transmitted via the Welsh Office, with the Secretary of State for Wales having responsibility to the parliament in Westminster for health, as well as other functions. Despite this, health policy had not greatly diverged from England, although health spending accounted for 34 per cent or £2.7 billion in 1999–2000, about 13 per cent more per capita than England. The projected budget for 2003–2004 was £3.8 billion. The elections for the new National Assembly for Wales threw up the same problem for the Labour Party as had occurred in Scotland, in that it did not gain a clear majority but was forced into a coalition with the Liberal Democrats. Again, as has happened in Scotland, the Minister and Committee for Health and Social Services have enacted changes from English policy. In health, this has resulted in an extension of free eye tests and free prescriptions and a greater emphasis on collaborative working between health, local government and the voluntary sector.

The Welsh Assembly Government is now responsible for policy direction and for allocating funds to the NHS in Wales. It started life with five regional health authorities but then planned to abolish them as 'an unnecessary bureaucratic tier' in its NHS Plan Wales (2001), given its new local health groups. In a break with English funding plans, The Assembly provided £420,000 to fund eleven nurse consultant posts, rather than leave trusts to find the money from existing budgets. The Welsh version of the NHS Plan, *Improving Health in Wales* (Minister for Health and Social Services, 2001), 'lacks the stringent targets of its English counterpart' but does give 'organisational form to a primary care led NHS', even if the hospital is currently very much the centre of Welsh healthcare policy (McLelland, 2002). Wales is also developing a very different agenda for mental health, not adopting the English National Service Framework for Mental Health but developing what is actually a more comprehensive strategy. It is also sticking with a locality model for community mental health teams rather than the fragmented, specialist model England has moved towards. Although the new Mental Health Act, if it passes through the Westminster parliament, will apply to Wales, Jane Hutt and Welsh clinicians made it clear very early after the draft bill's publications that it was at odds with the country's approach towards mental healthcare. As is the case with Scotland, the political networks and relationships between policy makers and clinicians are far closer than in England, allowing for swifter decision making and easier agreement in key policy areas.

Nurses face similar issues in Wales and, despite having a more devolved form of government, often hear familiar ministerial refrains. This was true when it came to pay and conditions, as well as clinical and educational development, although Wales' largely rural communities meant there was less opportunity to establish large teaching hospitals than would be the case in England and the Welsh Assembly's national strategy for nursing was aptly titled, *Realising the Potential* (The National Assembly for Wales, 2000). With a view that nursing in the country was 'backward and isolated', recruitment drives were necessary both in Wales itself and London. Arguably, the decision not to develop the role of the nurse in primary care within the NHS Plan Wales was something of an own goal in this context but *Creating the Potential* (The National Assembly for Wales, 2001) was then hailed as the first strategy for education for nursing, midwifery and health visiting, combining a strong clinical component with administrative, research, negotiating and planning skills. The national vacancy rate was only 5 per cent in late 2002 and, although staffing establishments were historically set at a relatively low level the Welsh health minister, Jane Hutt, announced the Executive's intention to recruit an additional 16 per cent, or 6,000, nurses by 2010, with an emphasis on enticing nurses to return to the service, in the process placating the RCN's earlier criticism of a lack of targets for nursing numbers. Nonetheless, it was not clear exactly how this might be achieved and the promise was dismissed at the time by Unison's head of health, Dave Galligan. For the problem of retaining experienced nurses was another of the key challenges facing Welsh nursing which, again, came back to its funding problems as much as any perception about its nursing practice being 'backward,' misplaced or not. While some academics had argued that Wales should actually plan to be an 'exporter' of nurses i.e. training more students than are needed for the country, the RCN estimated that establishments are so low that an additional 2000 nurses were needed (Lipley, 2000: pp 20–1).

However, declaring that devolution is a process rather than an event, Assembly members supported health minister, Jane Hutt's, determination to make the NHS a 'family friendly, flexible employer' emphasising partnership working, particularly with social services. With staff representatives to take their place on NHS boards, the Welsh were following in Scottish footsteps while another significant difference from the English NHS Plan was the Welsh decision to retain Community Health Councils.

▶ Devolution: Northern Ireland

Devolved decision making was already established in Northern Ireland by 2001, with its assembly having been adjudged by local health workers to have been 'a very positive move', offering the opportunity to lobby its members and feed into the political process in a way previously impossible. With a cross party health committee whose meetings are open to the public, the opportunity for a dialogue about health and nursing matters is inevitably far more likely than was ever the case when politics was run from Westminster. Thus the assembly was developing its own version of the NHS Plan with attempts to 'move away from the medical model'.

One key area of difference for Northern Ireland is its history of sectarian violence, which permeates its healthcare system as it does every other aspect of life in the province. Even long after the ceasefire, with the Northern Ireland Assembly established, nurses and other health workers were facing death threats by both breakaway Loyalist and Republican paramilitaries (Munro, 2002a: p 8). Supporting staff enduring such difficulties is one of the things that unites Unison and the RCN, but it is a problem that can and does spill over into the workplace to affect relationships between staff themselves (Davis, 2002: p 14). This has been a backdrop to the public life of Northern Ireland for more than three decades now. Painfully slow progress has been made in bringing the communities together and inching towards a political settlement, but less progress has been made in incorporating the six counties into the kind of modernisation process that has characterised the rest of the UK's healthcare system, with the RCN alleging that Northern Ireland has the worst record in the United Kingdom for promoting the career development of nurses. *Developing Better Services* (Department of Health, Social Services and Public Safety, 2002) was issued by the Northern Ireland Executive, but its main focus was organisational and managerial structures and change. Northern Ireland is also the only part of the UK that will not have its own equivalent of NHS Direct, which have been established in both Wales and Scotland following the original success in

England. The development of nurses and nursing is not an issue that Unison has directly addressed but the RCN have responded to *Developing Better Services* (op. cit., 2002) with a manifesto for nursing in Northern Ireland, *Commitment to Care* (*www.rcn.org.uk*, 2002). The College's argument was that meaningful reform could not take place without gaining the support of, and fully involving, nurses, midwives and community practitioners. The Department in Northern Ireland had failed to realise nursing's potential and continued to marginalize them.

The Acute Hospitals Review was published in 2001, setting out a vision for the next fifteen years, with 'ambitious targets for implementation'. It was acknowledged by the minister for health, social services and public safety, Bairbre de Brun, as having taken place 'against a background of many years of under-funding of health services, which has undermined and weakened their capacity to deliver the quality of service demanded of a modern hospital system' (DHSSPS, 2002). Recommending that the existing four health and social services boards and nineteen trusts be replaced by a single strategic authority and three health and social care systems, it received a very mixed response. While much of the review was, implicit within its title, concerned with what was, essentially, a re-organisation of hospital services, there were some workforce issues addressed, such as a planned increase in nursing staff of 20 per cent or 2300 nurses, along with the usual nods to family friendly and flexible employment practices while, as with other UK countries, there is a surplus of applicants for every training place. There were also plans to increase and develop the number of midwife-led services and clinics. Important in the context of future relationships with Irish health services, working in collaboration with the Republic of Ireland was regarded as essential, building on existing cross border interchange, with patients to be offered access to treatment at the most convenient location, irrespective of whether it is in the North or South (Bradley, 2002: pp 6–10).

Dissolutions of the Northern Ireland Assembly inevitably delayed any attempts at reform or, indeed, policy making generally, much to the annoyance of many local nurses and the RCN. Despite opportunities to exploit the local policy interface, many nursing critics saw Northern Ireland as lagging 'at least two years behind Great Britain', in key areas such as establishing primary care groups, nurse prescribing and 'nurses' involvement in planning their own areas and organising how their resources should be spent', as well as career progression (Duffin, 2000: p 12). Moreover, as the process of change progressed, there was a unified protest from the RCN, RCM and BMA, who viewed the introduction of the fifteen Local Health and Social Care Groups as 'perverse', introducing 'unnecessary bureaucracy, undermining patient care, threatening nurse led clinics and threatening jobs'. The RCN complained that, far from local networks delivering on policy, 'It is evident what we put forward has been ignored' (Munro, 2002b: p 8).

It is in the very nature of devolution that it will both take on aspects of the previous political relationships in each of the devolved countries while progress will differ sharply. This is as true for nursing as it is for anything else. It does, however, tell us much about the nature of decision making and undermines that notion that politicians so often use to justify their policy making: that there is no alternative. We are now witnessing four alternative approaches to the NHS specifically and healthcare systems in general. Although much of the remainder of this book will focus on the English model, where the opportunity exists, contrasts with other models will be made.

Given the very recent nature of devolution, it would be neither helpful nor wise to assess each country's policies in relation to health and nursing a success or failure. It is sufficient to note that a great experiment has begun and the challenges it faces and opportunities it throws up may have just as great an effect on nurses in England as in Scotland, Wales or Northern Ireland.

▶ Are nurses part of the problem or part of the solution?

Long term gain has often been sacrificed to quick profit in the British economy, with the market and City financiers who make it work having absolute rights, while British workers have amongst the weakest rights of any industrialised country. Yet, 'the good society recognises interdependencies of claims and responsibilities, which is at heart the role of the welfare state' (Hutton, 1996: pp 1–2). This principle can be translated into almost every area of working life, particularly in the health service. Introducing a market economy, with its competitive rather than collaborative culture, exacerbated the already weak position of staff and increased the power of its decision makers.

Democracy is, in fact, in very short supply in the NHS. Its only elected representatives at any level are in trade unions, none of whom have direct responsibility for decision making. 'Democratic' practice rarely finds its way into decision making at lower levels either. Faced with directives about national policy, trust managers have little apparent choice about whether or not they are going to implement them.[7] More, it is a case of how, when and who will do the work.

Even when there is room for discretion, the process for involving nurses often seems to be unclear and/or inconsistent, whether it be to introduce change across the nursing workforce or simply for a single team. Inevitably, there cannot be one process for all decision making; nor would it be right to imagine that the health

---

[7] The question of discretion and how policy is translated into practice is an interesting one, which will be discussed in more detail later in this chapter. Suffice to say, at this point, that even when instructions are apparently clear, organisations and individuals within them can, on occasions, find room to manoeuvre, interpret and find some degree of discretion – especially when strongly motivated to do so.

service can function as a collective or with all staff being involved in agreeing every decision.

Yet, Hutton's point is easily recognised. Members of the Scottish Parliament's health committee 'attacked NHS organisation's for operating a "culture of secrecy and fear," criticising health boards for their lack of consultation over proposed changes, inculcating a "culture of fear among staff, who were afraid to speak out over issues such as bad practice" ' (Wright, 2000: p 10). According to the government, 'The biggest consultation of front line staff in NHS history' took place in May 2000. It was seeking the views of clinicians and members of the public alike in preparation for the NHS Plan. However, only five weeks was allowed to digest the views of a nation. This would allow hardly enough time for an army of civil servants to read all the written responses or reports from focus groups, let alone collate the information and prepare meaningful summaries for the politicians. Even were that to have been achieved, no time would have been left at all for those politicians to consider at any length counter proposals, new ideas, clarify issues or conclude the debate.

At a more local level, the matter of what constitutes consultation, when it is applicable and how it should be managed seems to cause endless confusion within the health service. Often, managers – even those at a very senior level – seem to think that giving their staff information about change before implementing it constitutes consultation. In some cases, proposals are circulated with a deadline for returning comments so close to the implementation date that, as with the NHS Plan, it is pretty obvious that, whatever the validity of those comments, nothing will change. Consultation is also now conducted on email. Indeed, a number of trusts now use the electronic media to circulate more information but have not taken steps to ensure that it is available to those who do not have ready access to it, which includes vast numbers of nurses, busy in their own clinical areas. In the words of Lord McCarthy's report, *Making Whitley Work*, quoted in Section 39 of the General Council's Conditions of Service (HMSO, 1984), 'It should be noted that the mere passage of information is not consultation. Consultation *involves an opportunity to influence decisions and their application*' [my emphasis].

What needs to be *negotiated* with nurses because it constitutes contractual change seems equally unclear. In part, a significantly reduced trade union presence within the workplace and subsequent lack of scrutiny of such principles contribute to this. The increasing pressure on managers to deliver change within shorter and shorter timescales – often with funding dependent on achieving impossibly tight deadlines – is another obvious factor. Inviting bids, in a very short space of time, for monies to implement centralised policy is another example of the way the New Labour government has adopted, and then built upon, the methods of its predecessor. However, it clearly contradicts the government's often stated intention to ensure that trusts involve their staff in the running and development of their own services far more than in the recent past. This is reflected in the summer 2000 edition of *National Health News*, whose headline boldly proclaims, 'Staff are "cornerstone" of radical plans for NHS', promising ten key roles for nurses as defined by the Chief Nursing Officer, a larger workforce, better training, improved conditions and fairer pay. The catch is that rewards are attached to a 'traffic light' system that means that 'extra investment and resources need to be matched by reform', with money going to trusts that achieve government targets (NHS News, 2000). Thus success – and subsequent reward for achievement – is regarded as integral to the implementation of policies that no one locally has had anything to do with developing or even having limited input into. In fact, this has created problems that only the most Machiavellian centralist could ever have forseen. More than £700 million allocated to the NHS was not spent in the financial year 2000–01 – enough to have built ten hospitals – because managers could not initiate the correct bids within the given timescales. A growing level of 'initiative paralysis' was blamed for 'keeping back reforms' (Ahmed and Hinsliff, 2001: p 2). In fact, while money was being made available for specialist or new services, managers were still expected to undertake all the work needed to meet the targets of 'cost improvement programmes' or cuts. Equally, the strings attached to the reforms were holding them back from getting the money they needed for the most basic services they were supposed to be managing. That £700 million could also have made an imaginative and significant contribution to recruitment and retention was not even on the agenda.

Government recognises staff must implement change but doesn't want them involved in shaping what that change will be. It certainly doesn't correspond with Christine Hancock's comment that 'Nurses are the "sleeping giant" of the NHS' and integral to both change and shaping the future of the NHS. At the same conference, celebrating fifty years of the NHS, then health secretary, Frank Dobson, 'told a full house of managers about the huge potential of nurses, *who should be seen as part of the solution and not the problem with the NHS*' [my emphasis] (O'Dowd, 1998b). In some respects, this seems to be an extraordinary comment for a health secretary to have to make, but it merely reflects the hidden reality that is virtually unchanged from the contempt and disdain shown by ministry officials and hospital committee members a half century earlier. It also highlights the scale of the problem from two ends: the apparent lack of insight displayed by nursing leaders coupled with the vain hope that, somehow, through the efforts of others or a kind of historical inevitability, a 're-awakening' of the 'sleeping giant' that is the body of nurses will occur and change will come; the other is that, if managers really do view nurses as 'the problem', it is no wonder that they should seek to exclude them from decision making and influencing the process of change.

▶ Issue networks or iron triangles? A policy framework and nurses' place in it

In fact, the more formal aspects of the policy making process has loosened up under New Labour, who tend to use more pluralistic mechanisms such as issues networks, involving interested parties on specific projects or policy issues, forming and reforming, dependent on the issue, with different participants. This works around the more rigid policy 'iron triangle' enshrined within the NHS in 1948, made up of key members of the medical profession, departmental officials and politicians. This iron triangle, as described by Hayward and Hunter (1982: pp 152–4), had as its framework a pattern of stable, predictable and relatively closed, private relationships. In part, this was disrupted by the Tories' move away from the largely rational model of policy making that had accompanied the broad consensus surrounding the NHS and conflict avoidance believed important to maintain stable personal relationships within the triangle (p 147) to the political model that they judged to be necessary to achieve more radical change. Yet it has undoubtedly survived, at least in part due to the medical profession's fierce syndicalist approach to trade unionism which makes it so difficult to introduce change to which they are opposed. Hogwood and Gunn (1984) put forward a strong argument that managers have forged a way through into this policy framework. If anything, this makes it even more difficult for nurses to find their own way through to the centre. In this context, nurses can – and do – play an important role in issues networks but remain excluded from 'core' policy issues that shape healthcare in the United Kingdom. This is despite the work of some excellent and committed civil servants who have established solid networks and imaginative ways of working, even in the face of the relentless political demand for new policies and their implementation – while Chris Ham (1992: pp 107–10) notes that they are still adept at both initiating and re-shaping policy when they perceive the need or decide it is in their best interests. Ham also highlights the use of 'non decision making' or the exclusion of key issues from the policy agenda as a means of consolidating the status quo and those who derive power from it (see 'below').

▷ A taxing problem: how can we afford to put more money into the NHS?

Another major problem for contemporary nurses is that their work is fashioned by a government that has adopted aspects of the old Conservative ideology towards the public services, economy and management of the health service, yet has a desire to push forward a programme of change at both a micro- and macro-level as significant as anything in the lifetime of the NHS. Change has been the only constant in the experience of NHS staff. The pressure to move onto the next target or objective, at times, can be relentless. Yet if this occurs in a service where there are severe financial restraints, there is not only the pressure of the new but also the problems accompanying the loss of services for which there is no longer any funding. Of course, controlling the purse strings is the ultimate means of dictating what happens, how and when it is done and by whom.

New Labour not only adopted the Tories spending plans before coming to power but their attitude to the overall means of funding the NHS, with rises in direct taxation ruled out. As early as 1996, political commentators were warning that 'Labour could be left with no choice but to raise taxes' if they were to fund their long term plans for the NHS (Wintour, 1996).

Two months into New Labour's first term, many of the unions were urging Gordon Brown, the new chancellor, to earmark extra cash for the NHS. The RCN argued that, by sticking to his predecessor's spending plans, Brown was making cuts while Roger Kline of the CPHVA warned of a crisis unless 'at least 2 per cent more in real terms' was added 'just to stand still'. Only Unison offered the chancellor unreserved support (Gulland and Porter, 1997).

By July 1998, even Unison's support was wearing thin as Brown announced to the House of Commons that the pay review bodies (PRB) would no longer be able to base their recommendations solely on the recruitment and retention needs of each profession but must base them on affordability as well as the government's inflation target (then 2.5 per cent). Concern was highlighted by the fact that public sector pay had fallen by a further 16 per cent since the last big, across the board increase for nurses in 1982. Even the Institute of Health Services Managers was worried that taking too restrictive an attitude towards pay might backfire when there was such a critical shortage of nurses and doctors.

Brown's third budget garnered more admiring headlines and health was again signalled as a winner. However, many pointed out that, given the huge budget surplus he had at his disposal, far more could and should have been put into public service spending and he was, indeed, 'projecting a cut in public spending' (Wintour, 1999). And despite the apparent windfalls blowing into the NHS garden, some were quick to say that the picture was not all one of blooming roses. London Health Emergency pointed out that:

> Trusts across the country will be stuck with a bill totalling at least £115m, on top of their requirement to make 3% 'efficiency savings' each year.
>
> The nursing pay increase averages out at 5.8% for 417,000 [nurses] covered by the PRB, costing the NHS an extra £380m a year. But NHS budgets had set aside only 2.5% for pay increases – equivalent to £165m. Even with the additional £100m Frank Dobson has taken from the so-called 'modernisation fund' to help cover the cost of the pay increases for this year, Trusts will have a total of just £265m towards the £380m required. This takes no account of the 10% increase in London weighting payments which was announced alongside the pay increases and which will add a further headache to Trust bosses in the capital (London Health Emergency, 1999).

Earlier in 1999, however, the government had broken with its pattern of spin and determination to make 'good news' announcements about the health service.

'Labour admits NHS in crisis' declared the headline on page one of *The Guardian*. In fact, it was a crisis brought about by the shortage of nurses that was hindering hospitals' ability to cope with the influx of patients in the midst of a 'flu epidemic'. The issue then became one of which government was to blame – New Labour or the Conservatives, when they were in power prior to May 1997. *It also highlighted the issue of nurses' pay as a key factor in recruitment and retention* [my emphasis] (Brindle, 1999). It seemed that New Labour's love of 'joined up thinking' didn't extend to the matter of nurses' pay.

Public support for Labour's handling of the health steadily bled away in its first two years, but during the winter of 1999–2000 became a critical haemorrhage. Although Brown had a £12 billion budget surplus – one of the biggest in history – spending was constrained by the need not to upset the City (*The Guardian*, 15.3.2000).

Whether or not the government increased spending or increased funding for public services and social policy was not the issue. As far as they were concerned, until the late winter of 2001, the issue of increasing direct taxation was a closed book. This was despite the rational case put forward for it and the mounting evidence that, despite the big increases the chancellor was able to make within his 'self imposed constraints', it was the only way government ambitions, public expectation and nurses' concerns about service delivery were ever going to be met financially.[8]

This is not just an academic point. The use of power to control the political agenda and create a particular climate has to be understood. If the funding remains insufficient, the focus inevitably falls on how it is spent. On the one hand, those who spend it are vulnerable to criticism; on the other, rationing healthcare or alternative means of funding move up the agenda. Chris Ham, a health academic and professor of health policy and management at Birmingham University, argued that, 'Rationing has always been a feature of the service, but the NHS reforms [of 1991] brought it into the open.' Of five options put forward by Ham to resolve the NHS's funding problems, four considered forms of rationing, increasing charges for NHS treatment or greater involvement from the private sector. Only one mentioned the possibility of adjusting existing current spending priorities or increasing taxation but ruled these out as 'the political debate [is focused] on how public spending can be contained and taxes cut' (Ham, 1996).

New Labour has continually set about limiting the parameters of debate, both on the future and funding of the NHS, increasingly referencing it to the private sector. Indeed, in the midst of the 2001 election campaign, Tony Blair signalled another

---

[8] It wasn't until late 2002, with the country facing a war against Iraq and close to recession, that the prime minister and chancellor could advance a coherent agenda supporting the need for increasing public borrowing and tax increases.

policy change as he announced, with no advance indications, that his government would be looking to the private sector to become involved in managing and providing 'non clinical' services within the NHS. What did this mean? Both during and after the election widespread public concern as well as anger from nurses, doctors and other health workers was expressed. This was shared by the trade unions. In a show of outright opposition to the government almost unprecedented up to that point, they demanded – and got – a meeting with the prime minister. What gave the impression that Blair's view was more ideological than pragmatic was that ministers and government spokespeople all supported his assertion that the private sector had a role to play in providing healthcare – but were at a loss to explain how, in any shape or form.

The issue was due to come to a head at that year's Trade Union Congress (TUC) Conference but was not debated as the world reeled at the September 11 terrorist attacks, which occurred on the day Blair was to have explained his position in his traditional speech to the Congress.

Few, however, can have been prepared for the announcement four months later from Health Secretary and arch-Blairite, Alan Milburn, that it was time for the NHS to be 're-defined'. Milburn said he was using this groundbreaking speech to defend it from its 'enemies'. The NHS, he argued, should be 'decentralised with a plurality of providers operating within a framework of clear national standards regulated independently'. He dismissed any expansion of private health insurance as costing the NHS more money than it would save, equally scorning the Conservative favoured option of patients paying to see their GP, as well as European insurance-based systems, claiming European governments were shying away from them due to the scale of the funding burden placed on employers and employees. Yet the Health Secretary said the NHS, 'Still has the feel of the 1940s – both for those working for it and those using it. Queuing is endemic. Staff are run off their feet. Patients are disempowered, with little if any choice. The whole thing is monolithic and bureaucratic. Having been part of a government responsible for the state of the NHS for nearly five years, he went on to say, 'It is run like an old style nationalised industry controlled from Whitehall.'

But the health secretary saw an answer in 'recent research on high performing private sector organisations.'[9]

'Hospitals, whether they are public or private, will get more money for being able to treat more patients more quickly and to higher standards. Who provides the service

---

[9] The Secretary of State didn't elaborate on what he meant by this. However, evidence from mental health services supports the counter-argument that private services are very costly and fail to deliver high standards of service. London's private psychiatric hospitals were charging exorbitant rates to the NHS – between £250 and £345 per patient per day in 1998, with between £85 and £345 just to admit someone. Feedback from patients and NHS clinicians was that very little was done for patients by way of

becomes less important than the service that is provided. NHS healthcare does not need to be delivered exclusively by line-managed NHS organisations but by a range of organisations working within the national framework of standards and inspection. The task of managing the NHS becomes one of overseeing a system not an organisation. Responsibility for day to day management can be devolved to local services.

Within this new definition of the NHS, the franchise could go not just to another public sector health organisation but in time to a not-for-profit body such as a university or a charity or to some other external management team. As franchising progresses it is possible to imagine a number of local health organisations all being run by a single team of successful public service entrepreneurs. It is the management that will be franchised. This is not privatisation in any way, shape or form ... Some will see this as a very controversial step. I think it flows from the devolution agenda of the NHS Plan (Milburn, 2002).

Milburn had taken the view that this was the only way in which innovators and clinical leaders could get the opportunity to put into practice their ideas but could offer no real evidence for this assertion, nor any that these new reforms would be at all successful. Indeed, though he had dismissed the internal market, there were remarkable similarities between his reforms and those of the Conservatives twelve years earlier in that both had sought to get money flowing with the patient and create independent, self-governing trusts within an NHS framework. With this announcement, Milburn had simply gone much further than the Conservatives would have dared, by allowing the private sector to get access to NHS funding and its managers to take over NHS hospitals. To suggest this overtly ideological shift in an apparently non-ideological way was inherently misleading. In failing to differentiate between the importance of franchising healthcare from who might run a McDonald's outlet, the health secretary beggared belief.

Suggesting this would not create a market economy in health was highly disingenuous on Milburn's part. Given that there is a fixed sum of funding for the NHS, if one hospital or trust gets a larger slice of the cake, another inevitably gets less. Inevitably, many critics saw this as the end of the NHS and the final triumph of the

---

contd.

treatment and even less when it came to nursing care. The bill for having insufficient mental health provision in London and our major cities was running to millions of pounds in the 1990s, money that was pouring out of the NHS, at the cost of opportunities for the development of staff and services. It was also draining the NHS of experienced staff, most of whom had been trained at great cost by the health service. Nor did Milburn indicate where managers experienced in running multi-million pound, highly complex organisations would be found. Given some of the spectacular failures of private sector ventures such as Railtrack and Enron, the disgraced US owned multinational, perhaps he was hoping for some cut price recruits.

private sector Bevan had thought banished, along with hospital flag days, in 1948.[10]

Intriguingly, Milburn's earliest and most informed critic was his predecessor as health secretary, Frank Dobson, who delivered a withering attack from the back-benches. Citing 'recent private sector disasters', Dobson noted that few managers from the private sector had the required experience and questioned the wisdom of abandoning the public sector ethos just as increased funding might have an effect.

▶ A model for understanding power

Politicians exert power. As do doctors, as well as civil servants and managers. But so do nurses. Power is rarely a word used in a neutral way. The exercise of power might be described as 'corrupt', 'sexy', 'abusive', 'decisive', 'wrong' but rarely 'right'. But, while there is opportunity to use it, that is what the powerful will do.

We have already seen that controlling the way consultation is carried out is an exercise in power. For example, in his speech to the New Health Network, Alan Milburn was able to say that, as a result of the consultation exercise carried out in May 2000, the public and clinicians alike supported the NHS Plan even though it's unlikely any of the comments made through the exercise ever influenced the final document. The health secretary certainly didn't see the need to produce evidence for his claims. Equally, holding meetings called with little notice or making it difficult for people to attend, not giving people advance information about key issues on the agenda, setting the parameters for discussion, are all an exercise in power.

But what exactly is this thing called power? The Oxford English Dictionary defines it as, 'The ability to do or act; vigour, energy; particular faculty of body or mind; Government, influence, authority (over); political ascendancy'. To what end, however, is not defined. Does this exercise of power at a national, even at ward level, actually matter? Changing massive organisations is, after all, a near impossible task. Even Tony Blair admitted this when talking about 'the scars on his back' from his attempts to change the public services.

Within an NHS trust or PCT, it is clear that boards, chief executives and their managerial teams on occasions struggle to successfully implement change as they want it to be implemented. For even the relatively powerless have one key element of power at their disposal – the power to do nothing.

It is not, then, a straightforward issue and needs further examination if we are to understand its role in decision making. There are many models of power, some

---

[10] Indeed, Blair and Milburn were only prevented from allowing the new Foundation Hospitals to borrow money on the market – which would have taken them irrevocably into the private sector, and outside Treasury control – by a rearguard action from Gordon Brown, in a momentous behind the scenes row that, at one point, threatened to split the government (Freedland, 2002).

relatively well established – although no less contested for that – with postmodern approaches entering the debate and disagreeing with almost every model that has gone before, arguing that there is no single way of examining a phenomenon, so there cannot be any single truth or reality, but that all things exist in a state of relativism (Wilkinson and Miers, 1999). While it is important for nurses to explore their situation from a number of perspectives, moving forward the narrative of this book, one model will be used here to allow an in-depth examination of the issues as they affect nursing. This is a 'three dimensional model' put forward by the sociologist, Steven Lukes. He looked at pre existing models of power and concluded that these were too preoccupied with the more visible dimensions of power relations, as exhibited by individuals behaviour in decision making on issues, actual or potential, over which there is an observable conflict. Taking the view that there were less overt, or visible factors to be considered, he developed what he called a three dimensional view, arguing 'that men's (*sic*) wants may themselves be a product of a system which works against their interests and, in such cases, relates the latter to what they would want and prefer were they able to make the choice' (Lukes, 1974: p 34).

Lukes defined the concept of power by saying that A exercise power over B when A affects B in a manner contrary to B's interests. In this, it extends far beyond actual and observable conflict. A may exercise power over B by getting her to do what she does not particularly want to do, but also exercises power over her by 'influencing, shaping or determining her very wants', or the very things she thinks she should do. Thought control, he argues, 'takes … many mundane forms, through the control of information, through the mass media and through the process of socialisation'. He also suggests that the most supreme and insidious use of power is to prevent people, to whatever degree, from having grievances by shaping their cognitions and preferences in such a way that they accept their role in the existing order of things, either because they can see no alternative to it, or because they see it as natural and unchangeable or because they value it as divinely ordained and beneficial (Lukes, *op. cit.*, pp 23–4).

Reading back over previous chapters, it immediately becomes apparent how this view of power can be applied to nursing, nurses and their shared history. Angels, the need for self sacrifice, the common good, the needs of the service, the needs of the patient have all been used to tap into the altruism most nurses bring with them into their work. Moreover, we have already seen the control of information routinely used, as well as the process of socialisation. Nurses have many grievances but most often these are private 'feelings' that find little if any overt expression. Certainly, nurses tend to accept the existing order of things at least as much as any other group of workers. The 'wants' of nurses are shaped in such a way that they are pursued, despite the personal cost and effect.

A simple but graphic example can be seen when nurses are expected to stay on beyond their rostered hours because there is more work to be done that the staff can manage within their planned establishment for that particular shift. This is commonplace and all nurses have done it. Theoretically, 'time owing' or 'time off in lieu' is given to the nurse for staying on, or coming in early. However, there will be very few, if any, who have not worked numerous hours over and above their normal hours without getting anything in return. A special report commissioned by Unison, *First Class Team, Second Class Pay* (Unison, 1999) has estimated that nearly a third of NHS nurses work a full two weeks unpaid each year. Numerous reasons are trotted out to justify this. Nurses take no meaningful sense of grievance, as they accept their role and what is expected of them, either because they can see no alternative to it, see it as natural and unchangeable or value it as organisationally ordained and beneficial. And no trade union challenges it or even raises it as a serious issue that nurses could change relatively easily were they to take collective action.

This also happens with nursing practice. The dissemination of information about good practice is not an objective process. It is one that is highly edited in nursing journals, by department of health officials and within trusts or directorates within trusts. The same processes are used – whether consciously or not – with the result that nurses will never even know about some initiatives that would impact favourably on their practice, are given information that might make them think that some new practices are more beneficial than others. The demise of primary nursing – and the authority it was beginning to acquire for nurses – was an exercise in power, with the vast majority of nurses unaware of whether or not this was in their best interests. It just seemed to happen. Similarly, the unofficial down grading of nursing posts since 1988 seemed to establish a pre-ordained, unchallengeable reality.

▶ Nurse power

'Nurse power' has a context. It is a phrase that entered the nursing vocabulary in the late 1990s, essentially through the *Nursing Times*, but reflected a move that was being pushed with equal vigour by government and the Royal College of Nursing (RCN). Given this triumvirate's importance in the nursing world, it can be accepted that this thing called 'nurse power' was, therefore, important. But what was it? Where had it come from? How had nurses suddenly acquired it? This book has spent a great deal of time arguing that there are deep rooted reasons why nurses have been subjugated as a group, placed in a system where they are expected to subordinate their needs and take on a subservient role. The government, so this argument runs, has been among the key beneficiaries of this, but so, indirectly, have nurses' organisations. So what could this be about? Yet again, Lukes' model of power might be a useful vehicle through which to try and understand the process. For it was power acquired and to be used within a certain context, or set of unspoken rules. It was not about accessing the actual power that nurses have to develop an understanding of their needs with a view to articulating those and set about meeting them. It was to serve the 'common good' more effectively within a shifting socio-economic and political climate.

It occurred shortly before another term became highly prominent in nursing literature. This was leadership, a quality that was identified as key to nursing's future by the participants in the RCN's *Futures Project* (Gulland, 1998a). But, again, the question has to be asked: where does leadership come from? Is it related to power? Having looked at the way power is wielded by politicians, it might be expected that nurses who have become politicians might be in a position to provide both leadership and benefit from any power they have from their office. Yet the verdict from ward leaders in 1998 was that nurse MPs were 'out of touch' and not valuing nurses after that year's pay award was staged. However, the same nurses' criticism of a lack of leadership also extended to the RCN's general secretary, Christine Hancock (Kenny, 1998: p 12).

If leadership wasn't coming from MPs or the general secretary of the RCN, what of the chief nurses, the position for the leading nurses for England, Scotland and Wales? When Dame Yvonne Moores announced her retirement as Chief Nurse for England in 1999, her successor, Sarah Mullally was not on anyone's shortlist for the vacancy. With a background as nurse executive at London's Chelsea and Westminster Healthcare NHS Trust, which had included a spell as acting chief executive, and aged only 37, many wondered if she was both too young and inexperienced to take on the role of a key NHS civil servant. Moores was known for her continuing theme of 'nurses are the key to the future' and 'delivering the government's agenda' (Gulland, 1999b), much the same as Christine Hancock, but little of this seemed to be infecting nurses on the ground with any enthusiasm. It was also many years since Moores had worked in a clinical arena or carried operational responsibility. Mullally could lay claim to far more recent clinical and operational experience. She was moving into a civil service post which would undoubtedly influence clinical practice, yet has as its prime responsibility, as Moores had indicated, delivering government policy and getting nurses to do the same. This is a useful distinction and one which places the relationship between nursing hierarchies and nurses in context. It requires taking nurses where they might not otherwise want to go, or in a direction that is not necessarily in their best interests. That is part of the job. It makes, however, the title 'chief nurse' something of a misnomer, having far more in common with that of director of nursing services. Perhaps it accounts for why chief nurse is not someone with whom most nurses immediately identify and why the post holder is not a prominent national figure, as might be expected of the head of one of the largest workforces in Europe.

Undoubtedly the most interesting development in this area was the highly controversial decision by the RCN to appoint an American nurse to the post of general secretary. However, Beverley Malone came with a lot of other attributes that made her 'different'. She was the first black woman to hold the job, had previously been president of the American Nurses' Association and worked with the Clinton administration in Washington. Far more charismatic than her predecessor, her appointment had all the appearances of signalling a change of direction, even though the College was unwilling to do more than offer the bland 'best candidate for the job' line in response to the furore that followed her appointment.

After several years, Unison finally named Karen Jennings, one of its professional officers and one of the few nurses employed by the union, as head of nursing before she went on to become its first female head of health in 2002. However, as shall be seen in Chapter 7, in such a large and shapeless union, one person, or even the small team that represents Unison's health group, is only going to be able to make a marginal impact and restricts the potential for them to be able to provide real leadership. The UKCC, being 'rebranded' as the Nursing and Midwifery Council (NMC) is also in a position of providing nursing leadership. However, its perceived record is not one of success. It has often been heavily criticised on a number of fronts and is, again, not a body that most nurses in practice would be looking to for inspiration and examples of practical leadership.

If leadership and, therefore, nurse power, are not present on the national stage, where will they be found? Management is not an area many would recommend in the pursuit of the good leader. But, again, it is rarely as simple as a case of 'good' and 'bad'. Research from 1995 showed that top managers were working an average of a fifty-six-hour week, with detrimental effects on family life and a resulting loss in effectiveness. Partly, this was due to the misapprehension that 'being present' was the same as being effective. The pressures were attributed to tighter timetables rather than greater workload. Some of the reasons identified for the consistently long hours worked were a cultural expectation and a recognition that managers are unpopular and need to justify their position and pay (IHSM, 1994; Moore, 1995: pp 24–7).

In a separate survey, clinical nurse managers also identified that they had been inadequately prepared for their role in key performance areas. For example, '27 per cent felt insufficiently prepared to provide pastoral care for their staff'; other areas in which they perceived they had been inadequately prepared included developing audit, budgeting, 'acting up' for senior managers, dealing with difficult people/situations and clinical supervision (Gould *et al.*, 2001: pp 3–6).

To some degree, management – as opposed to individual managers – will always be unpopular, especially in a service as hierarchical and pressurised as the NHS. Moreover, in such a hothouse environment as the contemporary nursing team, where tensions between team members arise but are difficult to confront, partly because of the perceived need for team members not to have arguments or 'fall out' with one another, the external manager is a good target for the team's frustrations. However, there are sometimes good reasons for that frustration and for overt conflict. In 1998 the NHS Trust Confederation were claiming that recruitment and retention problems were not strongly pay related and that 'nursing is not a very badly paid profession but a respectably paid one' (O'Dowd, 1998b). Inevitably, management can only represent a view to the PRB and await the outcome of its recommendations. It has no control over that and, when told the pay award, has to find the money from its budgets. One, less overt, way managers can control this financial pressure is through the structure of the nursing establishment. By 2000, the RCN were reporting that the numbers of nurses at 'G', 'H' and 'I' grades had fallen by 13 per cent in eight years, with 9,000 'G' grade posts being lost alone. This loss of senior posts had several effects. It inevitably stifles career progression. The unions had already been able to present information to the PRB the previous year that, while 80 per cent of the cohort of nurses who registered in 1989 had moved beyond 'D' grade after five years, this had dropped to 55 per cent by 1993, with the proportion being promoted beyond 'E' grade being halved in the same period. The obvious knock on effect is on retention but, with the loss of experienced staff, goes leadership. Thus the lower graded posts are not only held by less experienced nurses – who have less authority to make key decisions and take on a leadership role – but know only too well why they are in that predicament. And while the government's popularity has undoubtedly been seriously damaged in nurses' eyes, so has the credibility of their own managers. Even the UKCC was moved to criticise managers for, in effect, using disciplinary measures as a means of 'management'. Mandie Lavin, the Council's director of professional conduct, said 'it was fairly typical to hear disciplinary cases that had been triggered by bad management decisions. "If nurses are working in fear it will impact on the care that is being delivered. We do hear stories where practitioners are working in very vulnerable situations"' (Coombes, 1996).

Those in senior nursing positions, however, report a whole host of problems, including tensions between their clinical and managerial roles, unrealistic expectations of what they can achieve, with little support or understanding from managers. 'Nurses have long passed the stage of feeling exasperated by the oblivious attitudes of some managers to their dilemma' wrote P. Burgess in the letters pages of the *Nursing Times* (Burgess, 1998). A particular concern has been about the development of roles and the expectations that go with those. When senior nurses – team leaders, nurse practitioners, ward sisters/charge nurses and so on – have operational responsibilities, they almost always report how these heavily impinge either on staff management or practice development. 'Supervision is always the first thing to go when it gets really busy' is a common, if guiltily spoken, comment from nurses. But with the creation of a multitude of new nurses' roles that might have alleviated some of the burden expressed by senior nurses, a lack of clarity about these can increase stress levels, blur boundaries and complicate practice and responsibilities. Equally, the failure to properly define roles within teams and to define the role and focus of the service as a whole, an essential managerial task, has been shown to lead to inefficiencies in both referrals and practice (Audit Commission, 1999; Furlong *et al.*, 1998).

Sound leadership is not, then, a feature of NHS management. The overall view is one of management not valuing its staff, a view reinforced by virtually every survey amongst nurses, when 'poor management', 'the way I am managed' or 'the attitude of management' are cited as a key reason nurses consider leaving their post. Little comfort can be taken from knowing that such a view is not the exclusive property of the NHS.

In a survey from the Institute of Directors in 1999, less than a third of the companies sampled calculated the cost of staff turnover; a fifth were convinced their workforce did not give them a competitive edge; and, astonishingly, half would not hire most or all of their staff a second time around.

> The 1998 Workplace Employment Relations Survey [WERS] covered nearly 2,000 private and public sector bodies. Of a selection of techniques labelled high commitment management practices – such building blocks as job security, training, family friendly policies and influence over work patterns – a minority of organisations had even half in place. None had all.

> 'At the same time, WERS underlined the growing body of evidence that these practices and better performance are linked. It is broadly accepted that organisations which manage people well are likely to have more committed employees; commitment feeds into higher productivity and thence into better financial performance'. Despite evidence that the best performing workplaces were those where high commitment management practices were well embedded, just 14% of organisations had a majority of them in place (Caulkin, 2000: p 9).

Moreover, in knowledge-based organisations, of which the NHS is one, experience, skills, creativity and innovation are the organisation's most highly prized assets. But they are the 'possession' of their staff. When those staff walk out the door at the end of their shift, a manager who has not put in place mechanisms to lure them back the next day is missing the point. It's not just the cost of covering vacancies and recruiting. The invisible cost is incalculable. Trust and commitment are rapidly moving beyond being an optional extra, even for managers and NHS trusts that have, in effect, seen their staff as a commodity for the past decade or so.

▶ The hidden costs of managerial failure

A study of community mental health nurses suggested that 'a very high proportion' experience 'extreme levels of stress' at work and that 'scores were significantly higher among nurses who felt their line managers were unsupportive' (Burnard *et al.*, 2000).

Sickness rates in the nurses surveyed averaged out at nine days each. In 1998, sick leave in the NHS was calculated to be costing the service a staggering £700 million a year. With NHS sickness absence running at 5 per cent, this is 1.3 per cent higher than that in industry. Trusts which recorded lower rates of sickness absence 'placed more emphasis on communication between workers and managers, devoted more time to staff training and allowed staff greater control and flexibility in their jobs' (Brindle, 1998a).

When all these factors coalesce, a story that is familiar to all nurses emerges. It demonstrates quite graphically that the concept of 'the common good', the needs of the patient or the needs of the service are blandishments that are used to conceal a sinister but unnecessary truth. One nurse, with five years post-registration experience, wrote an article for *The Observer*, explaining how the lack of nurses presents those working on the wards with major dilemmas about whose care to prioritise and of being unable to work in the way she had been trained:

> Each morning I wake up praying for the day when I never have to wear my uniform again. Each year the job becomes more intolerable, the pressures higher and the staffing levels lower. I work with colleagues whose eyes are dead, the spirit which drove them into nursing crushed.
>
> We make 'phone calls regularly [to our managers] when we are at breaking point in the hope that they can do something constructive instead of breezing about the wards with pieces of paper. Nurses who complain are gently persuaded that they are overreacting and unable to cope – and that perhaps this means they are unsuitable for promotion' (Anonymous, 1997: p 18).

In the face of these undoubtedly daunting problems, it is perhaps unsurprising that some managers shy away from becoming involved with their nurses and clinical work. They not only face the high expectations and demands from the nurses themselves; above them are perched their own senior managers and a trust board, above whom towers a government that is even more demanding, imposing ever tighter deadlines on new work, projects and reforms, dangling money but making it hard to obtain. In the process, it sets new standards, targets and objectives while insisting the manager improve the working lives of the staff and introduce a range of policies to create new consultation mechanisms and a staff friendly environment – regardless of how contradictory this is. Not only do managers face this fundamental obstacle to establishing a meaningful relationship with the staff whom they manage, very few will have had any training whatsoever in the art and science of managing people. They will possibly have been shown how to interpret and manage budgets, and will have brought with them experience from previous posts, whether they be in nursing, elsewhere in the health service or a completely different field altogether. Training schemes for managers established since the 1980s, have been taken up by relatively few and, once they are in post, few trusts operate development programmes. Long-term courses are regarded by many as a luxury, in terms of time they cannot afford, such are the operational demands of their day-to-day work. Mentorship and formal, organised supervision are also relatively scarce, leaving people in key jobs in an extremely vulnerable and unsupported position.

Once in post the pull towards a particular culture is strong indeed. Tasks are managerial. The majority of meetings are with other managers. The span of responsibility is invariably so large that there is little time to spend with the staff in particular teams. The pay and conditions are usually different, with few managers these days remaining on the Whitley contracts that determine nurses' pay and conditions. Many managers will also acknowledge that, within their managerial 'team', there is a competitive edge. The culture of long hours referred to earlier in this chapter is not an act of God, it is created by the managers themselves, and by their bosses. Parts of their previous working lives that might have counterbalanced this are often jettisoned, either along the path to promotion or when they get there e.g. trade union membership (and, perhaps surprisingly, until recently some level of trade union activism would not be uncommon amongst managers when they were in junior positions). To seek help is often seen as even more of a sign of weakness than it is for nurses. Most importantly, is the lack of direct, regular contact with patients and any direct involvement in the actual service that is being managed, leading to a genuine lack of understanding of the working reality of the nurses managed. The better managers can apply themselves to learning about the nature of the work in its detail, spread and culture, and empathise with the difficulties and share the satisfaction. In many cases, s/he can then manage as well as anyone who has progressed from a clinical post.

For those who are new to the clinical arena, it can seem a 'foreign land', strange and vaguely threatening. And it is, of course, the source of all their problems. It is the operational side, the managing of the clinical service, that generates overspends, conflict, problem staff and incidents. Perhaps it is no wonder that Frank Dobson had to remind his managerial audience that 'nurses are not part of the problem' – but in many ways they are *exactly* the problem; they are the ones who ask the difficult questions, who say that this or that policy is unworkable, that this or that difficulty has arisen – even when all the planning or the policy suggested it should not have – and always go on about how busy the service is, about the difficulties with the patients....

These 'core' problems, essentially how to provide a good, effective service to patients within the given resource, often appear insoluble from a distance. The common response of a managerial team is to review the operational procedures. To be busy. To hold meetings. To be busier. To write newer policies. Hold more meetings. To be busier still. To ask for reports and statistics. Attend even more meetings. To be so busy that one can't be accessed. To re-organise and re-structure and then re-review. If that doesn't solve the problem, it can all be done over again. There's plenty to keep an organisation and its managerial team busy. And, of course, the problems don't go away. Rather like those annoying fairground amusements, they just pop their head up from a different hole; no matter how quick the hammer slams down it fails to stop them, and up the head rises somewhere else. And every nurse in the country will be familiar with the next tactic, which has been termed maximum administrative delay. It is employed by overstretched managers to help them prioritise the umpteen priorities they find flung at them from clinicians across their sphere of responsibility and involves getting on with the most pressing task and not doing anything in response to other requests or problems for as long as possible, waiting to see if they 'go away'. And so it goes on, until those chasing the managers either give up or persist to the point where something has to be done. It is no co-incidence the acronym for this is MAD management. This approach creates its own difficulties, however. It requires the manager to further divorce her/himself from the problems the staff are trying to bring to their attention – it is an understandable safety valve for people who don't want to find out too much about the severity of the problem because, if they do, they will feel compelled to try and resolve it to the exclusion of other things that have been identified as urgent and equally important. Inevitably, many managers will feel issues passed on by their own manager should take precedence. It takes the task of problem solving to another level altogether if the manager is passing on instructions that are going to complicate the clinical work even more, such as freezing posts or calling for more statistics and so on. Thus the process of drifting further from the clinical arena, from the concerns of the staff, continues.

In the worst cases, it is at this point that dissent surfaces and the manager becomes part of 'management', a wholly alien group who act as if they are on a completely different side to the staff they manage and are, in actuality, responsible for. It was in this way that the worst of general management operated. Nurses were alienated and most definitely came to be seen as part of the problem. When problem solving and re-organisations didn't work, harsher disciplinary mechanisms, including 'gagging' clauses in trust policies and people's contracts were used. The dissent quietened. Compliance was – wrongly – assumed to be co-operation and concordance. The gap widened.

▶ Emotional intelligence – one way towards better management?

This government, like any other, wants good leadership in the NHS but of a particular quality. The management and leadership it wants is one that will deliver its agenda, which is to increase the 'productivity' of the workforce in defined areas of performance, a favourite theme of Alan Milburn's. Yet people like Christine Hancock are right. Nurses are the key to delivering change of any sort. There are so many of them that, whichever way they go, the service goes with it – which, ironically, means they have an enormous, if hardly tapped into, power. The 'hidden' price of disenchantment is a form of stagnation. It is this that has so frustrated Blair and his acolytes, yet is a problem of the government's own making. To engage with the workforce, leaders in nursing need to be working alongside them, sharing an agenda and trusting them to deliver, if not on their own terms then terms that are negotiated. The introverted culture which has submerged nurses, where ideas and creativity are stifled needs to be replaced, not by recreating the internal market, as Alan Milburn thinks, but something far more pluralistic. Discipline, control and keeping people in their place by holding down grades, removing senior positions and keeping nurses at arms' length in the decision making process has patently failed. Succession planning, comprehensive development and leadership training – albeit a very different kind of leadership – and authority being given to senior nurses (which are very much a part of the package that is being advocated at a national level but not yet finding its way into the workforce), as well as ways in which nurses can be empowered locally have to offer a more viable way forward. But only if those currently in power are willing to relinquish control.

Key to any such change is how nurses are to be led, as opposed to manage. Many good nurses currently want nothing to do with becoming a manager. They consider the rewards too few, the work undesirable and pressures too great. They want to retain clinical contact and work alongside their nursing colleagues. Moreover, the managerial culture can be, in itself, alienating.

Managerial failure is just as endemic in the private sector. But there is something to suggest that the health service has had the answer under its nose in the shape of its nurses. Whether nursing has denied itself the opportunity to resolve the tensions described above or, because of the prevailing power structures, been led to believe that it hasn't the wherewithal becomes, therefore, all the more interesting.

Research has shown how brain processes mean that 'the signal generating fear reaches the amygdala before the cortex', resulting in people being 'driven into defensive and non-rational behaviour by their instincts without being aware of it', which might account for why so many managers 'persist in making decisions that are bound to damage their [organisation]' (Syrett and Lammiman, 1999). Theorists such as US psychologist Daniel Goleman stress that 'emotional intelligence' may be an answer to this kind of problem. It has little to do with IQ – indeed, he claims that many conventionally intelligent people are emotionally immature – and is a much sought after quality by enlightened employers. It is characterised by self awareness and an ability to relate to others, or empathy. Those with these attributes influence and work well in teams, as well as provide sound leadership. It is not just about the end point but how that end point is reached:

> After more than 100 years dominated by the Aristotelian principle that intellect always triumphs over instinct, management recruiters are abandoning their worship of the high IQ and placing a new premium on emotional maturity. Goleman recently looked at the profile of top performers in 500 companies worldwide and found that a high IQ got the best managers only on to the first rung of their chosen careers. After that, personal qualities such as an ability to empathise with others and grasp of the big picture counted for much more than analytical skills.
>
> At Pepsi-Co, for instance, divisions whose leaders possessed such qualities outperformed others by 15–29%. British head teachers with these skills also got better results than schools with heads who were 'aloof' or dictatorial in their management styles (Syrett and Lammiman, 1999 *op. cit.*).

Emotional stimuli are registered by the amygdala. Conscious emotion is created both by direct signals from the amygdala to the frontal cortex and indirectly. The indirect path involves the hypothalamus, which sends hormonal messages to the body to create physical changes. These are then fed back to the somasensaory cortex which, in turn feed, back to the frontal cortex again, where it is interpreted as emotion. This process is integral to decision making. People who have lost the ability to gain bodily feedback find emotions indistinguishable from thought. They are unable to interpret their emotional response or 'gut feelings' and their decision making is grossly impaired. The work that has been done around the left/right brain split reveals that, while it is nowhere near as emphatic as some would have us believe, there are 'quite specific functions that are "hard-wired" to the extent that, in normal circumstances, certain skills will always develop on a particular side'. So the left hemisphere is analytical, logical, precise and time sensitive. The right is dreamier, holistic in the way it processes information and more involved with sensory perception than abstract cognition. Although the two hemispheres work harmoniously most of the time, occasionally one side dominates the other, or takes in information that the other has not, for some reason, processed. This can lead to acting on 'hunches' or instinct, or in an overly 'rational' way. There are also more sophisticated differences between the male and female brain than the shopping/sex dichotomy of popular folklore. The corpus callosum in the female brain is larger than in men. This is a band of tissue through which the two hemispheres communicate. The same is true of the anterior commissure, which again links the two hemispheres, which may offer at least part of the explanation as to why women can interpret their own emotions and empathise more than men, as well as incorporate emotion more easily into speech and thought. Women can also bring both sides of their brain into play more than men when doing complex mental tasks. When it comes to making decisions, women are then able to take a broader, more self aware and empathic perspective and consider more aspects of a problem, as opposed to the more focused view a man might have (Carter, 1998).

Perhaps, then, one reason that the existing, masculine managerial culture in the NHS has been unsuccessful, is that it is not sufficiently emotionally mature and disables its practitioners from taking a broader, holistic and empathic perspective and style, despite the fact that this would yield better results than the more 'aloof', focused and ultra rational approach currently favoured. Of course, this also reflects the dominant culture perpetuated by the medical profession. This, in part, stems from the differing roles of nurses and doctors. The latter are trained to focus in on symptoms, diagnosis and specific treatments. History taking is precise, ordered and systematic. This sharply contrasts with the way nurses both assess and care for patients, where training and practice have developed an increasingly holistic, patient-centred approach.

With a growing body of evidence that different organisational structures and a new approach to the way in which people work and are managed can reap great benefits, is there any genuine desire for change? Theodore Zeldin is a historian and intellectual who is leading a European Community funded project, trying to create new vision of work, driven by a form of education that is designed to broaden the scope of knowledge, helping people to step out of the constraining and uninspiring specialties which are a hangover from the nineteenth century in design and culture. He thinks there is a 'great desire for change – even among the heads of faceless bureaucracies' – but perceives a feeling of powerlessness, of not knowing how to change. While acknowledging it would not bring utopia, he believes such change would enable people to feel they're not so alone or despised, that they have something in them if only somebody would help them to develop it' (Flockhart, 2001: p 7).

▶ Republican management

These are the contradictions, the challenges that those responsible for the NHS must resolve if it is to function effectively. It is not about re-organisations, re-structuring or greater commercialisation. It is far more fundamental, and more difficult than that. An essential component of any such change will be a radically different form of management.

A story from Abraham Lincoln's second attempt to get himself elected to the Illinois state legislature perhaps illustrates the point. He had decided to eschew speeches and statements of principles in favour of a more direct approach. A typical example of this was a pitch he made to about thirty farmers. When told they would never vote for a man who was ignorant of field work, he reputedly took a farm implement and led the harvesters on a full round of the field, declaring that he should be sure of their votes and, indeed, did go on to win the seat easily. This was a literal translation of the maxim detailed by Thomas Jefferson and America's Founding Fathers that its leaders should be both professors and ploughmen. It was this that was the basis for the republicanism of the United States. This was not a recipe for the masses running the country – it was a desire for the people in charge to be truly representative and to know of the problems facing the people they ruled. It was clearly not to remain the case – increasingly, America's leaders were far more legislators than ploughmen, having less and less contact with them, either the literal farmers of the land or those who sowed the seeds of the nation's industrial and economic growth in the cities[11] (Cullen, 1998). But as an ideology, it was in stark

---

[11] The fragility of any system and need to safeguard it is exemplified by the US presidential election of 2000, which demonstrated that even a system designed to give everyone a voice and safeguard the democratic process can be systematically corrupted. Michael Moore gives a hilarious but chilling account of how this was taken to the status of an art form as Democratic presidential candidate, Al Gore, polled more votes than his Republican opponent, George W. Bush in the Republican controlled state of Florida but still found himself

contrast to the oligarchic and repressive regimes many of its people had fled – a not dissimilar view that some working within the NHS might have of the nature of the institution, regardless of the quality of their own direct line managers.

If the form, content and culture of management is to be different, it requires a new means of being delivered. Given that management is about people, it is apparent that this means either new people or helping those already in the system find within themselves a new way of doing their job and, perhaps, even helping them re-define that job. In part, the government has recognised this by initiating new leadership programmes but, as so often is the case, it then contradicts itself by saying that it wants the private sector to come in and manage the NHS. If it were to be truly radical – and, one could argue, serious – it would adopt a form of republican leadership for the health service. Within hospitals or community services, the principle of senior managers coming out of the staff groups they were managing is achievable. Moreover, in many cases, they could balance their management with retaining a clinical role (or developing an involvement with a clinical team if they have come from a non-clinical background), thus fulfilling the dual role aspired to within the Jeffersonian model. Immediately, the manager is talking the same language as other staff, subject to the same experiences and able to listen, first hand to the issues that concern clinicians and, most importantly, patients. It also offers the manager something else: the chance to be a leader. Some would query the difference between the two or suggest that leadership is managing without responsibility. Another way of looking at it is that managers have *effective control* of a subject while leading is conducting or guiding by being in front, while in the process of being with those s/he is leading. Thus leaders tend to be people of deserved influence, the same as those they lead but with something more.

The scale of the problem is that, unless there is a fundamental re-think to the role of managers and where they sit in the structure and organisation, it becomes almost inevitable that they compound the problem, simply because of their huge numbers and the tasks they generate. According to Revill (2002b: p 6), nearly 25 per cent of NHS staff is in management or administration, with the numbers rising from 168,730 in 1996 to 188,530 in September 2001. There are eighty-seven

---

contd.
'defeated', with the process ratified by a Republican controlled Supreme Court. Bush went on to be handed the US presidency despite, again, polling fewer votes in the country as a whole (Moore, 2002). Apart from the international furore that followed (with America's old Cuban opponent, Fidel Castro, apparently offering to send in impartial election observers to help them with their 'difficulties') many American nurses were left devastated, not just because of the contempt shown for the electoral process but because of the consequences for nursing and the American healthcare system, which many of them believed would suffer at Bush's hands.

different types of manager, working in 'new tiers of bureaucracy that are clogging up the system, slowing down work and interfering with [patient] care'. The number of senior managers rose by 50 per cent in the same period.

Yet managers are legitimately complaining of being unable to get through their work as it is, without having to retain or develop some level of clinical or service involvement. In part, the nature of that work has to be questioned, as well as how much of it is actually designed to support the clinicians and the essential work of the organisation. Arguably, if this becomes the key task of the new managers, not only will their workload be decreased but both it and they will be more focused, by their own experience and their direct involvement with their staff. Moreover, the number of staff within leadership positions can increase as some aspects of the clinical work are shared around. This inevitably means a change in management structures but offers an opportunity to complement the feminine characteristics of nursing into a managerial model, and diffusing hierarchies.

The current model involves many layers, fashioned into pyramidal hierarchies. These are essentially both bureaucratic and defensive structures in the sense that there are numerous channels of communication to be negotiated, with each layer generating its own mini structures, reporting mechanisms, bureaucracy and decision making processes. Even with the best of intentions, simply passing on decisions, seeking information and working between these layers creates its own work over and above the needs and work generated by the organisation's primary purpose. The age-old problem of layers within the hierarchy generating tasks to justify their own existence is also widely recognised. The defensiveness results from their static nature, with parties within one layer looking both up and down, perhaps not knowing all that is happening in the separate layers, driven by the perceived need to respond to potential problems and weaknesses within only their own 'line'.

The nature of the structures not only impairs clear communications and decision making, it also stifles the creativity of those lower down the chain of command as there are managers above them doing little other than 'acting down'. Those at the bottom of the pyramid, the largest number by far, often feel they know little of what is happening above, how decisions are made and invariably begin to feel distrustful as well as distant and devalued. Importantly, however, they know an awful lot more about what is happening in their section of the pyramid, which is where the effects of the decisions made by the managers at the top are most acutely felt.

Changing structures to something resembling concentric or interlocking circles involves more people in the task of managing or leading and allows for greater creativity and flexibility (see Figure 6.2). People can 'work across' rather than 'down' in times of crisis or difficulty. Leaders are visible and accessible. Information can be shared 'around' rather than passed down.

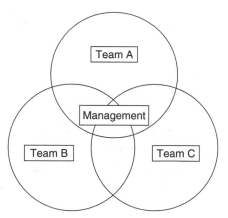

Figure 6.2 A new structure for management

Moreover, good leadership does not occur in a vacuum. It requires a framework, a set of 'rules' and boundaries, a clear focus and shared understanding of what is happening and why. Supportive structures have to be established so that staff can be involved from the outset in solving the problems facing them and remain so (see Figure 6.3). This might involve self-rostering on the off duty, looking at how a challenging patient can best be nursed or making changes to the ward timetable. Ideas can be acted upon more easily and the shared ownership creates less confrontational relationships. Senior management can 'hold' a strong, well-organised centre that relates to other parts of the organisation in a supportive and enabling way. It generates networks that can be activity or service based rather than a hierarchy that has to support the top of the pyramid regardless of the impact on the rest of the structure. The circles are far more like communities, with their managers at the centre, a part of, rather than at the top of. They can also move around more freely and, because they have opportunities to listen and participate both as practitioner and manager, can help people deal with the immediate problems while taking a longer term view. This can also facilitate staff working both collectively and collaboratively rather than in the insular, competitive way that has resulted from rigid line management. Thus they can maximise the knowledge, skills and experience of whole teams.

Nurses then have the opportunity to be involved in leading as well as managing, utilising particular areas of expertise, perhaps in cultural awareness, assessment or supervision of staff working with particular patients. The trust gets the added bonus of being able to build a culture based on the combination of empathy and self awareness that characterises nurses' clinical work. This can be both empowering and increase effectiveness and efficiency, with the result that 'productivity' or improved patient outcomes are increased.

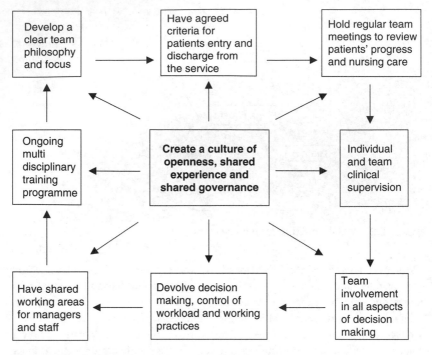

Figure 6.3 A supportive structure for clinical teams

That this type of approach can actually work has already been demonstrated in a study of successful women leaders, as well as the example of successful ward managers and team leaders (Helgesen, 1990; Lewis, 1998a: pp 30–1; Lewis, 1998b: pp 32–3; Hart, 1999: pp 48–9).

This also returns nursing to its collective, 'catholic' tradition of communal nursing in, and of, the world, which utilises a pragmatic concordance between theory and practice, of having power but sharing it and moves it away from the individualised, isolating culture that has successfully been forced onto nurses, who are then expected to worship a hierarchical and abstract nursing ideal, whether that be vocational devotion and obedience to the word of the matron, the common good or new gods such as evidence based practice.

Inevitably, such radical changes create a chain reaction and all involved would find it an extremely demanding process to go through; it is immensely hard work to shift organisations, both in their ideology and operational style. But it is also hard personally to face that level of change. For some, it involves giving up power, for others – and this can be as hard – it involves acknowledging that they have now got power, with the responsibilities and decisions that go with it. Moreover, for managers, there has to be an acceptance that other people have more information, knowledge, experience and skills, but that these can be tapped into and utilised in a way never before possible. If we are talking about emotional intelligence, we have to acknowledge that, in terms of our employment relations and structures, we are deeply immature at the most senior levels. Attempts to change are hampered by other aspects of policy that directly contradict them. That so many nurses and others involved in healthcare have made some progress in these difficult areas is both a great achievement on their part and reminder to others that it is possible. Even more demanding for those who have made the shift, or even begun the process, is the need to stay in touch with colleagues who are struggling. The beauty of the concentric circle approach is that it *can* spread its net far and wide, beyond line management boundaries and rigid hierarchies. Many nurses are waiting for the opportunity to make a change. It has to be recognised that the leadership being provided 'from the top' is inadequate and poor. It fails to articulate the genuine needs of nurses and nursing. There is often a mistaken assumption that there are situations where there is a lack of leadership. In fact, like power, leadership is always present: it can simply be very poor. And if people are poorly led they are, at the same time, being taught to lead poorly. However, little changes can have an immense effect on local conditions and these are the lessons that are being learned in areas where significant advances have been made. Nurses can do no more than lead amongst the people with whom they are working. If change for the better is affected at that level then the leadership has been effective in itself.

▶ Conclusion

The poverty of New Labour's election pledges to nurses demonstrates not only a lack of ambition but also an almost complete lack of imagination. Given the situation they inherited in 1997, with the hostility toward the outgoing Tory government and the massive fund of goodwill that was theirs, the scope for building a new, enabling and creative culture that would, in itself, have delivered a massive change agenda was immense. The failure to act upon that was not simply a missed opportunity. It was a profound failure of leadership. Like corner shopkeepers taking over a once grand but undervalued department store, they approached the task at hand with the sole objective of managing it better than their predecessors. Perhaps throwing in a new line of socks at the same time. When the issue of leadership, as opposed to management, is explored in a nursing or health service context, it has to be remembered that the overall thrust and direction will always come from government. If that is poor, mean spirited or anonymous, always aimed at saying the phrase that will get a headline, aiming no further than the next month or two, or seeking something for nothing, that will have its effect all the way down the line to each and every nurse working with her or his patients.

What stops nurses, this most powerful group, from exerting power? Divided, poorly led – and on occasions, misled – they are blinkered in elaborate structures that make it difficult to see what is happening or participate in decision making, let alone take control of their destiny. It is highly unlikely that nurses will find salvation through parliamentary politicians of any party. More centralised and controlling than ever, the government has power; it determines the funding for the NHS and tries to set the parameters of debate about the future of the service. That it is vulnerable to ever more global influences only means that nursing is more marginalised. The policy process is complex, travelling down different avenues but usually fuelled by politics, even when clinical considerations either seem to be, or are sold as, the only driving force.

Power, whether used by government, the medical profession, managers or senior nurses is essentially a means of exercising control, to affect people to behave in ways that are detrimental to their own needs, even to prevent them from realising what those needs are. It is not being used for the good of the service, the patient or to deliver an NHS that is more effective, responsive or any of the other buzz words of the Blairites. Marginalising the nursing workforce and selling them a culture and tradition that does them a disservice has a direct knock on effect with patient care. The fact that, locked within its inner workings and development, nursing perhaps has a potential solution and one that could create the kind of change the government claims to be seeking only adds insult to injury. The notion of an entirely new way of providing management and leadership is alien to those in power.

Certainly, no one is going to hand power to nurses on a silver platter. No one cares for nurses. At least, no group cares sufficiently about nurses *per se* to go out of its way to advance their cause. All too often, nurses have been sucked into accepting the 'common good' and sacrificing their needs to that uncommon altar. Doctors care but only inasmuch as their own agenda is advanced and supporting nurses and nursing issues will not have a detrimental affect on their overall position of power and influence. The public do care but are relatively powerless to do anything. They care not only because either they themselves or their loved ones will inevitably be patients at some stage in their lives but also because, broadly, there is respect and admiration for the work nurses do.

Given the relative powerlessness of both groups, some thought is needed about the possibility and value of any alliances in the future. There are those who argue consistently that nurses' future is in developing its 'caring' role rather than trying to hitch a ride on the 'curative' coat tails of the medical profession. This requires aligning the workforce with the vulnerable, the needy and those who are often poor if not dispossessed. To get that elusive seat at the decision making table, nurses will have to behave differently and think about themselves and the work they do very differently. An important issue in that quest is whether or not nurses' unions care about them. That we will seek to answer in the next chapter.

The story so far, as outlined in this chapter, might seem hard on New Labour, maximising its failures and contradictions rather than focusing on its achievements.

Given that it has an entire government department and one of the slickest political machines in the developed world doing that, readers should be able to find examples of New Labour's own version of its achievements. There is very strong evidence, however, that this government has failed nurses and the health service, as much by what it has not done as by its actual active decisions and actions. Yet, compared to the governments of Margaret Thatcher and John Major, indeed, many of its predecessors, it *has* achieved many things. It is far too early, for instance, to get a proper perspective on the effect of the different NSFs, Improving Working Lives, the development of PCTs, or the NHS Plan. Devolution, as has been noted above, has effectively ended the concept of a national health service for the United Kindom (although countries had already been developing services in a semi autonomous fashion before 1997). New Labour's achievement has been to oversee the transition to four nations which now have a health service of which they can take ownership, involving the people within their countries to varying degrees. In this respect, Scotland is probably further ahead on this agenda than any of the others and the English health service, facing an uncertain future with Foundation Hospitals, lagging behind. These have been bold, sweeping initiatives. New Labour has also excelled in some areas that are of no direct relevance to this book but have an enormous impact on people's lives and it may well be recorded by history as one of the better reforming governments. Which, of course, is the point. Politicians are faced with innumerable pressures, decisions, priorities and, ultimately, choices. Whether or not it is their intention to do the 'right' thing or act in a 'good' way – and there is no reason to doubt that many MPs in New Labour have sought to do that – it is almost inevitable that they find themselves drawn to doing that which is most expedient, responding to the greatest pressure. The powerful get their way.

▶ Further reading

Hayward S and Hunter DJ (1982) Consultative processes in health policy in the United Kingdom: a view from the centre. *Policy Administration*, 69.

Hugman R (1991) *Power in Caring Professions*. Basingstoke: Macmillan.

Lindblom C (1959) The science of 'muddling through'. *Public Administration Review*, 19.

Lukes S (1974) *Power: A Radical View*. London: Macmillan.

Niven N and Robinson J (1994) *The Psychology of Nursing Care*. Leicester: The British Psychological Society/Macmillan.

Obholzer A and Zagier Roberts V (eds) (1994) *The Unconscious at Work: Individual and Organisational Stress in the Human Services*. London: Routledge.

Pettigrew *et al.* (1988) Understanding change in the NHS. *Public Administration*, 66.

Wilkinson G and Miers M (eds) (1999) *Power and Nursing Practice*. Basingstoke: Macmillan.

▶ **Useful websites**

www.doh.gov.uk
www.n-i.nhs.uk
www.wales.nhs.uk
www.show.scot.nhsuk
www.unison.org.uk
www.rcn.org

7 The Great Divide: Trade Unions and Nurses

I dreamed I saw Joe Hill last night, as alive as you and me
Joe Hill, by Earl Robinson and Alfred Hayes, as featured in a performance by
Paul Robeson, 30 January 1942

▶ Introduction

In 1962, George Woodcock, then general secretary of the Trade Union Congress (TUC) turned to his colleagues on the TUC general council and asked, 'Why are we here?', or what was the trade union movement all about. The simple answer he got was, in essence, to 'fatten the wage packets of the members and not much else'. Woodcock was looking for more from his fellow trade union leaders, and wanted to develop a means of avoiding the apocalyptic future he saw, including free market excess, high unemployment and government legislation that would shackle the unions as they had been pre-Second World War. He didn't get it. (Aitken, 2000). Forty years on, there is little evidence the question is even in the heads of the leaders of the trade unions and organisations representing nurses. Apparently they are there, therefore they do.

It would be easy to suggest, given the enormous difficulties still facing nurses and the apparent inability to make significant progress with the so-called 'professional' front or significantly improve pay and conditions, that their representatives have failed in the most fundamental areas. Easy, but only a small part of the story. The trade unions made tremendous gains for nurses during the twentieth century, often at great personal expense to the individuals who took on leading roles. At particular points in our history the achievement was not measured in progress at all – during the 1980s, for instance, the radical right-wing governments of Margaret Thatcher were constantly threatening hard-won employment rights over and above those they snatched away. It was largely trade unionists working away behind the scenes at local and national level that managed to resist this. In the workplace, the efforts of trade union representatives are largely unseen but their protective wrap is felt by every nurse and health worker, whether they are a member of that union or not, as they negotiate agreements, amend policies in favour of staff interests, set 'case law' at a local level through the representation of individuals and protect the use of procedures so that staff retain their legitimate rights, whatever they have done. Often, this lack of awareness on behalf of staff, both members and non-members, is accompanied by a lack of gratitude, expressed as a 'what have you ever done for me?' attitude. Like nursing, the job is never easy.

As has been argued in the previous chapter, using Luke's model of power, there are a variety of reasons for nurses not actually recognising their true interests or pursuing them in any cohesive and consistent fashion. The vast majority of nurses who belong to any organisation are members of either the Royal College of Nursing (RCN) or Unison, with the Community Practitioners' and Health Visitors' Association (CPHVA) and RCM dominating health visiting and midwifery, respectively. Large, 'general' unions like the GMB also have some nurse members, while small, specialist associations such as the Community Psychiatric Nurses Association (CPNA) occupy a place at the other end of the spectrum. These organisations take their place alongside the British Medical Association (BMA) and a range of unions and associations representing staff from the Professions Allied to Medicine (PAMs) in negotiating with the Department of Health's civil servants at a national level and employers, e.g., trust managers locally. However, there can be no doubt that the world of *nursing* trade unionism is dominated by the big two – Unison and the RCN – and it is they who will be the focus of this chapter, along with the CPHVA and RCM where appropriate. By looking at the respective histories, policies, political positions and actions of the RCN and Unison – as well as their relationships with each other, the wider political community and, most importantly, their members – we can try and understand more about nursing and its current state.

In part, this will be achieved by a brief chronological account of events during the twentieth century, but which will pay particular attention to the hidden history of radicalism in nursing. In this early history, we will see how the origins of division were established. The contrasting fortunes of first The Confederation of Health Service Employees (COHSE) and then Unison, against those of the College will be explored, focusing primarily on the factors that allowed them to flourish or made it difficult for them to survive at particular times. How Unison was formed is an inevitable part of the story, as well as its struggles to establish an identity for itself as a public sector union while simultaneously promoting its service groups and occupational groups, like nurses, within those. The extraordinary grasp of the political that has always guided the College will demonstrate to readers the clear potential nurses have for influence: this begs a comparison with the more overtly politicised relationships favoured by the TUC and Labour Party affiliated unions which, for generations, have paid money directly to the party currently in government, questioning exactly what nurses get for their money.

Nurses' pay is examined again, this time in the context of local pay bargaining as it was introduced by the Tory Government in 1995, heralding a 'virtual dispute'. It makes for an interesting comparison with 1987–88. Finally, the pernicious effects of the split that was institutionalised in nursing trade unionism as long ago as 1948 is analysed, as is its legacy for contemporary nurses and what the future may hold for both the unions and their members, along with any potential for change.

▶ The origins of division

The division and lasting enmity between nursing's trade unions and professional associations is almost unique in labour movement history. It reflects nursing's position between a profession and skilled trade, as well as its many and varied strands and their different historical evolution. Social class was another determinant, not just because of the differences between the women who came into nursing post-Nightingale and before, but also the way nursing values were expropriated by the middle class and the relationship nursing had to those men who had quickly established control of their work.

From the earliest moves to form organisations that would support nurses and articulate their aspirations, key differences were evident. The British Nurses' Association (later to become the Royal British Nurses' Association (RBNA) was elitist, anti-trade union and unwilling to accept men into its ranks – but saw the advancing of its professionalising agenda as inextricably linked with the cause of advancing women. With the training and registration debate hotting up, The College of Nursing (later to be the RCN), founded in 1916 and with articles that strictly forbade it from becoming a trade union, was established on the premise that it would be the body to approve training schools, maintaining any registers of trained nurses and promoting nurses' issues in parliament. It was also able to absorb nurses who may otherwise have been attracted to the fledgling trade unions organising in hospitals and asylums. An immediate competitor to the RBNA, their bitter feud was eventually won by the College because of its willingness to compromise – notably in subordinating 'nurses' interests' to those controlling the healthcare system. However, in what was to establish a clear pattern in nursing politics, having tired of the inability of the nurses' organisations to agree on virtually anything, the government went ahead with its own legislation in 1919. In establishing the General Nursing Council (GNC), it wrong footed both Associations.

The College reacted swiftly, reconfiguring itself as a lobbying and campaigning organisation, and gained the majority of seats on the new GNC in 1920. Having a ruling body made up of senior medical staff, hospital administrators and matrons proved immediately advantageous. Such figures were inevitably able to exert influence on senior nurses, many of whom joined. They in turn had an even more significant impact on their junior nursing staff and the College's ranks swelled with new members. It set up the *Nursing Times* as its in house magazine and gradually tightened its grip on the nursing agenda, appropriating and building upon the Nightingale myth early on, identifying its own ideals with those of nursing as if the two were one (Abel-Smith, 1960).

Asylum attendants were working in what could have been another universe. Excluded from the main nurses' organisations, they attempted their own type of reform. This was based upon their desire to improve their pay and working conditions but took them on a different path altogether. They began trying to form trade unions in the 1880s. The regimes in which they were working were already brutal and brutalising; but in the face of fierce opposition from the employers, it wasn't until 1910 that they were successful, when a group of Lancastrian charge nurses founded the National Asylum Workers' Union (NAWU).

The political and industrial relations climate in the period leading up to the First World War was extremely volatile. NAWU's demands, for a shorter working week, increased pay and a slackening off of some of the more repressive working conditions, were comparatively mild; nonetheless, in the still wholly de-unionised area of healthcare, the threat was considered too great. Officials were victimised, the union opposed at every opportunity. The coming of war quietened NAWU's demands and, in common with so many organisations, also took away many of its leading figures, who did not return from the trenches. Despite the threat of revolution hanging over large parts of Europe, the end of the war saw no resumption of the turmoil that had coloured Britain's political landscape before 1914. Yet, NAWU staged its first strike in 1918, just as the Poor Law Workers' Trade Union (PLWTU) was founded (Carpenter, 1988). Both unions were grappling with similar issues although both remained specific to their own employers, rather than forming a general union, an approach taken by some workers in industry. They both accepted all staff into their union. Nurses joining these unions were roundly criticised by the professional organisations, not only out of a sense that they were betraying their vocational tradition but also because of an anxiety that, should they be successful, others would follow.

▶ A hidden history of radicalism

Although it may seem unbelievable to those who see nurses as conservative, compliant and subservient, there is a long and rich history of radicalism, struggle and campaigning that has been largely ignored or hidden in the telling of the nursing story. The early years of both the NAWU and the PLWTU saw recurring setbacks. In most cases, these were countered by outbreaks of radicalism. The Battle of Radcliffe, in 1922, marked the pinnacle of NAWU's attempts to secure improved pay balanced by a shorter working week against a recessionary climate and growing unemployment. Nurses and patients combined to resist the Visiting Committee at the Notts County Mental Hospital, Radcliffe, who called in police, bailiffs and strike breakers in a dispute that had started after the Visiting Committee had cut wages and actually increased the working week, then sacked all the staff as they waged a legitimate challenge to these decisions. The 'battle' involved the nurses and patients barricading themselves in the wards, turning fire hoses on their attackers and holding out for nearly four hours. It finished, with the nurses being ejected from the hospital, many of them to be blacklisted (MHIWU, 1931; Carpenter, 1988).

The Battle of Radcliffe was a dramatic episode that symbolised a conflict unresolved more than sixty years later. In the short term, it precipitated a loss of almost 2000 union members and saw the health unions gradually settle into a period of conservatism and consolidation. Trade unions merged as new legislation re-shaped services.

The conservative climate in nursing changed with the Spanish Civil War, which attracted radicals from across the world, drawn as much by the romanticism of the Republican's epic struggle with the Fascists as any deep ideological stirrings. British nurses were amongst those who travelled to the Spanish battlefields, the most notable being Thora Silverthorne. Despite her quite extraordinary exploits in Spain, it was her actions when she returned to London in early 1937 that left an indelible mark in nursing history when she formed the Association of Nurses. This was the first – and only – trade union that was exclusively for nurses. And these were nurses recruited from London's prestigious teaching hospitals. Relatively small and short-lived (Ms Silverthorne and her colleagues took the political decision to take their union into National Union of Public Employees (NUPE) within two years), it nonetheless articulated a radical nursing voice and confronted the leaders of the College of Nursing with its most serious challenge since the RBNA. Moreover, the National Union of County Officers (NUCO) started up its own Guild of Nurses as a consequence, with several of its leaders, such as Iris Brook and Doris Westmacott, standing on platforms with Ms Silverthorne.

In November 1937, the people of central London were presented with an astonishing sight. Like a feminine version of Banquo's ghost, nurses who were Guild members were marching through its streets wearing masks to hide their identity and prevent reprisals from the employers they were to continue haunting for the next fifty years. Their issues had plagued nurses throughout the previous half century – staffing shortages, low pay, a working week that was too long and working conditions that were widely perceived as not only exceptionally harsh but unnecessarily so. NUCO and the Association of Nurses succeeded in capturing the public imagination. Supported by the Labour Party and TUC, their calls for reform were impacting on government. After years of supporting the pay regime and number of hours nurses were working, as well as the rules, regulations and code of discipline imposed upon them, the College was changing its position to fall in behind the new consensus. The government bowed to the pressure and set up The Athlone Committee to investigate nursing shortages. It found that nurses' pay and conditions were key factors in the staffing shortfall. Against an unprecedented backdrop of discontent and protest, which was denounced in the pages of the nursing press but supported by national dailies such as the *Daily Herald* and *News Chronicle*, the committee recognised, as Florence Nightingale had nearly a half century before, that adequately training nurses in sufficient numbers and maintaining sufficient numbers of a trained workforce could not be achieved by a piecemeal system of private enterprise. Discovering that the local authorities and voluntary hospitals – the latter especially – were creaking at the seams and unable to fund their services properly, it made recommendations that national bargaining machinery be established, with local councils for every hospital. The arguments of those who had dared challenge nursing's traditions and vocational ideal were entirely vindicated when the Athlone Committee accepted that a 96 hour fortnight and increased pay for trained nurses were essential in the recruitment and retention of nurses, with government making grants to hospitals to fund higher wages and costs (Hart, 1994).

This was not far off the stuff of revolution. Implementation of the Athlone Committee's report would have laid the foundation for a nationalised health service and, almost inevitably, the government backed away. Yet again, at a crucial stage in nursing trade union development, war intervened. But neither the problems nor the arguments went away. With the likes of Thora Silverthorne, Avis Hutt, Norah Large and Iris Brooke still leading the way, nurses' protests continued through the early part of the Second World War as unemployment amongst the ranks of trained nurses actually grew, despite massive numbers of vacancies.

The roots of lasting change were, nonetheless, pushing their way through and, as the war came to an end, Labour secured a massive Commons majority, with plans for a National Health Service (NHS) one of the key objectives of the new government. The nurses' organisations of the period had already undergone significant changes. The College of Nursing had the title 'Royal' bestowed upon it by the King in 1939. Health service trade unions were planning a new merger to bring them all together as the Confederation of Health Service Employees (COHSE), which actually coincided with the inception of the NHS in 1948. It was COHSE and the RCN which were to dominate nursing politics in the new NHS, although NUPE, the RCM and HVA were all to exert varying amounts of influence through the years. NUPE exerted particular influence through its ancillary staff and transformation of its structures, developing the role of the shop steward and being one of the first unions to bring forward women into key positions, developing equal opportunities and recognising the importance of the low paid by enabling them to play an active part in senior positions within the union.

On the surface, it looked as if the NHS had taken nurses into its heart. The new Whitley Councils were established to oversee national negotiating that would cover all aspects of their pay and conditions. The trade unions and professional organisations were stronger than ever. But old rivalries were undiminished. The RCN had snared the largest number of seats of any individual organisation on the Nurses and Midwives' Whitley Council and, with the support of the other professional associations, had effective control of the staff side. It was, nonetheless, a hollow victory. After almost a century, modern nursing was still split down the middle both politically and philosophically and, above all, remained relatively powerless.

▶ The ties that bind, the ties that divide

These were not insignificant differences that were splitting the nursing organisations. The trade unions were coming from a position of having been explicitly excluded from decision making and having to force their members' agenda onto the negotiating table. Industrial action had been a legitimate tool, amongst its many others, to achieve its objectives. Having ancillary staff, administrators and other health workers in its membership, its interests were not exclusively those of nurses. Those members, many nurses included, often from families where parents or other relatives had been members of a trade union, identified themselves within a strong working-class tradition and drew upon collectivist principles. Distrustful of management and senior staff, their often oppositionalist stance became woven into their culture.

The so-called professional associations, on the other hand, came from a tradition of working within a power construct, no matter how limited and limiting. Industrial action was anathema. On the surface, this was obviously in keeping with the notion that patients must always be cared for and protected. But their leaders also realised it would alienate employers and government. Many of the RCN's leaders were also, of course, nurses responsible for maintaining the service. Defining progress as increasing status, and achieving improved status by increasing the scope and scale of the nurse's role within a given system meant that they were confined to working within that system, influencing and lobbying whenever possible. Wanting close ties to those in power, the RCN remained determinedly aloof from the TUC and political parties, the opposite position of the other trade unions, all of whom affiliated to both the Labour Party and TUC.

Given the difficulties in presenting a coherent vision of nursing and nurses' aspirations, it was all the more difficult for COHSE. Many of its nurse members' interests and issues were similar to those of other occupational groups. However, it was hard to create any space to address those concerns peculiar to nurses or create an identity which would appeal to nurses who were not yet members. There were simmering tensions between different occupational groups, with nurses often criticised for not wanting 'get their hands dirty' and campaign with and for other members. As privatisation took its toll on ancillary members in the 1980s, nurses became more prominent and their interests came to the fore, undoubtedly a factor in the surge of clinical militancy in the latter part of that decade.

The professional associations and trade unions also represented a fundamental difference in the way in which policy was formulated and delivered. COHSE took the traditional trade union approach, with its annual delegate conference – at least notionally – the supreme decision making body. This involved branches debating their own motions and then submitting them for the Conference several months in advance, where they would again be debated and voted upon. It had a detailed rule book, policies and procedures about how its business should be conducted at every level. These were all part of a structural approach its founders had taken to ensure maximum democratic involvement and to bind its membership to the principle that all would abide by the decision of the majority. Officials at almost every level had to be elected. In an age when decision making in the rest of the NHS was equally deliberate, there were not any major problems posed by this approach. Besides, the reality was that, whenever necessity, or pragmatism dictated, the unions' national executive council, which met every three months, could initiate action. Even in between that, COHSE's full-time officers would negotiate and act within a policy framework that left them varying degrees of flexibility. However, as the pace of change in the NHS increased and management became more ruthless, the limitation of this way of working became exposed as too centralised and cumbersome. Moreover, the system of deciding policy through conference motion may have had some attraction in addressing the union's concerns about democratic process, but had tremendous shortfalls in terms of allowing rational and cohesive policy making, with decisions being made in the hothouse of brief and impassioned – but not necessarily informed – debate, with delegates' votes being cast for a variety of reasons.

The hierarchical approach of the RCN mitigated against this. Its annual Congress was stage managed long before New Labour began the process. Motions were vetted beforehand and, if passed at the conference, only carried the status of recommendations to the ruling Council, which had an extremely close relationship to the College's paid staff. With the general secretary then having responsibility for delivering on policy decisions, far more autonomy was delegated to the leadership by the significantly less politicised members, the majority of whom, by adhering far more to nursing's traditions and ideals, were also more deferential and willing to subordinate their own needs, in this case to their organisation. The College could then be more responsive and pro-active, particularly in the 1980s, a period when its increasingly managerialist culture had already been reinforced by the experience of its senior members after the Salmon Report in 1966.

It was these traditions that influenced nurses in their choice of organisation as much as anything, although the RCN had another significant advantage over the trade unions in encouraging new members into its ranks. Given that many, if not most, senior nurses, including tutors in the schools of nursing, were College members there was an obvious incentive in joining the same organisation, as well as the simple consequence of the role modelling that was part and parcel of the apprenticeship style of training that nurses undertook. Indeed, many nurses would change their membership from a trade union to the RCN as they moved up the career ladder, particularly in education. Tutors would, in turn, use their influence to recruit students into the College (Bellaby and Oribor, 1980; COHSE, 1990). Reasons given in various surveys over the years have been consistent, with College members saying they enrolled because it is 'for nurses' and stood for professional issues (Smith 1982; Mackay, 1989). Joining one of the health service trade unions was considered an 'act of solidarity', usually with other nurses. Outside of general nursing, that solidarity ran across grades, from untrained nurses to senior managers.

The first twenty years of the NHS saw the two sides build upon their respective strengths. However, beginning in the late 1960s, considerable movement back and forth between trade unions and the College took place, particularly during periods of heightened workplace tension. Nurses shifted according to their preference, either towards more direct action and a confrontational stance towards either employers or the other way. Another major factor in recruitment of new members would be the local officials and whether they were viewed positively or not. With pay and conditions becoming more and more of an issue, while nurses were able to advance nursing developments within their own clinical areas, the role of the unions and professional associations was coming into focus – and under the scrutiny of nurses who were potential members.

By the 1970s, the Whitley Council negotiating machinery was 'failing abysmally' both to deliver satisfactory national agreements or meet the needs of staff and managers locally. It was being used to 'contain costs by depressing health workers' salaries' (Klein 1989; Sethi and Dimmock, 1982). Nurses were being radicalised not only by their concern over their own pay and conditions but also ward and hospital closures occurring up and down the country. The combustible mood of nurses only made the process of union recruitment that much easier while the dramatic explosion of industrial unrest then enabled the unions to get more stewards and branch officials into the 'front line' of hospital politics.

Looking at the fluctuations of COHSE's membership in the 1970s and 1980s, it is possible to discern a pattern that relates to its willingness to lead with radical campaigns and the perceived success of those campaigns. Thus, its nursing membership increased steadily in the 1970s as it took industrial action in pursuit of improved pay that did fulfil its members' aspirations to a degree, which continued until it peaked in 1982, the year of the largest health service dispute ever. After that, the union's membership drifted into a steady decline that was arrested only in the period of clinical militancy in 1987–88. Any lack of success – at least in the minds of the participants – was followed by a move across to the RCN. Whether this was by the same nurses who had earlier deserted the College for COHSE is not clear (and on some occasions, as in 1988, it was a case of both new nurses joining one of the organisations and significant shifts both ways rather than one way traffic), but from 1988 the flow was steady. From COHSE to the RCN. The financial and political cost of this was one of the key factors in the union's leadership recommending that it merge with NUPE and Nalgo to form Unison. All three had suffered steadily declining membership throughout the 1980s and early 1990s, as had many other unions. The College, meanwhile, was able to double its membership during the same period, announcing it had the astonishing total of 300,000 nurses either trained or in training, in membership by 1993. Within a decade, a further 50,000 had been added to the College's membership, which included 37,000 students (RCN Bulletin, 2003). The correlation and affinity of nursing organisations with the social trends and politics of a given period are further reflected by COHSE's expansion in the preceding decade, when it had virtually doubled its membership between 1973 and 1983, reaching its peak of 222,000 members.

▶ A new dawn – or evening gloom gathering?

The great success of the RCN has been, for good or bad, to establish itself at the very heart of nursing practice. This has been through a combination of influences, not always complimentary. Its managerialist wing has worked to see that nurses deliver a service. Its 'professionalising' wing, made up of nurses working in education or occupying senior positions where clinical developments could both be nurtured and disseminated, dominated the education and practice agenda. In this latter aspect, an alliance between professionalisers and mangerialists – not something that always occurs or can be taken for granted – is also important, offering the opportunity to spread good practice. Because of its success, the College can attract the most gifted nurses and this, in turn, has enabled it to become one of the key training resources in the United Kingdom. Some members cite the use of its library and educational facilities as the only reason they joined. The effects ripple out through research, education and practice, meaning it has as much influence on nursing practice as any other body in nursing. It would be unthinkable for any nursing committee that wanted to be taken seriously not to have RCN representation on it and this would be true at almost any level within the NHS as much as it would be at the Department of Health or devolved organisations within any of the other UK countries. The same would be largely true of the other specialist organisations, such as the RCM, in their own area of expertise while Unison does the best it can, given its very limited resource.

Yet, this is like the house built in sand. It lacks the solid foundation that sustains progress and consolidates good practice on a global basis. The developments in nursing practice, training and education are subject to the storms of economic, political and strategic change and, in those testing moments, the College lacks the power to hold onto its gains. Much the same is true of Unison in the field of industrial relations. It shares some of New Labour's agenda and has been able to make the running on matters such as shared governance and *Agenda for Change*. But, for the same reasons as the College when it comes to clinical developments, it cannot bridge the gap between getting its members' needs and its own key objectives met unless it has the agreement of politicians, civil servants and, on matters that affect *its* members' interests, the medical profession.

On one level, it could be argued that the RCN has, at least, always been able to keep up with the evolving political world of nursing, if not remain one step ahead.

It used its position, as an organisation run by the senior nurses in that world, and the ideology it helped shape and perpetuate, to maintain its primacy and reproduce itself. Its independence gave it political flexibility. Having gradually accepted men, enrolled nurses, students and mental health nurses into membership, perhaps its biggest about turn, after years of opposing the inclusion of untrained healthcare staff, was for its leadership to recommend they be brought into the fold, with no convincing explanation for its changed position. Similarly, Rule 12, which forbade College members from participating in any form of industrial action and was considered '...a means of defining our behaviour...the real importance of which [was] symbolic' was abandoned amid high moral fanfares (Clarke, 1988).

If the 1980s was a pivotal decade for nursing, the same could be said for their trade unions, and one from which the reverberations still echo loudly in the new century. The RCN had steered its internal organisation and direction with little interference from government or the employers. In mirroring the consumerist trend of the times, it was one of the first unions to develop membership services that were unrelated to trade union or direct employment activity, ranging from car insurance to financial services. It further extended its educational wing and publishing arm, resurrecting its magazine, the *Nursing Standard*, and moving into publishing with Scutari Books.[1] It introduced direct mailing, keeping its members up-to-date with its activities and views, and sought new ways and new areas in which to recruit, with the result that it saw a rapid growth in members who worked part time, virtually all of whom were women, with many coming from the private sector. Its increasing membership reflected its growing confidence and many nurses' weariness for any further industrial conflict.

COHSE and other TUC affiliated unions experienced significant membership losses and political defeat as privatisation trundled through the NHS. Industrial action against cuts and closures in services was often equally unsuccessful and resulted in a loss of confidence and poor morale amongst activists. The defeat of the miners after their bitter strike of 1984–85, the print unions in Wapping in 1986, and the almost total loss of influence on the part of the TUC at government level added to its woes. For the RCN, the only overt setback during this period – serious as it was – came with the introduction of general management and the effects it had on its senior nurse members. The College was even able to turn the aftermath of the 1982 pay dispute to its advantage, claiming the Pay Review Body (PRB) was a reward for its moderate position and negotiating skills, an assertion supported by the prime minister no less.

The first industrial relations legislation under the Thatcher government was passed in 1980 and followed by subsequent Acts in 1982, 1984, 1988 and 1990. Amongst other things, these placed increasingly severe restrictions on picketing, restricted the 'closed shop', removed blanket immunity from trade unions,

---

[1] The College had long since cut its ties with the *Nursing Times*.

imposed election timetables on senior union positions, made unions regularly ballot their members to retain any political fund, prevented unions from disciplining members who refused to strike or who crossed picket lines, made them repudiate unofficial strikes and, finally, have to get existing members to periodically sign forms to state that they still wished to be members of the union they had joined in the first place (Marsh, 1992). Although some 'reforms' were widely recognised as welcome and overdue, others were perceived as imposing practices that were alien, highly restrictive and carrying a crippling administrative burden. Amidst these enforced changes, not only did COHSE and NUPE, and then Unison after them, have to worry about their own position, they also had to maintain a corporate position of unity within the TUC, whether or not it was in their best interests.

Particularly difficult and damaging was the need to get everyone to 'sign up' to stay in the union. Anyone who could not be contacted directly and signed their form would have to be taken out of membership. If the member paid by direct debit from their bank account, this was relatively easy. One of the key administrative shifts the RCN had made was to move virtually its entire membership to pay by direct debit, but for unions like Unison, with over a million members, many of whom had their subscription paid directly out of their wages, it was a mammoth task that had to take priority over all else.

The greater political intensity of the 1980s also drew the nurses' organisations closer together in a number of ways. COHSE began to make public statements that signalled a shift from its conservative position in relation to patient care and clinical development, reflecting the attitudes of younger members who were beginning to exert real influence. This was supported by its decision to make inroads into the 'professional' domain previously exclusive to the College, employing two professional officers, adopting more progressive policies towards community care and advances in mental health nursing – still its strongest membership base – particularly.

The RCN was able to stay at the forefront of nursing developments because it was often their members who were involved, whether the new initiatives were occurring in education or practice. This approach to new ideas and innovation, no matter how small the scale, was undoubtedly another element that was so attractive to students and younger, junior nurses. But it also enabled the College to define itself – as much as its historical attachment to Rule 12 – while maintaining its position within the corridors of power in the worlds of education and practice. It might not have had a high backed, comfortable armchair in the old boys' club of doctors, civil servants and politicians, or a place reserved at the policy making table, but it walked effortlessly through the corridors of the anonymous empire of decision makers, whispering its influence, throwing knowing glances and making every effort to make its presence felt. With Labour's collaborative relationship with the unions having collapsed in acrimony and recrimination, to be succeeded by the open indifference, if not hostility, of the Thatcher government, for all its efforts, COHSE, as with the other health and public sector unions, stood outside in the cold, looking in, despairing of ever finding the key to the door, let alone getting into the corridor.

▶ All for one or a free for all?

If the 1980s were a high water mark for nurses in bringing together their clinical and industrial aspirations, why were the unions and nurses' associations unable to capitalise on the relative strength, radicalism and coherence in their ranks? The battle for members was a significant factor. The entire dispute before, during and after clinical grading was conducted by both the main organisations with at least a partial eye on recruitment, each watching their own and their rivals' fluctuating fortunes like hawks. Every member was fought over. Nor was the rivalry simply between COHSE and the RCN. The dividing line between the College and COHSE went beyond the issue of tactics. It was deeply philosophical and political. But other health workers could be tempted into different trade unions if they felt COHSE was concentrating too much on its nurse members. Similarly, NUPE or Nalgo branches could try and outdo COHSE's radicalism in this period – regardless of their national union's caution – and win members in the process. The HVA, as it was then, or the RCM, were not particularly in a position to make major advances in attracting members. Indeed, the HVA was drifting into a period of crisis, while the RCM was trying to react to the unexpected disadvantages following clinical grading.

This competition for nurses was driven by a number of concerns. Partly it was a straightforward matter of 'my army's bigger than your army', with each organisation wanting to sell itself as the biggest nurses' union, equating size with quality and effectiveness. Members, however, brought money. This was of increasing importance as the union's emphasis moved from seeking to organise members in the workplace to providing extraneous services. With its members paying more in annual subscriptions than any of the unions, the College benefited even more from every new member brought into its ranks. Money, inevitably, could be invested in campaigns, membership services and the organisation's infrastructure, thus enabling it to maintain an effective and high profile.

There were also structural problems that stemmed from the very nature of the organisations themselves. The RCN, while accommodating people who had radical ideas clinically, was both politically and industrially conservative. Senior figures like Tom Bolger, as well as some activists and branches, may have been critical of Trevor Clay's leadership during the clinical grading dispute but enough nurses in key positions within the College also occupied senior positions in the NHS. The majority would accept the leadership provided on such issues. Because of this close relationship between the College's leadership and the NHS, its vested interests actually went beyond keeping up a cordial relationship with government and the health service employers. It was actually instrumental in helping to maintain the status quo or, if change were to happen, helping to manage the process of that change.

COHSE had gone out on a limb in the late 1980s but, as its membership slipped back into decline, facing, at best, an uncertain financial future, its political room for manoeuvre was severely constricted. The other unions were following the 'line' that the best way to support the Labour Party in its efforts to get elected was to maintain a relatively low profile and not 'rock the political boat'. Moreover, in the aftermath of clinical grading, trade union officials had had their hands full with appeals; as activists fell away, networks were breaking down and the relentless nature of the political climate was taking its toll.

The RCN never actually had strong local networks of stewards and activists to collapse. Its membership support was built around the work of relatively few lay officials in the workplace, but good communications into and out of its head office, that could be accessed by members directly, with full-time officers or seconded stewards carrying out a lot of representation of members. This was, therefore, another significant change of the period that did not affect the College. Like its counterparts in the trade union movement, however, the RCN was strongly centralist in its philosophy and did not want to relinquish any control. It was protective of its work within national negotiating committees such as the Whitley Councils and unwilling to cede any decision making from that level, which inevitably posed problems when trying to adapt to the challenges posed by the introduction of the internal market and the threats and opportunities that came with the potential for local bargaining. Moreover, the struggle for control within nursing was still far from over. Although there was a need to mend fences after the fractious arguing of that late 1980s, with COHSE and the College continuing to share duties on the Nurses and Midwives Whitley Council, both were still vying for, but could not achieve, overall dominance. The divide was as wide as ever and the weakness was being ruthlessly exploited by a government that had been seriously damaged by nurses when they had briefly managed to pull together, finding common cause in the aspects of *their* work and values.

▶ Unison – dangling in a tangled web

There was a historical inevitability about COHSE's decision to join in the faltering negotiations taking place between Nalgo and NUPE, with a view to forming a 'super union', a public sector union that would have a combined membership of over 1 million. A number of other unions had already merged to increase their critical mass and consolidate their finances. With the closer movement of health services to other public services, it followed the tradition of earlier health service union mergers.

Unison had so much going for it compared to COHSE in terms of size, resource and opportunity. There was a health group which encompassed all health branches and their members nationwide, with a lay committee responsible for providing leadership and a team of full-time officials at its national head office. Within the health group, a nursing committee was formed at a national level. Although there was no increase in the number of ex nurses to work alongside its professional officers, Paul Chapman and Karen Jennings, they had far more resources within the overall group, as well as access to staff working in communications, education, research, campaigns and legal services. The union divided its membership into thirteen geographical regions across the United Kingdom, each having its own council of delegates drawn from branches, forming the main link between branches and the national executive council, the union's supreme decision making body outside its annual national conference. A regional committee is responsible for leading the union within the region, again working alongside a large team of full-time officials. A team of full-time officers specialising in health worked within the regions and, although very few of the ex-NUPE and Nalgo staff had previous nursing experience, most had worked alongside nursing stewards and were familiar with the key issues facing nurses and other health workers. The British Association of Occupational Therapists merged with the union within weeks and in 1996, the Scottish Health Visitors Association completed a merger with Unison. When New Labour romped to victory in 1997, as the country's biggest union and largest political donor in the labour movement, Unison seemed poised to reap their rewards.

Yet, something had gone wrong. The merger negotiations had been extremely fraught as the three unions tried to satisfy their members' often very different aspirations and their full-time staff's concerns over their employment; the contrasting histories, cultures, structures, policies and procedures meant complex compromises were necessary. Activists wanted decision making as close to the shop floor as possible. Service groups, such as that for health, had to be accommodated alongside different councils, executive committees and specialist groups that would operate at a national and regional level. When Unison came into being in July 1993 its protagonists had created a multi-layered, tangled matrix that, through sheer size and complexity, inevitably suffocated spontaneity and leant even more heavily on procedure and bureaucracy. It was almost immediately gripped by tensions between branches, regions, the national structures and service groups. The devolved, lay activist led ex-Nalgo culture was incompatible with the centralist, full-time officer dominated culture that had developed in NUPE post-1979. All of these factors dogged attempts to forge new relationships needed at all levels of the organisation. Nor was any of this happening in isolation. The political climate at the time of its inception was deeply hostile and every part of the union was facing the most demanding challenges imaginable.

Ironically, the health group itself was perhaps most successful in forging a new identity. But it was increasingly marginalised within the union's wider structures. Before long, lay activists were drifting away from meetings lacking a health focus and even Unison's regional health committees had a lower attendance than either COHSE or NUPE had enjoyed individually pre-merger, despite the far greater number of members in the new union.

Concern about the relationship of the health group to the rest of the union grew steadily through its early years until a research project was commissioned to explore the actual reasons for key activists withdrawing on the scale they were. Only 20 per cent of those surveyed believed the health group had enough influence at a regional and national level and that many representatives from health had never 'opted in' to Unison structures in the first place, instead feeling distinct and separate from it. Some saw Unison 'as an entity separate from branch activity' with 'evidence of some resistance among active members of the health group towards further involvement in Unison as a whole' (Unison, 1998b).

Although deciphering union membership claims is an art in itself – the RCN reputedly never takes anyone off its membership lists, even after death, and senior figures within Unison privately acknowledge that their membership lists have long been wildly inaccurate – there are some indications that Unison has seen at best a steady state, but possibly some decline in the number of trained nurses in its ranks.[2] The general decline in membership that hit the trade unions so hard since the early 1980s has almost certainly been reversed as the expected increase in union membership under a Labour government has again occurred.

At the heart of this lies a great confusion about what sort of union Unison wishes to be. Its declared objective is to be an organising union but an internal survey 'suggests that the union has a long way to go before achieving [*its*] goal'. It continues to pour millions of pounds into membership services yet only 2.2 per cent of members cited this as a reason for being in the union, while 82.2 per cent was in it to receive support should a problem arise at work. Worryingly, and only partially within its control, the number who join because they believe in trade unions and want to take part stood only at 27.5 per cent although 57.2 per cent wanted to help get better pay and conditions (Kerr and Waddington, 1998). It has a similar dilemma about its nurse membership. Karen Jennings' elevation to head of nursing was almost universally welcomed but occurred at a time when the union, as a result of its strategic review, was diluting the service groups. Coinciding with another round of cost cutting in the face of continuing membership losses and financial difficulties, senior officers moved out of the health team at a national level. More important, as a result of a strategic review ordered by the National Executive Council, was the effective loss of the most senior health post in the regions, with their deputies being given a range of other tasks as well as managing the health groups within their patch. At the same time, many of the regions scrapped using full-time officers who specialised in health work, moving instead to a generic model. The direct relationship between the national and regional health groups was also effectively severed. Despite being deeply unpopular with health

---

[2] The exception to this would appear to be Scotland, where health membership is reported to have increased by 2000 in the period 2001–02 in the light of several high profile and successful pay campaigns.

members and prominent activists, the union ploughed on with its strategy, described by its then president as heralding, 'The "real Unison" replacing five years of "compromise structures" in the wake of the merger' in 1993 (Unison, 1998c).

It is not simply that Unison, the United Kingdom's biggest union, has virtually no profile amongst large groups of nurses, health workers or those associated with the NHS. Despite the efforts of those working at a national level in health, the union apparently has little to say that will engage its members in partnership, no coherent strategy that will help articulate nurses' needs and enable them to be met.[3] If it has, it has spectacularly failed in its attempts to communicate it. Even campaigns such as that for safe needles that will prevent needlestick injuries, and its 'Be Safe' campaign for better standards of care fail to make a significant impact. Unison's national conference has very few nurses or health workers playing an influential role, of great concern to the union's leadership and concerned membership, but a problem it has been unable to resolve; moreover, its health conference is increasingly becoming less important in the day-to-day realities experienced by those working in the NHS. It is now barely reported at all. Its presence in hospitals and other health service workplaces is solely due to the diligence of good branch secretaries, where they still exist. Perhaps, most importantly for a trade union, few of its key members can identify with it. Fewer still make any acknowledgement of liking it. Perhaps the most revealing comment about the relationship between the union and its members comes from some senior lay officials working in health who claim that dealing with Unison is similar to dealing with their own management in terms of bureaucracy and an apparent lack of understanding of the issues they are grappling with in their own work.

Yet, where a clear and identifiable presence in health has been maintained, it has yielded results. Within each region, there are success stories. Of interest has been the experience in Scotland, where Unison has developed a strong relationship with the Scottish Executive, albeit in a very different political climate to that of the English regions. Its officers and members have been co-opted onto working parties and committees and the union has easy access to interested ministers and civil servants. Nonetheless, where there have been genuine differences on industrial relations issues, Unison has not shied away from representing its members' interests, even to the point of industrial action, with its health organiser, Jim Devine, and

---

[3] One of Unison's great success stories has come from the work of people like Tony Chandler, in making major inroads into the area of lifelong learning, forming partnerships with employers to co-sponsor educational programmes for staff, particularly those who have not participated in any formal educational activity since leaving school, and working with government at a national level. Although Unison's education team has also developed innovative education and training packages for stewards and representatives, these have not been able to bolster the union's organisational decline in the workplace.

officers maintaining a high profile in the national media. Another exception has been the union's stand on student nurses, which has been an example of the type of leadership and campaigning it seems unable to replicate in other areas. It is rarely out of the nursing press as it pushes for improved conditions for students, an end to bursaries and educational reform (see Chapter 8). In some respects, this is similar to Paul Chapman's work with Healthcare Assistants (HCAs) and issues concerning their role, training and education.

Dave Prentis was elected as Rodney Bickerstaffe's successor in the middle of the furore over generic working of regional officials and the undermining of the health groups as a result of the strategic review. Despite associating himself closely with the review, he insisted that he was mindful of nurses' and other health workers' concerns. He took a higher profile than the then head of health, Bob Abberley, on nursing issues despite being tragically struck down with stomach cancer soon after his successful election, spending long months in treatment before making a welcome recovery. Prentis has since established himself as one of the clear leaders in the union movement, skilfully occupying the difficult position of 'critical friend' to the government but, at the time of writing, being pushed further and further into being critical by the government's stance on the fire fighter's dispute and war against Iraq. That he has been unafraid to align himself more with his members on these issues than New Labour and gained a far more prominent position on the national stage as a consequence has, in some respects, only served to underline the impression that Unison is increasingly a generalist union. The distance from the vast majority of its members working in healthcare remains undented, although members in other service groups report similar problems.

Whatever its relative strengths and weaknesses, COHSE was a remarkably 'well integrated union', on the evidence of a detailed survey published in its final months (Whitston and Waddington, 1993). Unison seems to find it hard to reach out to the average nurse, perhaps because of its own internal structures. The difficulties health members had with their union manifested regularly at health conferences when decisions recommended by the health group executive were rejected time and again by activists on the conference floor. It was so bad in 1996 that the then general secretary and a visitor to the conference, Rodney Bickerstaffe, had to 'warn delegates to "get their act together"'. (Payne, 1996). Many, however, took this to be a warning to the union's leaders in the health group as much as anything.

Even Unison's apparent successes have to be re-examined in the light of actual achievement. It has forged a far closer relationship with government than any of the former partner unions could ever have hoped for, and does have immediate and ready access to senior civil servants and ministers. But what tangible outcomes have come from that? Probably the key issues for Unison in health have been pay and conditions, the Private Finance Initiative [PFI] and keeping the private sector at bay. The 2002 pay award was announced to universal anger from nurses. Non-PRB staff seems almost at the point of giving up protesting. Health workers' response to virtually each pay award under New Labour has been largely one of disgruntled acceptance. PFI remains as a key plank of government policy, despite Unison's claims that it has won significant concessions. Both Blair and Milburn have repeatedly slapped the unions collectively in the face over the private sector, despite then coming back apologetically. There is no substance to this new relationship, they say, let's try and make another go of it – and, by the way, please keep on handing over the political fund donations. And then they go and repeat the process, as witnessed by the health secretary's statement on foundation hospitals. Bob Abberley may have stated that 'he sees Alan Milburn as "often as needed" and special advisors on an almost weekly basis', adding, 'We're part of the family now' (Cole, 2001: pp 24–7). But if this is true, it has all the ingredients of an abusive relationship and is a family seriously in need of therapy.

▶ The RCN: facing both ways at the same time

The last decade has been far from plain sailing for the RCN. Trevor Clay announced his impending retirement as general secretary during the clinical grading dispute and went the following year. With its usual prescience and willingness to do the unexpected, the College appointed Christine Hancock as his successor as general secretary. Significantly, at the time of her appointment, she was not working as a nurse at all but was a general manager. As outwardly cautious and reserved as Clay had been flamboyant and charismatic, Hancock faced almost as many challenges as her counterparts at Unison, albeit for very different reasons. Although it was not directly bearing the brunt of the government's hostility, the College was not being showered with much more than platitudes. While it was in accordance with government policy, there were no problems. On key issues where it disagreed, no quarter was offered. This had most visibly been the case at each year's pay round but also, crucially, on the loss of senior nursing positions post-Griffiths and, along with everyone else involved in healthcare, when the decision had been made to introduce the internal market and, even more antithetical to the College's philosophy, local pay bargaining.

With the emphasis that had been placed on membership services during Clay's reign, there was insufficient infrastructure to support a solid and comprehensive industrial relations initiative and this had to be beefed up rapidly. Hancock also undertook an internal re-organisation that proved less than popular with some of the staff re-organised.

The College had to be prepared to punch its weight over some political issues with the Tories when they were in power. It constantly disputed government claims about nurse numbers and was highly critical of staged pay awards. Again, it has taken the same position with New Labour. Indeed, at its 2000 Congress, Christine Hancock went so far as to argue that the government had only six months to save the NHS. It would do this, she said, by turning targets and deadlines into action and introducing a new pay structure that would reward nurses 'properly' (Munro, 2000a: p 5). However, history forced Hancock to lead the RCN into two policy changes that would have had her predecessors rending their uniforms in disgust.

The greatest nurses' pay dispute that never happened took place in 1995. The background to this was the government pushing forward with its agenda for local pay bargaining within its internal market. NHS trusts were using a minimum offer, based on a PRB recommendation, and choosing to add to it or not. Having made no progress in negotiations with the government, the decision was taken to ballot the membership on changing Rule 12 – to allow RCN members to take industrial action that would not be harmful to patients – and was supported by a 95 per cent majority, with 39 per cent of eligible members voting, then ratified at an emergency general meeting, when the announcement was greeted with 'whoops of joy' (Carlisle, 1995: pp 5–6).

Historic, yes. But why a change of the policy that had defined the organisation up until then? The membership was ready for it. Nurses everywhere were fed up with the market, the changed culture in which they were being forced to work, the way in which nursing and nursing care were secondary to financial and contracting issues. But, put simply, local bargaining would probably have signalled the end of the RCN as it had stood for the past seventy nine years. Had it been successfully introduced, local pay bargaining would have required a branch-negotiating framework within every NHS trust. Whether or not that was manageable, it would have fundamentally changed the nature of the relationship between members and their individual union. Alliances would have to have been developed with other unions in the workplace to ensure that negotiating committees worked collectively within their trust and used the necessary tactics to secure the best deal possible. The position of the national union on the key issue of pay and conditions would have been far less important and, therefore, they would be less important overall. Nurses would, by necessity, have to re-define their relationship to other health workers within their own workplace. The College suddenly found itself facing the contradiction of its position as a professional organisation and trade union – albeit, one which did not allow itself recourse to the full armoury of a trade union, including industrial action. After the trench warfare of clinical grading appeals, it had very few branch activists, no comprehensive industrial relations strategy to develop strong local organisation and, indeed, had nurses as members partly because they had been convinced that this was *not* the way nursing should develop. Local pay bargaining would, at best, create a new breed of RCN activist. At worst, it would have produced a haemorrhage of members into unions that had the infrastructure and willingness to represent their members locally.

Of Unison's partner unions, only COHSE had developed a policy that saw local pay bargaining as offering any advantages. NUPE had remained opposed to it. However, despite the obvious difficulty it would have provided for their main nursing rival, Unison's opposition to the government's strategy was just as solid, just as was the case with the other unions. The RCN could heave a sigh of relief and the election of New Labour less than two years later seemed to have ended the threat.

The other major event during Hancock's period of leadership was admitting (HCAs) into membership. Unison professional officer, Paul Chapman, a long time champion of HCAs, observed on numerous occasions that the elitist attitude and snobbery of the College would put HCAs off joining, even if they had the chance, a point emphasised by RCN members urging colleagues to vote against admitting them into membership because it would damage the organisation's credibility with the BMA (Gulland, 1998b: p 5).

Having been debated at Congress and rejected numerous times, Council in 2000 finally agreed to ballot the entire membership on whether or not to admit HCAs, but not into full membership. They were to be given voting rights but barred from standing for president, deputy president, the ruling council or having automatic rights to join any of the specialist clinical forums. Nor would they be able to nominate anyone for Council membership or president. Even were they to become stewards, they would not be allowed to represent registered nurses. Nor was membership to be thrown open to all HCAs. Only those with an National Vocational Qualification (NVQ) level 3, the equivalent of two A-levels, and numbering an estimated 8000 would be eligible to join. The membership, predictably, did not suffer the same angst as their representatives. An overwhelming 78 per cent voted in favour. But, despite a personal plea from Christine Hancock in the form of a post card to all its members, only 14 per cent actually voted.

Admitting HCAs meant jettisoning another of the College's defining principles that it was solely for nurses.[4] The RCN's leadership was pushing the issue again and again because of the increasing prominence – and numbers – of HCAs in the NHS and the evolving nature of the nursing workforce. Project 2000 meant students were no longer contributing to patients' care as part of the healthcare team. Competency-based NVQs meant managers knew exactly what they were getting with their HCAs. HCAs were also much lower paid and, therefore, more affordable than their registered colleagues. Their role was expanding to include work that would previously have been the domain of the registered nurse. A paper circulated through RCN Council and committees argued that, 'As long as healthcare assistants deliver a considerable amount of hands-on care, *and are outside the control of nursing*, they will present a dangerous, cheap and unregulated rival to nursing that could enable employers to wrest control of care delivery from the profession' [my emphasis] (Naish, 1998: pp 26–8). Just as it always has, the RCN was willing to adjust its course according to the prevailing winds. The apparently unshakeable tenets upon which it is built are no more than part of the mythology it has always

---

[4] The RCN had fought a long running dispute with Unison in the mid-1990s about whether or not untrained staff could carry the title, 'Nurse', with the College arguing vehemently that untrained staff were *not* nurses.

skilfully employed to control its membership and nurses. The political nature of the decision to admit HCAs is perhaps best underlined by the comments of the RCN's president in 1996, who told Congress delegates in her keynote speech that 'nurses could not be treated like other health workers and that the RCN was not, and never would be, a royal college of health workers'. These sentiments were endorsed by Christine Hancock, who commented, '[Nurses] are not like other health workers and we won't apologise for saying so' (Cassidy, 1996: p 20).

The opportunity to increase subscription income was thought by some to be another motivation for bringing HCAs into membership. Having paid out £15 million to renovate its already plush headquarters in London's Cavendish Square, money has often been a source of discontent for the College. Repeatedly, criticism was thrown at Hancock for what many thought an already over inflated salary that went up in sizeable chunks. In 1998, the College's accounts showed the average RCN salary at just over £24,000, the equivalent of an I grade nurse, with its general secretary earning £78,651 – considerably higher than Rodney Bickerstaffe at Unison – and an increased number of staff earning in excess of £40,000. The following year, plans were announced to scrap all face-to-face teaching programmes at the RCN institute because they were no longer affordable. With a 5.1 per cent pay rise set for College staff in 2000, stewards and activists were again critical of their leaders. However, these views were not shared by RCN staff, who threatened industrial action after an expected 5.7 per cent increase was not forthcoming in 2001. This was against a backdrop of a new general secretary negotiating for improved terms and conditions after being offered a salary with a maximum of £99,000. Members' resentment exploded in 2001, when the details of the package Beverley Malone, the new general secretary, would be receiving, as well as confirmation that junior officers in the College were receiving £27,000, while senior managers were getting between £55,000 and £72,000, paid by subscriptions from nurses, the vast majority of whom were earning well below £20,000. The furore that followed a further request for members' subscriptions to be raised in 2001, after a £16 increase the year before, was wholly predictable.

The argument was not just about money, however. Support or criticism of the organisation's spending was shaped by concerns about openness and priorities. Being left out in the cold when it came to decision making, many activists were worrying about whether or not a self-serving elite was taking advantage of this 'distance' and lack of involvement of the vast majority of their members. This had become increasingly pronounced during the latter part of the 1990s, never more so than when Council decided to withhold 5 per cent of any legal settlement won for RCN members – a decision taken by an organisation that purported to be a trade union but, in a naked use of its power, did not allow its members to decide on something so fundamental to their concerns.

These issues emerged openly during the College's presidential elections in 2000, when the status of the president's position was questioned. The president is senior to the general secretary, as the position holder is elected by the entire membership rather than appointed by Council. Yet the president actually ends up playing second fiddle, by a long way. Ray Rowden put himself forward as the candidate of the 'rank and file', as opposed to the 'RCN hierarchy' and criticised the way in which closed committees made decisions. He wasn't voted in by the rank and file, but there was a surprise result as the incumbent, Christine Watson, was voted out. Rowden argued this still represented a vote for change. The membership suggested it was happy to be managed rather than led and only marginally more interested than deciding whether or not HCAs joined them. A mere 16 per cent voted. However, it could be argued this was a case of a sophisticated audience recognising another pre-written script when it saw one, deciding that, whoever won, little would change.

Emphasis on leadership in the RCN is so pronounced because, as an organisation, that is how it maintains its public profile. With its already small number of activists diminishing still further, nurses don't often have local figureheads. Its regional officials tend to have little contact with members because there are very few meetings and no infrastructure for them to have ongoing involvement with. Although there are some prominent lay activists who will appear fairly regularly on the pages of the *Nursing Times* or its own *Nursing Standard* (which does give exposure to its views and personalities), they don't generally gain a profile with the national media. This is partly because Christine Hancock, like Trevor Clay before her, was not one to bring colleagues into the public eye. Although renowned as a skilful political operator, Hancock was far less comfortable in the public arena than Clay, resulting in the College's profile dropping considerably outside of nursing. However, the emphasis on the general secretary also reflected the organisation's hierarchical underpinning – something that is a genuine principle that has yet to change. The boss is just that. The boss.

For once, the new boss was definitely not the same as the old boss. When it was announced in early 2001 that an African-American woman, who had never nursed in the United Kingdom and wasn't a member, was the new general secretary of the RCN the nursing world was turned upside down. If Hancock had been the College's choice in the face of general management, what did Beverley Malone's arrival signal? Amidst the hullabaloo about exactly what she had demanded by way of salary and relocation expenses from the United States, some facts emerged. Having undertaken a master's degree in psychiatric nursing and doctorate in clinical psychology, she had gone on to become president of the American Nurses' Association. After that she worked in President Clinton's administration, at one stage occupying the most senior position ever held by a nurse in the US government. She had also been married to the drummer of the 1970s soul band, The Spinners, hanging out with the likes of Stevie Wonder and Aretha Franklin (O'Dowd, 2001: pp 10–11). Given that it wasn't her musical contacts that got her the job, the fact that she understood the workings of a private healthcare system, had worked closely with government and brought with her trade union, academic and clinical credentials can be taken as a view about where the most senior figures within the College thought British nursing might be going. Certainly, many felt that, for all her links and networking within the political establishment, Christine Hancock hadn't made a strong enough impact on New Labour. Indeed, insiders reported that Ms Malone immediately impacted upon New Labour's corridors of power, apparently tearing into one junior health minister in an early meeting, in a way that none of them had been used to from any senior health union official throughout their time in government.

Ultimately, the controversy about Malone's appointment was not about her as an individual. It was yet more concern that the RCN was so removed from its membership that this had been such a surprise, as well as an unequivocal verdict on British nurses, none of whom were deemed good enough for the job. The real issue was how and why the appointment was made. For those who did not want that discussed, the furore over Ms Malone's terms and conditions actually took the heat off them.

From the outset, Ms Malone had a consistent message that she put across in every setting possible: nurses must be more political. There is nothing new in this sentiment but, again, the dual role of the RCN and the way in which it has worked against the type of development and organisation that would promote political involvement among its members, means she faces an enormous task if she is genuinely determined to change the institution which she now manages.

It seemed also that one controversy would replace another as RCN members – some of whom were in a very senior position – continued a debate of sorts about Beverley Malone. Criticism followed a restructuring that saw three London based executive directors appointed at an annual cost of almost £300,000. It was claimed this was devaluing College members in Scotland, Wales and Northern Ireland as the secretaries of boards in these countries would report to the new executive directors. With several prominent staff suspended within the College, calls from lay activists in the regions for a vote of no confidence in her 'controversial leadership' grew (*Nursing Times*, 1998, 25: p 5). The College's chair of Council, Pat Bottrill, had to resign two weeks after making a reference to the Agatha Christie novel, *Ten Little Niggers*, while recalling members into a meeting after a break. Most thought that Ms Bottrill had made an unfortunate but unintentional faux pas and done the right thing by resigning. However, although it was unclear whether or not she had made the decision on her own, the *Daily Mail* used it as an opportunity to attack Ms Malone's leadership 'as extraordinarily rigid'.[5]

---

[5] The situation was confused when, three months later, RCN life vice-president Baroness Cox, claimed that Ms Malone had refused her offer of resignation after the Baroness had hosted a launch and written a foreword to a book – which she had not read – that contained homophobic material and condemned abortion (*Nursing Times*, 1998, 44: p 6). Bottrill's resignation also came just three years after Congress voted against a resolution aimed at getting nurses from ethnic minorities involved in College affairs. It was something of an irony that there were some who

▶ The wider trade union and political context – the Labour Party and the TUC

The RCN's excursions into the wider political world are selective. It may not want to fraternise with the comrades of the TUC but politicians of every hue beat a path to its door, which is open to all. The Tories have received an exceptionally frosty reception for some years now. Although Christine Hancock was more charitable, William Hague's first and only appearance at Congress, a couple of months before the 2001 election, drew sustained attacks from delegates and a wholesale rejection of a Tory government again running the NHS. Alan Milburn, on the other hand, got a 'rock star's welcome' (Ryan, 2000a). But by the end of that year the College was involved in a major row with the government on nurse numbers, claiming official statistics were seriously flawed and that, even if targets for recruiting 57,000 new nurses over the next four years were met, with 110,000 due to leave or retire on current trends, there would still be a shortfall of 53,000. This is, of course, the reason why nurses never seem to experience any let up from chronic shortages despite government success stories of hitting recruitment targets.

But the College's position of being courted by governments yet free to criticise them, even if it is only in marginal terms, is not one that has been open to Unison or other affiliated unions, who were firmly locked out under the Tories because of their relationship with the Labour Party. Yet, having talked up the 'special relationship' with New Labour, they have found this rather like Britain in its relationship with the United States under George Bush, pretty much one way traffic. Both PFI and the government's involvement in the firefighters' dispute of 2002–03, have clearly tested Dave Prentis' loyalty and patience. After eighteen years of Tory rule, Unison members had high hopes of a close relationship and seriously influencing policy with a Labour government. The relationship was there, but as already noted, Unison had to acknowledge the new government remained wedded to PFI, was side-stepping the issue of pay, not addressing equality issues, long-term funding of the NHS, public provision of NHS services or its democratisation (Unison, 1998d). The minimum wage was introduced early in New Labour's first term and the government signed the social chapter. Its Employment Relations Act 1999 introduced

---

contd.

thought that Ms Malone's appointment was also a means of digging the College out of the hole it had dug for itself, having to acknowledge its institutional racism after the Congress vote in 1999 (although this would have been an exceptionally extravagant means of doing so). Ironically, Unison's lower profile with nurses served it well when, in 2002, first the secretary to its Welsh regional secretary won £90,000 compensation for alleged harassment and Chris Humphreys, its regional secretary for London was suspended for several months while 'a certain number of complaints were being investigated' (Synapse, 2002: p 13). Both men subsequently left the organisation.

the right to trade union recognition in the workplace and a raft of other employment rights, both individual and collective, as well as family friendly policies. But the government had not gone as far as the unions had hoped, particularly with the minimum wage, and the scope of union recognition was watered down after pressure from the Confederation of British Industry. Moreover, much of the scope of the White Paper actually concerned individual employment rights, benefiting workers regardless of union membership. The overall result still left 'Britain with the harshest legal climate for unions of any major western economy' (Kellner, 1998).

The question that has increasingly vexed a growing number of Unison activists, however, is whether or not the vast sum paid over in political contributions to New Labour is actually worth it. Until 2001, such an attitude was mocked by the union's leadership. Indeed, it was New Labour that was making noises about abandoning the historic link. The first indication of its thinking came in 1996. The then Shadow Minister for Employment, Stephen Byers, allegedly told journalists that Tony Blair might ballot party members on severing the link if a Labour government faced a wave of strikes. If serious, it was a bold move. More than half the £12.5 million funding it received in 1995 came from the unions and, despite a considerable weakening of their position within the party since Tony Blair's arrival, they still had 50 per cent of the vote at party conferences, a one-third stake in the election of the party leader and sponsored the majority of Labour MPs. No such ballot occurred. But any pretence of partnership was dropped. Blair and his team, like a flighty dinner date at an expensive restaurant determined to hang on to her honour but have a good time, set out to continually stay several steps ahead of the trade union barons paying the bill. The likes of Rodney Bickerstaffe, John Edmonds of the GMB and Bill Morris from the Transport & General Workers' Union had to massage their bruised feelings, conceal their outrage or just wonder what is going on and why they don't know. Like the RCN, the TUC affiliates are as much in the decision making loop as the government want them to be, but are paying a small fortune for the privilege.

Paradoxically, Unison scores over the RCN in not having such a rigid 'professional' agenda. So it was seen as more flexible on issues close to New Labour's heart, like a new pay system. But its close ties also limit it in being able to serve its members best interests when those are not shared by government. Its leaders will be well aware that history amply demonstrates that public services, trade unions and their members generally fare better under Labour than Conservative governments. They do not seem, however, to be able to make the leap of imagination and seriously consider the benefits to both New Labour and themselves were *they* to break the link.

The ruthlessness of the government when dealing with the unions can be seen in its dealings with the CPHVA. Despite immense pressure from its membership, which threatened to split the organisation, its leadership was unable to secure the title of health visitor in the new Nursing and Midwifery Council (NMC), despite the widely held view that health visiting is a distinct entity in itself. With members' concerns that this was yet another step towards the margnialisation of health visitors, and possibly even towards their total demise, CPHVA director, Jackie Carnell, had to argue that not being named had been a concession to, in effect, allow the continued registration of health visitors and the inclusion of specialist community practitioners on the register.

▷ Case history 6: Nurses' pay – a little local difficulty

In 1982, the health service unions were campaigning for a 12 per cent increase, with a clear strategy in place if the government did not pay up. Twenty years later, the demand was for a 'substantial increase' for nurses. If anyone could decide clearly, what that was and it wasn't forthcoming, well, no one was quite sure what would happen next. But it would not involve nurses and nor it would not involve any form of protest. Increasingly, as nurses have been more and more enraged by their treatment under New Labour, their unions have failed to react.

In between those two extremes came the 1988 dispute and the 'virtual' pay dispute of 1995, which effectively trickled through into 1996. Apart from that, calls for action, arguments that nurses are hard done by, bitterness and disappointment have featured with depressing regularity.

The events of 1995 were almost a textbook case of how not to conduct an industrial dispute. It was during this pay campaign that the RCN made its landmark decision to change Rule 12 and permit its members to take industrial action, just as did the RCM. What had pushed the unions over the edge, however, was not that nurses and midwives were being offered too little by way of an annual pay increase; it was the introduction of local pay bargaining. A national offer of 1 per cent was made, with anything over and above this to be topped up by local trusts, with a government expectation that this would average out to 3 per cent. The PRB had accepted government policy on local pay bargaining and recommended a 1 per cent increase but with a recommendation that this be supplemented by a further 2 per cent locally, which the government then readily endorsed. Had a national award of 3 per cent been made, that would have been readily accepted.

Local pay bargaining had taken a long time making its way to the negotiating table, having been an integral part of the White Paper, *Working for Patients*, that introduced the internal market in 1990. The opposition of the RCN and RCM was inevitable once it became clear that trusts were not, as some had expected, prepared to offer 'sweetheart deals', giving preferable terms and conditions to organisations who agreed to no industrial action. Money was far too tight and the market had not given the relatively new self-governing trusts the financial freedom many had envisaged. They were still dependent on government funding, albeit through allocations dispensed by health authorities or commissioners. With no increased managerial resource, it was as unpopular with many trusts as it was with the unions. Unison's ideological opposition was, on the face of it, more difficult to understand. There had been cautious enthusiasm for it in COHSE and prolonged experience of it for all the health unions from the 1970s, when incentive bonus schemes for ancillary staff had been introduced. This had prompted an explosion in trade union membership and participation, with new members supporting their stewards as they negotiated directly on their behalf, and any remedy to outcomes they did not like lying in their own hands rather than having to be referred to any cumbersome national bargaining machinery. What Unison had in common with the RCN and RCM was a fear that, were its national negotiating role lost, so would control of its membership. After several years of relative impotence, many nurses and other health workers also worried that they would be no match for strong employers and would find themselves losing out on what was being achieved through the national process.

The unions thus had the difficult task of convincing members that 3 per cent was not a satisfactory increase if 2 per cent of that came from a 'local top up'. In this scheme of things, more than 3 per cent, which some trusts were offering, was unacceptable. Three per cent as a result of a national offer, however, was fine. They had to ensure that their local officials *did not* sit down with management to negotiate anything on pay. While demanding a national settlement of 3 per cent, they were seeking a critical mass of trusts to offer the magic figure with no strings attached, i.e., no variations to local terms and conditions. However, as the weeks rolled on, the unions' apparently united front crumbled. First, the RCM bowed out, calling off a ballot for industrial action and seeking 'peace talks' with the NHS management executive that they thought would advantage midwives.[6] RCN members were calling for action as loudly as they had been in 1988. Health minister, Gerald Malone, was accusing the College of becoming 'just another trade union' by changing Rule 12, as well as making veiled threats to scrap the PRB. The College backed away from the action that was being planned by the joint trade union side. Amidst confusion and acrimony between all the unions, vital positioning was going on. The RCN feared Unison was trying to introduce the notion of a new single pay spine, while both feared the other was looking for a means of blaming the other if

---

[6] Far from it. Midwives remained a long way behind nurses in the grading structure and it was several years more before the RCM could lay claim to getting its members anything approaching a decent deal, with all midwives starting as an F grade, which was part of the 1995 deal recommended by government but not implemented by the vast majority of NHS trusts. It was only late in 1999 that D grade midwives were finally eradicated in Scotland. During its 1999 campaign, the RCM had promised militant action if that was what it would take to change the government's mind about resolving their grievance.

the dispute failed. Unison had conducted an 'indicative ballot' to find out whether or not its members wanted to ballot on industrial action, but was plagued by inaccurate membership records and an unwillingness on the part of its branch officials to spend time updating records they were paying their national union to maintain. What they wanted was to ballot immediately on taking industrial action. As it turned out, the indicative ballot did show a willingness to ballot again for industrial action but on a predictably low turnout. With 71 per cent of the public saying they would support a nurses' strike on the issue, Unison finally re-balloted its members in July, for a 24-hour strike due to take place in September.

Despite having revised Rule 12 in the middle of all this, the RCN condemned Unison's plans, as well as personal attacks being made by local Unison officials on Christine Hancock and Scottish secretary June Andrews. This was in the light of the College indicating it was side-stepping the issue of local pay by recommending acceptance of 3 per cent offers with no strings attached.

The 'dispute', such as it was, ground to a stalemate as the year wore on through a complex, Unison brokered, face saving 'pay framework', provided effective protection of nurses' pay by allowing for all pay deals to be uprated to an increase of 3 per cent on 1994–95 levels. But the unions were left bitterly and hopelessly divided, with confused and impotent nurses finding themselves unsure of what had ever been the expectations of their 'leaders'. Most trusts offered 3 per cent, made up of the 1 per cent national award and a further 2 per cent locally. A small minority offered below that and a smaller number still actually awarded more than the 2 per cent local increase. The more radical trusts really took local pay bargaining to heart. Taking advantage of the unions' instructions to local officials not to negotiate, and already having introduced local trust contracts for new starters, with different terms and conditions to those employed on the existing Whitley Council terms and conditions, separate offers were made, with more being offered to staff on local contracts. Local bargaining, despite the unions' attempts to stop it in its tracks and many trusts' reluctance to have to bother with it, was a reality.

The following year, the RCN, still smarting at Unison's role in resolving the 1995 dispute, got its retaliation in first by demanding a 6 per cent increase before the other unions had even met to discuss the announcement of a 2 per cent national increase, with no recommendation from the PRB as to what should happen locally.[7] Health Secretary, Stephen Dorrell, rebuffed nurses' screams of indignation by saying that 2 per cent was not the deal. The deal was local pay bargaining. The national media, as it had the year before joined in the outcry, broadly condemning the government's offer. Unison and the other unions decided to top the RCN's demands by seeking a 6.5 per cent increase – although Unison was actually

---

[7] The 2 per cent national figure was described by Philip Hunt, director of NAHAT, as too large to give the flexibility that trusts wanted to set local pay. The same Philip Hunt, now Lord Hunt, became a minister in New Labour's health team.

dropping its original demand of 8 per cent in the process, without consulting its members, which prompted its then head of health, Bob Abberley, to admit, 'We make mistakes'. As the row about the 1996 award rumbled on, Powys Health Care NHS Trust saw the reality of local bargaining when it was finally forced to cave in and pay an overall 3 per cent when the hospital's unions balloted on industrial action, with the RCN supporting this for the first time since revising Rule 12.

The arrival of a new government signalled the death of local pay bargaining, which was just as well for the unions, as their inept leadership could never have achieved that on its own. Despite their clear agenda of avoiding local pay bargaining, neither the RCN nor Unison had the wherewithal to organise their members to achieve that objective, relying instead on events heading that way, given that the management of most trusts had neither the capacity nor will to go down that road. Christine Hancock and her senior officials were at pains to insist throughout that the change to Rule 12 was not linked to the dispute and never articulated any clear objective. Were they seeking a 3 per cent national pay award, 3 per cent as a combination of national and local awards? Even delegates to Congress that year weren't sure. As for Unison, seeking a 24-hour national strike in September, seven months after the initial announcement of a 1 per cent offer, by the time most nurses knew they were being offered 3 per cent, was cynical in the extreme. In 1982, September had seen the culmination of a six-month campaign.[8]

Immediately New Labour were in power, Bob Abberley publicly returned to the theme that had first surfaced in the 1995 dispute, a new pay system that would bring all NHS workers together in a single pay spine. The RCN supported the principle for all PRB staff but did not want to find itself back in with ancillary and admin workers. The medical profession was determined to maintain its own PRB. However, Abberley had persuaded government and *Agenda for Change*, the framework for negotiations on a new pay system emerged. However, just in case nurses started thinking their organisations might be determined to finally crack the problem of low pay, Unison's head of health warned 'a new national pay system would not mean pay rises for all. "There's no way we will get a new ... system if it's going to lead to a significant increase in the NHS pay bill"' (*Health Service Journal*, 1997: p 14).

When New Labour staged the 1998 pay award, again following the Tories, nurses were angry but union leaders placatory. Frank Dobson, having been the darling of the RCN Congress the year before (though not, interestingly, Unison's) was booed that year, despite having the usual jamboree bag full of goodies to announce, such

---

[8] One of the few trusts to rush headlong towards local pay left an interesting if unresolved conundrum for Unison particularly. The union at Homewood NHS Trust negotiated such a good deal that the staff was receiving performance related pay each year, which was costing embarrassed managers at its successor body a considerable sum (Healy, 1997: p 6).

as millions of pounds to fund nursing posts, enhance the role of the nurse and extend nurse prescribing. The joint staff side, representing all the nursing unions, continued to make detailed submissions to the PRB, both separately and collectively, emphasising cycles of nursing shortages, increased workload, stress and time off through sickness. *The Agenda for Change* negotiations were ongoing and New Labour held true to its commitment not to stage any more awards. It also developed an approach of having at least one headline grabbing increase, such as an increase for some 'D' grade nurses of almost 12 per cent or the introduction of nurse consultants with an upper earning limit of £42,000. Discretionary points for grades 'F'–'I' were introduced despite union reactions varying between caution and outright hostility. When cost of living supplements (COLS) were introduced in 2000, the unions reacted as if they had post-traumatic stress disorder, condemning them as a form of regionalised pay. Attempts to increase pay by the back door are being made by different unions through claims for equal pay for work of equal value but are extremely complex and take years to resolve. By 2001, Maggie Dunn, chair of the Nursing and Midwifery Staffs Negotiating Council, was summarising the staff side position as wanting 'quite a bit more than the 3.7 per cent of last year' (*Nursing Times*, 2001: p 4). By 2002, Unison and the RCN were more outspoken in their reactions to another pay award that was generally reckoned to fall short of the mark, although other union leaders were more welcoming. All, however, accepted. Nurses were far more forthright, as they were left lagging far behind newly qualified teachers, police officers and £10,000 behind junior doctors. Ninety-three per cent of nurses who responded to an internet poll by the *Nursing Times* condemned the offer. Most were appalled with the reaction of their unions.

In other countries, it was a different story. As British nurses were trying to decipher their unions' position on local pay, their Irish counterparts were rejecting government offers, culminating in serious threats to go on strike while providing emergency cover. Their employers more than doubled the amount on offer for pay, and promised to honour the findings of an independent commission, which included the Irish Nurses' Organisation's (INO) general secretary, and recommended a radical overhaul of nursing and midwifery and a new career grade. Still not satisfied, the INO put in a pay claim for 15–20 per cent. The following year, in 1999, the INO led its nurses onto the picket line when the Irish government had still not met nurses' demands in pursuit of a 23 per cent claim at the same time as nurses in Quebec withdrew their labour for several weeks to force their employers to increase their pay. This followed industrial action by nurses in almost every Australian state in a dispute reminiscent of their United Kingdom's counterpart's clinical militancy of the 1980s in that it was not only about pay but also staffing levels and standards of care, with nurses in Western Australia undertaking a six-day strike to secure their demands.

American nurses see politics as part and parcel of their work, with the American Nurses' Association (ANA) and other key nursing organisations adopting a political position, seeing which presidential and congressional candidates are prepared to support it and then, in turn, endorse the candidate and get on the campaign trail on his or her behalf. But the decision is made by members, who are provided with information about the candidate's views and then balloted about prospective endorsement. Nurses are far more active in lobbying their own state legislatures and are prepared to take action when necessary, although the California Nurses' Association broke away from the ANA as it felt it was too conservative and has gone on to secure improved deals for its members. Similarly, the American Psychiatric Nurses Association (APNA) was formed by ANA veterans who wanted a smaller, more focused organisation to progress their agenda, and which might offer an interesting model for British nurses (see Chapter 8).

▶ Is reform within the unions possible?

British nurses have been increasingly outspoken about their own union's performance on pay. There has always been a highly vocal element within each organisation which has taken a far more radical position than the majority, attracting lots of attention with their views. Unison has had more problems with members who are also in Trotskyist groups – not a likely problem for the College – who have taken an anti-union stance whenever possible, attacking the union's leadership and seeking to undermine their relationship with the wider membership and, with the lack of a clear political direction and industrial strategy within the union, they were increasingly successful in the latter half of the 1990s. But the level of criticism and disapproval has heightened in recent years. Much of this has focused on pay, although, in many respects this can be interpreted as symbolic of a deeper malaise or unease. Nurses wrote to the *Nursing Times* after the 1998 pay award, denouncing the RCN leadership and declaring they were switching to Unison. RCN stewards called for strike action later the same year and Mike Hayward, one of the College's leading critics, despite remaining loyal, noted a range of converging factors, from nursing shortages to widespread support throughout the country for nurses to take action against an image-obsessed government, and called upon the leaders of the RCN and Unison 'to pull the nation's nurses together. It is time that nursing's highly paid trade union leaders put their necks on the line for the people who pay their wages.... The mood is right for a more public show of strength. No longer should we fear to take industrial action' (Hayward, 1998). Again, in 1999, RCN stewards were calling upon their leaders to reject the pay award. This time, Christine Hancock's defence was that nurses had no choice but to accept it as the other unions were not even bothering to consult with their members over the award. Spuriously, she claimed that if they didn't accept it they would get nothing. Nurses were clearly fed up with the approach of high awards for relatively small groups while the majority got rises close to the rate of inflation. Health visitors planned to resurrect the Radical Health Visitors Association, a highly influential if small organisation from the late 1970s.

That the RCN and Unison are moving closer politically and philosophically, then, is unlikely to be a source of much comfort to nurses given that there are strong indications that both are moving away from *them*. Unison supplemented its professional department to work on UKCC cases and related matters. Any College attempts to increase its political profile will mean resolving at least some of its internal conflicts. These are exemplified by the decision to admit HCAs. Now they will have to negotiate on behalf of non-PRB staff, as well as finding themselves drawn into a whole new arena of industrial relations.

Both organisations concentrate a lot of energy into good, glossy leaflets that represent national campaigns and exploit direct mailing to good effect so that members know exactly what each organisation wants them to know. Indeed, many Unison branch officials complain about the amount of information sent through to them, which makes it impossible to sift through and decide what is important and what is not. Much of it, they say, ends up in the bin, unread.

Will they ever truly join forces? It is unlikely unless Beverly Malone is to fundamentally change the College, whose lay leadership would find the idea of being in a union with ancillaries, admin workers and the like beyond the pale. Equally, many in Unison would find it unimaginable to join forces with the 'old enemy', although such sentiments were probably more common in COHSE than either of its partner unions and are far more dissipated in Unison as it has lost much of its historical and ideological baggage over the ten years of its lifetime. Nurses have long been fatally weakened by the divisions between the key organisations, as witnessed in crucial periods such as 1982, 1988 and 1995. Yet, there is not even any practical support for a separation of responsibilities, with Unison providing a trade union role while the College concentrates on clinical and educational issues. The inability of the key nursing unions to even engage with them now and provide the effective leadership required in such difficult times only adds to the problem. Although the climate in the NHS has changed considerably from the oppressive period of the Thatcher and Major governments, the challenges facing nurses are, in many respects, as great. Perhaps it could be argued that the nurses who might carry a radical agenda forward are no longer there, that their problems are only those witnessed in wider British politics. Radical nurses are around but not finding anything in the trade unions to attract them. Instead, their energies are being directed into single-issue politics, supporting causes such as animal rights, human rights, anti-capitalitism and the environment.

Most unions have excellent training programmes for stewards and branch officials. But the failure to invest time, support and energy into supporting and developing branch organisation has resulted in weakening local branches, the lifeblood of any voluntary organisation. Unison's local government branches, many of which have tens of thousands of members, despite their declining membership in the latter 1990s, are often wealthy enough to employ their own staff, as well as having activists on full-time release from the employers. These are luxuries very few health branches experience. The nature of a steward's role can be both complex and difficult, representing members who are alleged to have committed a variety of offences, with all the procedural, moral and ethical dilemmas that come with that. Despite the apparent demise of local bargaining, in reality they will be involved in negotiating issues of importance to their members, such as staffing levels, shift patterns, the nature of the work people do, policies and even major contractual changes.

In the way that NHS unions mirror their host organisation, both have their own websites and have introduced a variation on NHS Direct. For the RCN it was a straightforward managerial decision and a top-down initiative, funded directly through subscription increases over a two-year period, and launched in early 1998, providing a 24-hour advice and information service to all RCN members. Telephone advisors were able to access computerised databases, Citizens' Advice Bureau resources but could also put the caller in touch with RCN officers. The path to Unison Direct was more torturous. First mooted long before the RCN's by full-time officers who had been amongst the first to realise the potential of the internet and new telecommunications media, the project went through pilot schemes, prevarication from the NEC and senior figures within the union. Eventually launched in the same year, it was more ambitious in scope, with its initiators seeing it as a means to put members in touch with branch officials easily, as well as get more basic advice than that being provided by the College. It also provided a service for stewards, who were all issued with pagers and participating branches were encouraged to use laptop computers to enable them to access email. With 25 per cent of union members already seeking advice about workplace issues *outside* the union because of being unable to access anyone from their branch, the importance of this minor revolution could not be underestimated. Both services were well received by their respective members with one vital caveat. When it was necessary to pass the caller's problem to a local steward, often the response was perceived as being slow in coming or didn't happen at all.

For all unions, trying to keep pace with people's increasing expectations was similar to that which nurses experience in the NHS. Providing more and better financial or leisure services has to be at the expense of something and cannot be a substitute for local organisation and structures that engage with local staff. Given that the RCN is not an organising union and doesn't want to be means that it will always drag Unison and the other unions further down the road of service provision in a race they cannot win. Moreover, for all the changes in society, the undoubted reason nurses and other health workers join trade unions is for local representation and to get better terms and conditions at work. That they are less engaged in the process of actually working to achieve that is down to the mixed messages the unions give out.

Entropy is a measure of the degree of molecular disorder existing in a system, just as time is the path from order to chaos. The process is irreversible. The trade unions, by their nature, try to 'put things back' and maintain a sense of order. This is like cosmic King Canutes helplessly facing the tide. Perhaps it is a part of the legacy of the onslaught of the Thatcher years that the unions appear stuck, looking inwardly at their internal machinery but unable to acknowledge their problems, instead projecting them 'out', onto the government, management, the members. They seem to have forgotten that it is necessary to look outward and forward – but not solely to see things as they are but to imagine how they might be, and show their members how they can get there. What will the future look like? How will we nurse? How will we create solutions to the problems of today and prepare the way for progress? If there is such a thing as a collective consciousness in nursing, it has shifted considerably. It is far more imaginative, creative, empathic and holistic than that of the trade unions that no longer represent but constrain them. The political world in which nurses live is larger, more complex, more intractable than ever. Constantly trying to appease those in power will not succeed. Nurses can move to a place where they view the problems differently, but need to understand their position now first. It involves a revolution in their own heads to help them make the external changes a reality. The national stage is not necessarily the one upon which they should act out the drama of their working lives. It is closer to home. Not even necessarily in their trust. For some the change is needed in the team in which they work. It will be to directly address their real concerns, gain some degree of control over their work, matching authority to responsibility, working in an environment that nurtures them and enables their caring role, with parameters about where that role begins and ends. And gives them a sense of not only being valued but also of being paid fairly for the work that they do. That is what nurses want from their trade unions but they will get it only when they are a vital part of those organisations.

There have been periods when the unions have done this and provided effective, engaging leadership. The Transport and General Workers' Union and NUPE gave rise to the organic growth of the shop steward movement in the 1970s. COHSE took on the mantle in the 1980s, when it allowed nurses their head to articulate clinical militancy. If the major nursing unions cannot pick up that historical baton, transform it into a vision for the future and rise to the challenge in the twenty-first century, it will not only be nurses who are the losers.

▶ Conclusions

Nursing trade unionism has been through tremendous changes in the past two decades, much as have nurses and the NHS. These directly reflect not only the wider political changes of the period but also the changed perception within nursing and that nurses have of themselves and their world. Nurses are certainly damaged by the long standing differences between Unison and the RCN, as well as the growing divide between themselves as an occupational group and their unions.

The nature of the major nurses', midwives' and health visitors' organisations, of course, reflect their histories and can still be traced in their current structures, decision making processes and culture. However, none have proven themselves to be particularly adept at adapting their relationship with their members or internal structures. This is of growing importance in an age of a mass media and communications revolution. The TUC-affiliated trade unions were severely weakened by the Thatcher and Major governments, a period when the RCN thrived, but they all failed to capitalise on the profound advances nurses made in the 1980s, both clinically and industrially.

Unison, as a general public service union incorporating health workers, has been a serious disappointment, with the service group structures having been considerably weakened since its inception in 1993 and the profile it has given to health workers' and nurses' issues increasingly submerged. Moreover, it has clearly failed to integrate its health activists into the wider union. The RCN has still not overcome its internal contradictions, thrown up by being both a professional association and trade union, and has never even begun to address the issue of how a trade union can be for *nursing* rather than nurses, wanting to participate in the management of the organisation in which nurses work, when we have seen the conflict that exists between the two. The College has accommodated major policy shifts that were important for its own survival, such as changing Rule 12 and bringing HCAs into membership but, again, these pose as many questions for its future as they answered at the time.

Being a TUC affiliate, Unison has wider relationships to consider, but the TUC has continued to struggle to make a wider impact on British society even with the election of New Labour, a government which has manipulated its relationship with the trade union movement and appears to be exasperating trade union leaders almost – but never quite wholly – to the point where they consider cutting their ties altogether. Both Unison and the RCN have strong relationships with civil servants and politicians now, but neither is able to use them to deliver on key issues, most particularly pay. Indeed, it is pay which now divides nurses and their unions more than any other, with the trade unions' evidence to the PRB being fundamentally the same as it was more than a decade ago and little progress having been made on delivering fair pay to all nurses.

The quality of leadership arises. With a workforce so clearly demoralised and often hopeless about effecting change, it is incumbent upon its representatives not only to articulate this sense of despair but to provide a vision of how things could be different and how nurses can achieve this. Given that the primary source of nurses' despair is the government and its policies, it is no good trying to get ever closer in the blind hope that the relationship is going to, by some miracle, yield some fantastical change. This is not a recipe for never-ending conflict, for it is also up to those who represent nurses, as it is with those who manage them, to again look at what may not change, and help nurses work with the consequences of that.

To lead them on, however, is both dishonest and damaging in the longer term and is the antithesis of real leadership.

Given the enormity of the political process, it might seem wholly impossible to effect any change. But if the analysis of those such as Michael Hardt (2000) is correct, there is no longer any clear place of power. The very complexity and enormity of the apparent challenge faced is what creates the conditions for nurses to resist those processes that are inimical to their needs and best interests. Because if nurses are the 'exploited' in the system, they do have common cause. The new political shapelessness offers opportunities for nurses to re-discover fragile values like their own rights, freedom, creativity, an independence that allows a position of partnership and reflects the truly interdependent nature of healthcare, and enables nurses to gain something very different from status – self-respect and a degree of control and authority over their own work, as well as reward, that is commensurate with their efforts and commitment.

There was a time when the great divide was between the RCN and the trade unions affiliated to the TUC. That has narrowed considerably in recent years, but the gap between the unions and their members is growing by the year. If it gets much greater, perhaps the obituary for nursing trade unionism will read: 'What do we want? Quite a bit more. When do we want it? Some time in the future'.

▶ Further reading

Cowie V (1982) Organised labour. In: Allen P and Jolley M (eds) *Nursing, Midwifery and Health Visiting Since 1900*. London: Faber & Faber: this is short on analysis and lacks a political grasp of some of the events described, but nonetheless offers a useful view of history from the then secretary of the staff side of the Nurses' Whitley Council.

Carpenter M (1980) Asylum nursing before 1914. In: Davies C (ed) *Rewriting Nursing History*. London: Croom Helm.

Carpenter M (1988) *Working for Health*. London: Lawrence and Wisehart: an excellent account of COHSE's history, almost in its entirety, told with passion and intelligence.

Cowell B and Wainwright D (1981) *Behind the Blue Door. The History of the Royal College of Midwives 1881–1981*. London: Bailliere Tindall: very much an 'in-house' view of the RCM, but containing some interesting material about the College's early years.

Hart C (1996) The great divide. In: *The International Journal of Nursing History* 1, 3. London: Royal College of Nursing.

Hart C (1996) United Voices. *Nursing Times*, 92 (29), pp 40–1.

Hart C and Walker M (1997) High-flying activist. *Nursing Times*, 93 (51): articles that describe Thora Silverthorne and Avis Hutt, two of the most remarkable women to have worked as nurses, both leaving an indelible mark on history.

The former also features the short-lived but influential Association of Nurses, the only trade union exclusively established for nurses.

Marsh D (1992) *The New Politics of British Trade Unionism*. Basingstoke: Macmillan. Interesting background material on trade unionism in Britain.

▶ Useful websites

www.rcn.org.uk
www.unison.org.uk

8 What is to be Done?

And always keep a-hold of Nurse
For fear of finding something worse.

'Cautionary Tales' by Hilaire Belloc

▶ Introduction

If the lines from Belloc's poem were actually to be applied to nursing and nurses, how should we interpret them? Nurses are valuable and should be retained. Nurses would agree with that. Managers, trusts, government – everyone – would signal their approval, although those with the power do not necessarily translate that into action. In so doing, however, they *do* have to hold on to nurses in a different way. If nurses are not to spin out of control again, as they did in 1988 and many times in the years before that, yet also not simply continue to vote with their feet and leave, a careful job has to be done to keep hold of them in a very different way, controlling them and the culture in which they work, their perception of themselves and their world.[1]

This last chapter could be given over to trying to draw things together and arrive at some conclusions. Yet, understanding nursing is not a static exercise. Power, politics and practice are a process. By the time conclusions are drawn in any of these spheres, time has moved on, a little more chaos has evolved from the order that went before. Indeed, does nursing people not remind us everyday that life is no more than a continual process of change, very little of which is within our control and to which we have to adapt? Which is not to say that conclusions of a sort cannot be reached.

Michael Hardt and Antonio Negri (2001) persuasively argue that there is no longer any 'centre', that the new global economy is a 'non place' unlike the homes of the great powers in earlier centuries. In this sense it replicates the internet, one of the things with which it links – and exploits – seamlessly. There is no single controlling power – indeed, power has no one place in the global economy. Old systems and principles for understanding politics, economics and power are having to be re-interpreted. Rather than taking the view of many 'left of centre' thinkers and politicians that the postmodernised global economy is all powerful, that global corporations have an irresistible grip on power, Hardt and Negri hold that there is still a historical sweep towards progress, that we are a creative and enlightened

---

[1] Of course, this was the great feat of the matrons pre-1948.

species who can use the circumstances of the new economy to seize power from those who exploit it.

If this can be true on a global scale, can it be said to be the case for healthcare in the United Kingdom? Given the uncertainties and shifting position of the 'centre', it becomes necessary to make real political choices. The rediscovery of older concepts or values such as 'freedom', rights, responsibilities, creativity, autonomy within a containing collective identity become possible – all the things that nursing, at its best, can boast. Nurses currently at the forefront of clinical and educational innovation are often looking back to our past to retrieve and adapt aspects of our work that were successful but lost because of external changes, pressures on services impacting on good practice or simply not continued after experienced practitioners left.

This chapter will not avoid looking for conclusions, but they will be framed within an evolutionary and dynamic process. Practice influences politics; politics impacts upon practice; the use – and abuse – of power continues. But the future, which is the key theme of this chapter starts with our students, in whom we inevitably place much hope. Recruitment and retention will be discussed again – as well as the government's arithmetic. This will involve not just looking at how many nurses there are currently working in the National Health Service (NHS) and other sectors, but how many are being recruited, how many are leaving. It is also necessary to think about what these nurses could or should be doing, as well as what they are actually doing and how many are actually needed. The Private Finance Initiative (PFI) is a major part of nurses' future, as is the Nursing and Midwifery Council (NMC) and are thus covered here. For perhaps the first time, a link is established between long-term concerns in nursing: health and safety, whistleblowing, bullying, stress and violence are all interrelated, as will be shown in this chapter. Pay, the relationship between nurses and their trade unions and patient involvement are also featured once more. As with the other issues considered here, it is because they will inevitably continue to have some impact on nurses and nursing. Yet, as has been the case throughout the book, they also have to be viewed as symbolising the struggles facing nurses and to extract the principles necessary in resolving them, as well as how power might be seized back from those who have it. As part of that debate, the book will consider shared governance and how nurses might re-instate themselves at the centre of their trade unions. From that, we might learn how nurses could exert some degree of control over their local circumstances rather than simply be the victims of apparently unknown, external forces, whatever the issues, whatever the situation.

▶ Learning for the future – education and training

Being a student has never been easy but the twenty-first century is far from the golden age envisaged by the educationalists and professionalisers who fought for educational reform in the shape of an academic, university-based training such as Project 2000. Yet, despite the poor image of student nurse training, the number of applicants has continued to rise in recent years. Partly as a result of government advertising programmes, there was a 20 per cent increase in 1999 from the previous year – with applications for Project 2000 training expected to be around 70 per cent higher. Nursing was even more popular than computer training. About 2700 students embarked on a degree course in 1999 and 14,834 were taking part on Diploma courses, increased from 12,567 in 1998. But 2000 also saw a five-year high in drop-out rates for nursing and midwifery students in Scotland and 14 per cent dropping out across the United Kingdom.

▷ Education and training: student bursaries

Student nurses occupy a peculiar position. They receive a bursary but are expected to maintain a demanding work schedule alongside their academic programme. The bursary has been a running sore since Project 2000 was introduced and student nurses were taken out of NHS employment. It is another issue that splits the nursing unions, with Unison campaigning for students to be paid within the NHS and the RCN supporting the bursary system. Unison estimated in 1999 that if students had remained as NHS staff from 1988 they would have been earning twice as much, as well as having employment rights, superannuation and sick pay. It would also encourage a responsibility on the part of trusts to give students jobs at the end of their training. The response from the chair of the Royal College of Nursing's (RCN) Association of Nursing Students was to equate change with the loss of both academic and supernumerary status – something Unison had never called for (Coomes, 1999b). Defenders of the current system usually make the same association – spuriously – and have argued that bursaries should be increased *while access to social security benefits and hardship funds should be made easier* [my emphasis] (Hale, 2000). In such thinking, the old vocational ideal and the College's pre-war ideology of nurses working longer hours for less pay, lives on.

Students themselves have campaigned vigorously for a change to their bursaries, pointing out that they have a different academic year, no long holiday in which to earn extra income, have clinical placements on numerous – and often distant – sites and often have to travel at times when transport is, at best, difficult. Finding affordable accommodation is a problem, while working excess hours not only affects attendance for lectures but also writing assignments. Academic pressures are greater with Project 2000 and students often complain of a lack of support both in their academic work as well as from mentors in clinical placements. But, for many, the bottom line remains money. The year 2000 saw Unison's Jim Devine head up a campaign for students' bursaries in Scotland to be doubled, highlighting a national 25 per cent drop out rate as proof that students couldn't survive on the average £5000 bursary, reasoning the Scottish Executive rejected. Arguments that the current system protected students from the 'abuse' of being used 'as a pair of hands' were dealt a blow when it emerged that 45 per cent of nursing students were regularly left unsupervised on wards and 54 per cent had been left to cope alone on more than two occasions, during their training to date. In the same Unison survey, the 1000 students questioned complained of lessons being regularly cancelled and 94 per cent thought the Common Foundation Programme (CFP) hadn't prepared them for their branch programme (Coombes, 2000a).

In January 2000, with the government having demanded that the NHS exert more influence over nursing education – with £1 billion being spent on health professionals education annually – and sixteen universities changing their training system to increase practical skills' training, 78 per cent of students surveyed by ICM and the *Nursing Times* thought students should be employed by the NHS (*Nursing Times*, send students back to NHS, 27 January 2000). When the *Nursing Times* repeated the survey in August, 60 per cent said financial hardship had made them think about leaving their course, 95 per cent were doing extra work to supplement their income while 67 per cent wanted the bursary replaced by a salary (Ryan, 2000b). In the face of its members' overwhelming view the RCN *still* supported the current system – and what it perceived as the interests of nursing rather than nurses.

▶ Education and training: is it effective?

As noted earlier, there have been growing concerns about the nature of student nurse education. But, again, it is not as simple as looking at *a* curriculum, for there are different types of training and these have their own supporters and detractors. Degree nurses, for instance, have been estimated as being able to develop key skills more rapidly, which is highly valued by employers. Nevertheless, Lord MacKenzie – formerly Hector to his friends when he was general secretary of Confederation of Health Service Employees (COHSE) – is only one of a number of Lords who have criticised modern nurse training as too academic. The branch structure has also been criticised, with inadequacies highlighted in both the learning disabilities and mental health branches. The Sainsbury Centre for Mental Health had already identified a huge gap between the training of mental health nurses and the needs of the service in its report, *Pulling Together, The Future Roles and Training of Mental Health Staff* (Duggan *et al.*, 1997). The ENB would not accept the thrust of the Sainsbury Centre report yet reached a similar conclusion. *Fitness for Practice* (UKCC, 1999) noted the concern 'that newly qualified nurses do not possess the practice skills expected'. Frank Dobson, when health secretary, added his disapproval during the 1999 winter bed crisis, linking an overly academic Project 2000 not only to nursing shortages but the inability of hospitals to cope with higher numbers of patients during the winter months, and leaving newly qualified nurses unprepared for their clinical role. It was all the more galling that Virginia Bottomley, a former Health Secretary in the Conservative government that introduced Project 2000, echoed his comments. Moreover, a whole host of 'unqualified' commentators in the largely conservative press were quick to add their tuppenyworth. Brian Sewell, the art critic for the *Evening Standard*, summed it up: 'Nurses now achieve academic levels that far exceed those of many university courses – an appalling waste when applied to their work at the bedpan level'.

'Well educated' nurses will notice that this resonates with the debate about clinical practice from Chapter 4, and echoes the long debate about religion and science. It misses the point by an equally wide margin. There have been major problems with Project 2000 and it has, by the standards set out for it, failed. But this is yet another example of nurses, as students, practitioners and educators being blamed for matters that are beyond their control. Nurse training is about getting bodies through an educational system as cheaply as possible. Yet, the government wants a nursing workforce that can take on the work of junior doctors, as the latter group see their working week decline and role evolve. This requires highly educated staff with a strong academic background. However, it – mistakenly – presupposes that nurses will not be required to undertake their caring role, which is exacerbated, as they also need to pick up work from other health and social care staff as those disciplines are re-organised or face cuts.

Hence the dilemma. For it would seem to be pretty straightforward to organise a training that would deliver a workforce with a clearly defined role. Barristers and solicitors don't suffer the same ambiguity. There are no headlines about the adequacy of the education and training they receive for their job, or whether or not they should be doing the work of chartered surveyors. Nurses are squeezed because there are so many of them to educate, which makes it an expensive enterprise, and because policy makers lack clarity about exactly what they are being trained for. Professor Phil Barker from Newcastle University suggests:

> If nurses are losing their caring focus, if not caring capacity, the answer does not lie in criticising them. Education in caring is needed – not training – recalling the root of the word *educere*: to draw out from within. We were all born with the capacity to care. However, the complexities of the (dis)organisation of healthcare environments (and training) often suppress this potential .... The development of a human science of caring will require resources and ingenuity (Barker, 1999a: p 24).

It's actually a wonder that student nurses managed to learn anything. Project 2000 placements were usually for one or two days a week, for a very limited period, which left many students finding it difficult to become involved with, and settle into, a team. These difficulties were compounded if they found themselves in a pressurised service with few trained staff or mentors with little time to guide them through the placement. With cohorts varying between 50 and 500, lecturers have to talk *at* people about the nature of being human, health and illness, as well as describe the skills needed to carry out this complex and ever changing work that we call nursing.

242 Nurses and Politics

Most universities have to negotiate contracts with their local workforce confederation for vastly increased numbers of students to meet government targets, with no increase in resource, particularly in the shape of more lecturers. Students use lecture halls that won't accommodate their number, and many teachers acknowledge that for particularly large lectures they rely on numbers of students staying away. There is not the time for pastoral care, individual academic supervision, small group work or skills sessions where much of the nature of nursing can be practised. The need to process large numbers of students, as well as the pressure to achieve 'results' means that two components of a different type of learning are lost to nurses. The first concerns emotional intelligence. As Evans and Allen (2002) note:

> Giving students information without the affective skills to act upon it creates a great sense of dissonance and disharmony for a student, contributing to intra-personal difficulties, making it harder, not easier for them to nurse well. A major part of nursing is the use of self that requires self-awareness. The key to self-knowledge lies in intra-personal intelligence or having 'access to one's own feelings and the ability to discriminate among them and draw upon them to guide behaviour' (Gardner, 1989).

> An emotionally adept person who knows and manages their own feelings well, and who reads and deals with other people's emotions effectively, is at an advantage in any domain in life, but is perhaps especially suited to the caring professions. There needs to be a balance between thinking (cognition) and feeling (affect). Intellect cannot be used to best effect without emotional intelligence. (Evans and Allen 2002)

The second is developing critical thinking. Indeed, far more than was the case with the older style training, the circumstances and structure of P2K and its variants actually hammer critical thinking out of the student. Critical thinking involves the application, analysis, synthesis and evaluation of information so it can be used to construct personal meaning. Without this ability, students cannot go beyond the mere collection of information to weave threads of information together to create knowledge. Critical thinking is a particular process, which requires time and reflection and encourages in-depth focus on a topic, promotes problem solving and reasoning, as well as critical analysis and evaluation. It enables nurses to get a deeper understanding of the problems they and their patients face, as well as equipping them with the skills to resolve them. Critical thinking cannot thrive in hierarchies, while status creates a pedagogy and didactic position, acting as a barrier to its growth. Lecturers and practitioners are engaged in any number of attempts to provide students with high quality education, most of them being organised, in spite of government policy and resource difficulties, such as the use of critical learning incidents and small group workshops, which are conducive to the development of conceptual skills in critical exploration and problem solving (Smith and Russell, 1991: pp 284–91). Involving practitioners in delivering education was a government target (Department of Health, 1999a) and enables students to have access to an educative process that is grounded in clinical practice. Problem-based learning has been developed as an alternative to didactic lecturing. It is an instructional methodology that allows learners to 'acquire knowledge and skill in nursing by encountering real practice situations as the initial stimulus for their learning...learners grapple with the complexities of the situations, search for connections...and use existing and new knowledge to generate outcomes'. Possible outcomes are debated and justified, with learners collaborating through analysis and critical reflection (Williams, 2001: pp 18–26). E-learning offers enormous opportunities for students to access the Web and new technology, although there is an equally daunting potential for problems (Blair, 2002). It could pave the way for a widening gap between those providing education and those receiving it. Were its creative application harnessed by educational institutions, it could provide lecturers with more time to combine it with the kind of initiatives identified above.

The pressure that lecturers are under is lost on many nurses; they are no longer 'nurses' but employees of educational institutions, on completely different terms and conditions and largely removed from the healthcare site. They have been subject to even more radical changes than many nurses working in clinical practice. Schools of nursing were closed down and staff transferred into higher education at the same time as Project 2000 was being introduced, with tutors trying to accommodate a new educational philosophy at the same time as fighting to secure their own livelihoods.[2] Phasing the new training in over five years instead of ten, as had been originally planned, made matters worse. Moreover, as well as having to accommodate massive increases in pre-registration student numbers, they also have to devise, administer and teach on courses for the rapidly changing world in which registered nurses find themselves. For almost every clinical innovation, such as prescribing rights, needs to be taught. It is right to argue for lecturers to retain a clinical role but, again, overlooks the conditions they find themselves in. This kind of dual role offers a great deal but it requires sufficient numbers of lecturers to make it possible and a co-operative and imaginative relationship between the university and NHS trusts. Equally, there is a strong argument to suggest that opportunities should be made available for experienced nurses to develop a limited, well-defined academic role. Both initiatives would benefit the individuals, the service in which they work and students' education. As well as bridging the practice – theory divide, such moves would bring academic and NHS organisations together.

Moves such as slimming down the CFP from eighteen months to one year, allowing more time to be spent in branch programmes, will undoubtedly help, as will the reforms to education such as those piloted by the Faculty of Health and Social Care Sciences at Kingston University and St George's Hospital Medical School.

---

[2] As education funding was cut by the Tories, ENB figures showed the number of nurse lecturers fell by 19 per cent between 1993 and 1996.

These saw the introduction of a 'post P2000' training that arose out of the United Kingdom Central Council's (UKCC) education commission report, *Fitness for Practice* (UKCC, 1999), with the CFP reduced to one year, students beginning their clinical placements after just eight weeks and a shift in the emphasis of the training to half practice, half theory rather than the two-thirds theory that had characterised Project 2000.

▶ Education and training: genuinely making a difference?

The options the government put forward in *Making a Difference* (*op. cit.*, 1999), such as 'hop on, hop off' options for post-registration education, developing continuing professional development programmes, strengthening the link between vocational training and pre-registration education and developing more flexible career pathways into nursing all hold out promise.[3] Yet, at its heart, there is still ambiguity about what kind of nursing workforce it is seeking to create. For these changes still don't solve the problems of increasing numbers, inadequate resources, bursaries, a lack of clarity about the nurse's role – or recognition that if it is to become increasingly 'flexible' then the educative process needs to help students accommodate that. The government doesn't recognise that a well-educated, academically sound workforce can also be one that is well equipped to undertake the key role of providing nursing care, in all its complexity. For the dichotomy about a capability to care versus academic ability is a wholly false one. One informs the other. The nurse's role is not one that will ever be explicitly defined or have clear boundaries in the way that a surgeon's, or a radiographer's or a lab technician's is. It is one that evolves, changes and incorporates parts of several others at the same time. Caring is a relatively simple task, if one has the capacity to do it, but nursing is an incredibly complex job. Some aspects of it could – and should – be much better defined but flexibility and adaptability are necessary, partly because nurses' roles are dependent on their setting and those settings are already highly variable and evolving.

Adapting to change is, therefore, one of the key elements of nurse education. It needs to be added to communication skills, emotional intelligence and critical thinking, to help nurses develop the core skills they will need in their work when other elements are added, such as the ability to undertake assessments, problem solve and use decision making techniques suited to a variety of clinical and managerial situations. This will also assist them in developing collaborative approaches to nursing, using group work and collective learning assignments that can also

---

[3] Although this is yet another example, that can be dated back to the introduction of the old General Nursing Council (GNC), of government's impatience with nurses' organisations to deliver a suitable strategy.

allow for the application of leadership skills from the outset. With these skills we begin to prepare a workforce for the future.

A single educational spine, that does not preclude people on the basis of a lack of qualifications but allows students to progress at a pace that suits them, from pre-registration training into a career of lifelong learning is not only more democratic but enables the NHS to capitalise on the talents and abilities of a larger pool of recruits.[4] There is no reason that Health Care Assistants (HCAs) could not have an educational pathway that takes them from National Vocational Qualifications (NVQs) to registration if they have the aptitude. Their ultimate career path may differ from students that come in via a more defined academic background, but the argument that nurses should be discriminated against because of their background was lost in the 1930s and 1940s.

Unison is entirely correct in arguing that ditching bursaries in favour of a salary does not mean a concomitant increase in the abuse of students' supernumerary status. Moreover, there are times when it is right and useful to the student and her/his education to be a 'part' of the clinical team. In conjunction with an improved education programme and lecturers having manageable groups to teach and work *with*, it would almost certainly improve retention rates. The real problem is that no government to date has been confident it can manage a well educated, stable and organised workforce.

Nurses have long realised they don't have to be passive recipients of education but this needs to become the norm rather than the exception. They have skills and knowledge that they can pass on to one another, by bringing in colleagues from different areas and then reciprocating the 'favour'. Clinical teams can undertake their own educational needs' audit, identifying individual's training needs as well as those of the team collectively, in order for it to progress and improve practice. The same audit can also identify areas where particular nurses can teach others, providing a community of skills for mutual learning and development. They *can* take the time to educate themselves collectively over an extended period. Indeed, there is no reason that nurses cannot have protected study time in the same way as medical staff do – it is essential if nurses are to be expected to develop. The shortcomings highlighted earlier can be addressed in any number of creative and positive ways with a different attitude and determination not to be treated in the same way any longer.

---

[4] The NHS University, announced by Milburn during the 2001 general election campaign, may deliver something of this. At the time of writing, details are unclear. He and British Medical Association (BMA) Chief Executive, Jenny Simpson, one of its prime movers, have talked about it, not only as a centre for lifelong learning, a means of equipping all NHS staff with core skills, such as communication, but also for instilling a corporate ethos into staff – even regulating who has the required 'skills' and 'capabilities' to work. Whether or not staff can expect a traditional university education is unclear – but it seems unlikely.

▶ How many nurses do we need?

Anybody who actually bothered to add up the number of nurses the government claims have been newly recruited or returned to practice since 1997 would conclude that there are now more nurses than patients. However, most would recognise that, as has been the case with NHS funding, New Labour has simply refined the practice of its predecessors and stretched a gallon out of a pint pot by regurgitating announcements over and over. The first of the big promises followed its comprehensive spending review in 1998 – when that famous '£21 billion' was announced as new money for the NHS (see Chapter 5) – and Frank Dobson announced 7000 more doctors and 15,000 new nurses would be recruited before the next election. At this stage there were an estimated 8000 vacancies. New Labour had already promised to increase student intakes by 12.5 per cent in 1998 and 1999, which would bring 4000 new students into training (Brindle, 1998b). Reductions in the numbers of student nurse places under the Conservatives in the early 1990s contributed to the shortages of trained staff in the late 1990s. There was an enormous chasm between vacancies and actual posts to be filled before the issue of inadequate establishments could be tackled. The depth of the problem was revealed when Income Data Services surveyed seventy-three NHS trusts and found that 78 per cent were experiencing recruiting problems, which had more than doubled in three years (IDS, 1998). Almost inevitably, Tony Blair waded in. Nurse shortages equated with longer waiting lists. The Prime Minister feared these, in turn, would fan public disillusionment with his government. News of an 11 per cent pay rise for nurses was leaked, although the detail that this was only for relatively few nurses at 'D' grade, was omitted from the government's spin.

A £5 million recruitment campaign was initiated and a year later, Alan Milburn was able to claim that 2700 additional whole time equivalent nurses and midwives had been recruited, along with another 2000 students in nurse education. Only a week later, questions were being asked. NHS Direct had swallowed up 600 nurses into brand new posts and 3568 of 17,954 new nurses registered with the UKCC had come in from overseas. This could actually indicate a net loss. Indeed, the Department of Health was putting vacancies at 6900, a reduction of only 1100 from when New Labour had taken office, although the RCN put the figure at 15,000 and many NHS trusts were reporting vacancy rates of at least 10 per cent.

Having failed miserably in its pledge to increase nurse numbers by 15,000 by the 2001 election, New Labour decided to renew its vows to the populace that had so soundly re-elected it. It would recruit 20,000 extra nurses and midwives as part of its National Plan for the NHS.[5] Something wasn't working. A paltry ninety-eight nurses were recruited in Scotland in the twelve-month period ending in September 2000.

---

[5] Although the government did now have a strategy it was aiming to deliver through a host of policy initiatives such as *Improving Working Lives and Making a Difference*, it was still not acknowledging the scale of the problem or its wider

Spending on agency and bank nurses in Scotland was £25 million – which then rose to £44 million in 2000–01 (O'Dowd, 2002c). Nonetheless, Alan Milburn was able to announce a UK increase of 20,740 nurses and midwives between September 1999 and September 2001, built on a dramatic 15,000 increase in the second of those years. He couldn't resist claiming this met the target set in the *NHS Plan*, although this was actually for an increase between 2000 and 2004 to build upon those already recruited by the millennium. New Labour's success was, however, tempered by a set of figures as alarming as these were gratifying. Almost 9 per cent of the workforce was leaving annually. In 2001, this would equate to more than 31,000 nurses and midwives, leading to an RCN claim that 115,000 new starters would need to be recruited over the next two years if that government pledge was to be met by July 2004 (Mullholland, 2002a). Moreover, the huge hole created in student nurse placements in the 1980s and 1990s, which resulted in a steady decline of newly registered nurses up to its all time low of 12,000 in 1997, had left as its legacy an ageing workforce, 73,000 of whom are set to retire between 2002 and 2007. This promoted one senior civil servant to admit that the 20,000 students entering nurse education each year 'would have to double "just to stand still"' (Akid, 2002b: p 7). However, even the extra 20,000 didn't take into account drop-out rates of up to 38 per cent at some universities, and 34 per cent of nurses qualifying not coming into the NHS in 1997–98 (Finlayson *et al.*, 2002: pp 538–41).

The pool of registered nurses *not* working and, therefore, available as potential returners stood at 65,00 in 2002, but with no details available about their skills and likelihood of coming back into the NHS. Which was why trusts increasingly cast their net over foreign shores to increase nurse numbers. In 1998, more than 600 nurses were recruited from South Africa, despite the fledgling democracy's attempts to build its own health service. Amid growing protests about taking nurses from some of the poorest countries in the world, concern over recruitment agency costs, estimated at £350 million in 2000, also surfaced. Foreign recruitment is not a new strategy. It offers the most temporary of solutions to a structural problem. Yet, it nonetheless remained unchanged. The Phillippines became the biggest source of

---

contd.

parameters. In the United States, salaries were significantly higher – registered nurses could be earning $35,000–$65,000 (approximately £23,000–£43,000) according to qualifications in 2000. Yet, with industrial relations between nurses and private hospitals deteriorating steadily in the face of many of the problems that had afflicted British nursing in the 1990s, vacancy rates were even higher. Predictive studies were forecasting that by 2010 there would be a registered workforce of less than 650,000, with an expected 1.8 million registered nurse posts to fill (Buerhaus P *et al.*, 2000). American nurses were clear that status was not a solution and nor was pay alone. A good working environment, job security and involvement in decision making that affected work matters was also of vital importance.

recruitment in 2000–01, with 3396 being taken onto the register, but for some countries it was an issue of deep concern: Nelson Mandela had to add his voice to those asking Britain to stop recruiting his country's nurses. It was to no avail. South Africa lost more than 1000 of their nurses to Britain in the same year (UKCC, 2001).

The problems of recruiting and retaining sufficient numbers of nurses are compounded by the absence of those actually employed. In 1995, sickness rates among trained nursing staff was second only to that of ancillaries and closely followed by HCAs, averaging out at 5 per cent, compared to a national average, in all occupations, of 3.5 per cent. The cost to each NHS trust was estimated to be £1.4 million a year (Health Education Authority, 1995). The figures had risen to 5.6 per cent absence, costing each NHS trust an average £1.8 million per year by 1998 (Gulland, 1998c). Both surveys revealed that nurses did not take time off sick lightly. As seen in Chapter 6, contributing factors in staff sickness include a perception of being badly managed, poor communications and a lack of involvement in decisions. Doing agency or bank shifts on days off leaves staff feeling drained and needing sick time, as do the stresses of shift work, particularly internal rotation, when nurses work a mix of day and night shifts. These factors combined with the emotional exhaustion and chronic anxiety of working with the distress and disturbance of the sick and the dying creates the phenomenon often referred to as 'burnout', predicating sickness. However, for a small majority, it can also be a rebellious act, taking something back for oneself from an ungenerous employer. Nurses get sick pay, a concession won by the unions long ago, and it is undoubtedly, at times, used by some individuals as a means of compensating for low pay, lack of overtime and a feeling of being hard done by.

The whole debate about nurse numbers has been shrouded in claim and counter claim. What is clear is that nurses, at some stage in the near future, are going to have to press the government either to bite the bullet and set the conditions for nurses to stay in their jobs or re-define the work of an increasingly small number of registered nurses planning care for large numbers of an untrained workforce to carry out.

▶ What does the NMC have to offer nurses?

It's not a complete caricature to suggest that most nurses thought the UKCC took too much of their money for placing them on a register they were entitled to be on by dint of passing their exams. It was not a 'popular' institution. A tiny minority of nurses bothered to vote to elect nurse members onto its board.[6] Few mourned its loss

---

[6] Even when the unions openly campaigned for 'slates' of their own candidates, as in 1997, the turnout was a mere 13 per cent – was this apathy in the face of a vibrant democratic process or a cynical response to a body that was seen as having little relevance to the working lives of nurses and, when push came to shove, while carrying out its role of protecting the public either could not or would not act to help them maintain collective standards and develop their practice?

when the government decided it should be scrapped and replaced with the NMC. The UKCC started life in 1979, along with the separate national boards of Scotland, England, Wales and Northern Ireland, replacing the General Nursing Council, which had been the regulating nursing body since 1921. These new institutions were charged with the responsibility of working together to improve standards of training and conduct and regulate practice, with control and responsibility over all forms of training as well as placing all nurses on the appropriate register or roll (UKCC, 1999). The boards could inspect training establishments and the workplace and, if unhappy with standards, suspend training status, as well as validating training courses and programmes.

The Council, made up of forty nurses, midwives and health visitors elected by the wider workforce, and twenty appointees of the Secretary of State, communicated with nurses through its quarterly bulletin, *Register*, while publishing various pamphlets and guidelines on practice. Some of these were specialist, e.g., *Guidelines for mental health and learning disabilities nursing* (UKCC, 1998) while some, like *Guidelines for the administration of medicines* (UKCC, 2000) or *Guidelines for records and record keeping* (UKCC, 1998), were generic. These were put together by full-time staff but after 'extensive consultation with nurses, professional organisations, carers and service user groups' (UKCC, 1998a). It would also set up working groups and commissions, such as that initiated to examine the future direction of preparation for practice, as well as look at *The Scope of Professional Practice* (UKCC, 1992) and develop a revised regulatory framework for post-registration clinical practice, in *A Higher Level of Practice* (UKCC, 1999).[7] 'Democratic participation' stopped at the electoral process and individual consultation exercises, but limited places were always available to observe Council meetings and the Professional Conduct Committee, while open days were also organised. Events were organised to explore issues such as professional development and would be taken to venues across the United Kingdom. It was also accessed by enormous numbers of nurses via its advice line, which was taking up to 5000 calls daily in 1999, as well as contacts by email and letter. These contacts were also analysed on computer, in order to identify key concerns being raised by registered nurses, then fed into other areas of UKCC working, for instance the issue of disguising medication in patients' food and drink (UKCC, 2000a).

The UKCC was receiving the equivalent of £1 per month from every registered nurse, with a cool £4.3 million, or 49 per cent of its annual budget, having to be spent on professional conduct matters. Remaining funds were shared between maintaining an accurate register and professional standards and development

---

[7] Interestingly, *had* the UKCC enforced the concept that nurses should have to prove their competence before taking on an extended role or moving into areas of advanced practice, nurses may well have been better protected from having so much responsibility thrust upon them with no authority, reward or status to accompany it.

(UKCC, 1996). When the Council commissioned a survey of nurses' views, 77 per cent of those surveyed in 2000 thought it was an effective regulatory body, with 97 per cent agreeing that it was important to have a body like the UKCC in existence (UKCC, 2000b). There were, however, other indications that all was not well.

It didn't start with rumblings about self-regulation, but that was where the criticisms of the Council's performance led. This boiled over into a major controversy when a 'series of decisions resulted in convicted rapists and child abusers remaining on the professional register and, in some cases, continuing to practice as nurses or care assistants' (Editorial, *Nursing Times*, 1997). The issue of the UKCC's performance in dealing with professional misconduct was to dog it until the end. Despite criticism of its procedures, and even some of its bedrock principles, such as the code of conduct, its leaders usually took a defiant stance. Alison Norman, the Council president, exemplified that in defending the code against charges of being 'unrealistic, clumsy, unwieldy and placing unreal demands' on nurses, 'reducing the nursing profession to a state of fear', countering that 'its principles underpinned the educational preparation of nursing students' as well as 'being used by practitioners to develop local clinical standards'. Of the 1000 complaints received each year, the vast majority were dismissed as frivolous or pointing to organisational rather than individual failings, with around 140 cases coming to a full conduct hearing and about '100 nurses being struck off, with 65 per cent of charges relating to the physical, sexual or verbal abuse of patients or instances of cruelty and neglect' (Norman, 1998).[8] One of the problems with the Code is that it is inevitably open to interpretation. Given the enormous range of activities nurses are engaged in, the different circumstances in which they find themselves nursing and the fact that, although they may be highly competent practitioners, their performance may fall below somebody's expectations in a given situation, all are potentially vulnerable. Moreover, nurses are also liable to be held accountable for certain activities outside of work should they fall foul of the law. Whether or not the Council would actually take a case all the way to a conduct hearing, the anxiety of such an eventuality inevitably weighs heavily on some nurses.

The UKCC was also wrestling with another, larger dilemma. Many of its ruling Council members held a senior position, either in a managerial or educational post. The Council thus 'understands' the problems of the employers. It may have occasionally been critical of managers – rather than the culture of NHS management and institutions – but it has never acted upon those who have placed nurses in a position when 'professional standards' have been seriously compromised. It

---

[8] Two-thirds of nurses struck off are men, while nearly 60 per cent of complaints are against male nurses. The figure for all nurses struck off reached an all time high, at 104, in 2001, with complaints also hitting a peak at 1142. However, this is significantly lower than the 4500 complaints against doctors in the same period (Munro, 2001a).

presided over the individualisation of nursing, using the *Professional Code of Conduct* (UKCC, 1983 and 1992) and *Exercising Accountability* (UKCC, 1989) as its tools. These defined good practice and the web of rules that was being woven around nursing practice. They might have been able to cite all the benefits Alison Norman used in its defence, as well as the protection of the public, but the net effect was to emphasise and reinforce the message that nurses were on their own rather than part of a larger group working to collective principles and shared responsibilities. Moreover, when nurses really needed the protection of their ruling body, as they faced gagging clauses and increasingly authoritarian regimes in their trusts, the revised version of *Exercising Accountability* fell far short of expectations. The very fact that Unison had to launch its 'Be Safe' campaign in the late 1990s was a reflection that the UKCC was not meeting the needs of its nurses. When NMC President, Jonathan Asbridge, wrote in the first edition (NMC, 2002) that, 'Public protection can only be delivered if the NMC is able to earn the confidence of the registered nurses and midwives whom we regulate', he was discrete enough not to comment on how that was a goal that has eluded the NMC's predecessor.

▶ The NMC: what does the government want for nursing?

If the UKCC was doing a good job and the majority of nurses supported it, why did the government commission an independent review? The outcome, published by JM Consulting, called for its abolition. It also called for health visiting to be absorbed into nursing and midwifery separated out altogether. Its principle aims were to reduce bureaucracy, instil a harder professional edge and greater focus on the core purpose of the regulatory body. Perhaps the two most contentious proposals were that nursing be regulated in a much larger body providing the same function for all health professions, doctors included, while a role was suggested for the RCN in defining routes for professional development (JM Consulting, 1997). Unison, predictably, blasted the latter proposal, supported by many others who shared a concern about a commercial educator and trade union having anything to do with the content and delivery of statutory qualifications. The review sat on ministers' desks with leaks that it was planning to implement legislative changes by Order, a device that bypasses the usual processes of parliamentary debate and scrutiny. Then, in February 1999, came the announcement that the UKCC and national boards were to be axed and replaced with the NMC.

Perhaps one of the final humiliations for the Council was that it had to increase its fees by 67 per cent, from £36 every three years to £60, the first rise in seven years, to pay for the changes that included its abolition. The inevitable outcry from nurses was about both the increase and what they were getting for their money. Disquiet about the government's rush into changing the system also emerged. Achieving a balance between reducing bureaucracy and maintaining a group that could represent the concerns and issues of all nurses, midwives and health visitors is a key problem. The NMC's membership was reduced to twenty-four, including the president, seven 'consumers', two employers, two from education and four nurses, midwives and health visitors from each of the UK countries. The proposals for the new NMC would give it:

- Greater powers to protect the public by increasing its ability to deal with poor performance as well as misconduct;
- Increased lay participation;
- Greater transparency, including a responsibility to consult more widely;
- Allow it to impose conditional registration;
- Have a slimmer register – with three 'live parts', registered nurses, registered midwives and registered health visitors, instead of fifteen;
- A statutory protection of the title 'nurse,' with stiff penalties for impostors.

Ultimately, it was not so much a case of looking at the detail of what was being done but considering the implications. The government had picked up the ball, ran with it and kicked it straight into the open goal that nursing offered it. It would have been unthinkable for any government to have imposed its agenda on the medical profession in the way New Labour did with the NMC, which was about tightening its grip on nursing as much as anything else.

However, Deborah Glover, former clinical editor of the *Nursing Times* could not have been more wrong when she wrote, 'What nurses must realise is that self-regulation is not a right, *it is a privilege*' [my emphasis] (Glover, 1999: pp 30–1). It is a right, earned by the nurses who fought tooth and nail to get a register for nurses almost a century ago, and those before and after, who fought their own battles to raise the profile of, and give dignity, meaning and integrity to, nurses and the work that they do. It is maintained by nurses who carry out extremely demanding work in the most difficult circumstances. Like all rights, it requires democratic involvement to be maintained and needs to be defended by nurses. They ignore that at their peril and it could be argued that nurses continue to be punished for swallowing the notion that they await salvation by dint of privilege rather than through rights for which they actually have to fight, both to win in the first place and then maintain.

▶ The NMC: how well are nurses prepared? PREP

Post-registration education and practice (PREP) is a little bit like nasty Aunt Pertunia. She's around somewhere. She keeps threatening to come and stay and an uneasy feeling is generated in the whole family whenever the subject of a visit is raised. But no one is actually clear at all about what would happen were she to arrive on the doorstep. For PREP has been 'arriving' since the mid-1990s. In fact, it was in March 1995 that Mary Uprichard, then UKCC president, wrote to registered nurses, 'It is with pleasure that I write to you about the implementation of the UKCC's standards for PREP.' An extensive document identified the purpose of PREP as being, 'To improve standards of patient and client care, both directly and indirectly' (UKCC, 1995). This would be achieved through nurses meeting four requirements to maintain their registration:

- Complete a Notification of Practice every three years or if the area of practice is changed;
- Undertake a minimum of five days of study or equivalent every three years;
- Maintain a Personal Professional Profile with details of professional development;
- Undertake a Return to Practice programme if out of practice for five years or more.

If nurses are using more than one registrable qualification in their practice, they still only have to undertake a five days study. Maintaining a professional development plan is expected to involve a self-assessment of strengths and weaknesses, setting learning objectives and an action plan. The recording of study time and learning outcomes is another part of this process. By 1999, the term continuing professional development was associated with PREP and by March 2001 nurses could receive a request from the UKCC to audit how they had met the requirement – with which they would have to comply. However, another requirement was that nurses would have spent a minimum of 750 hours or 100 days in practice before being able to re-register or undertake a return to practice course. Anyone wishing to retain dual registration as midwife and nurse would have to do 100 days in each. Given that a whole range of activities qualify as educational and involve professional development, meeting the requirement is nowhere near as daunting as it appears. Teaching sessions, reading articles, journals and books, clinical supervision, journal clubs, clinical review meetings all contribute as learning activities and are as valid as conferences and formal educational courses. The work comes from maintaining the professional profile. PREP initiated a cottage industry, with study aids being published, nursing journals cramming their pages with articles that were described as being suitable for PREP and fancy portfolios being put on sale. One matter that periodically punctured the sales' pitch was that of obtaining study leave and funding, which was left to the individual nurse.

PREP's efficacy was never seriously questioned until the Bristol Royal Infirmary inquiry report into the care of children receiving cardiac surgery. Between thirty and thirty-five children died unnecessarily as a result of substandard treatment. Although surgeons were clearly identified as being responsible for the deaths, Professor Ian Kennedy, the inquiry chairperson, stated that nurses, with all other healthcare professionals, should have their fitness to practice externally reviewed by a range of people, including members of the public. Having completed a 525-page report, Professor Kennedy threw a shot right across the bows of PREP, stating that it was no more than 'a piece of paper' and 'not sufficiently rigorous'.

His proposal, he acknowledged, 'places demands on nurses, but properly so. From that demand will come recognition of their role' (Mullholland, 2001a).

► Last among equals – nurses' struggles for equality

The fundamental problem that has bedevilled nurses' attempts to achieve both financial and institutional equality – that they are women – is now being recognised and equal pay claims may be the way in which they begin to finally overcome the obstacles so neatly placed in their way for the last century and a half.

Even within that large body of staff that are nurses, however, there are still those less equal than the majority. Racism has permeated nursing ever since Mary Seacole was denied official access to the Crimea, despite her experience in caring for victims of cholera and yellow fever, as well as surgical skills developed in treating people with knife and gunshot wounds (Alexander and Dewjee, 1984).

The sight of a group of young white men charged with the murder of Stephen Lawrence, a black teenager, swaggering in and out of court, smiling gratuitously into the cameras were the most overt and sickening reminder of the problems that lurk deep in the depths of the nation's psyche. The conduct of the police in the case, inept and insensitive at best, something far more sinister at worst, was systematically exposed by the campaign mounted by Stephen's parents, Doreen and Neville Lawrence and their supporters before being documented in the McPherson Report (1999). After the guilty escaped justice – and arguably it was more than Stephen Lawrence's murderers who were guilty – notions of unwitting and institutional racism became the topic of national discussion.

The *Empire Windrush* was the first ship to bring people across from Jamaica to seek work in the United Kingdom, including women who would go on to train as nurses. In fact, the majority of people coming into the NHS from overseas were pushed into ancillary posts but a sufficient number were recruited into nursing to ensure the survival of the NHS. Their reward was to be treated with suspicion, hostility and outright discrimination, finding themselves exploited and marginalised in their economic and social lives. Their presence was required but aroused widespread hostility at all levels, from landlords and shop owners to employers, from patients to trade union branches. Many were encouraged to train as enrolled nurses even if they had the obvious ability and qualifications to gain their registration and get a foot on the career ladder. By 1975, 20.5 per cent of all students were from overseas, with many being directed into mental health, learning disabilities and care of the elderly, all of which were having particular recruitment problems. Most people from black and ethnic minorities remained in low paying, insecure jobs, with unsocial hours in unhealthy or dangerous environments (Solomas and Back, 1996). Nurses were no different and many found it hard to gain promotion or move into more attractive areas of nursing.

COHSE full-time officials began to recognise trends in the grading process in the late 1980s, with minority ethnic staff being placed into lower grades than their white counterparts, even when they were working alongside one another. Moreover, there was some evidence in the late 1980s that minority ethnic staff were overrepresented in those being investigated by the UKCC (Carlisle, 1990: pp 25–9). However, given that the UKCC – and most NHS employers – were not conducting any ethnic monitoring, much of the evidence gleaned from that period was inevitably anecdotal. Black and Asian nurses have reported clear harassment and difficulties with patients over long periods. In 1995, *Nursing in a Multi-Ethnic NHS*, a government report, found that 60 per cent of 'black' nurses and 58 per cent of Asian nurses had experienced similar problems of racist attitudes among patients (Beishon *et al.*, 1995). Black and ethnic minority staff face racism and are blocked from promotion (Coker, 2001). Just to prove that there can be some equality in discriminatory practice, 'A study by the Medical Practitioner's Union found that white consultants in England and Wales were three times more likely than those from ethnic minorities to get distinction awards, which can add up to £62,815 a year to their salaries' (Carvel, 2002).

Even before the McPherson Report there was a growing acceptance that, even if direct racism may be decreasing, institutional racism remained a problem for the NHS. The issue has been subject to a number of political and policy initiatives. The NHS Executive ordered managers to take a proactive and positive approach to tackling racism although concerns that the decline in numbers of people with an ethnic minority background joining the NHS had reached crisis point were not founded. The decline was real, but not from all minority groups. However, many nurses from ethnic minority groups are a significant part of an ageing workforce. Many will leave nursing feeling little has changed, despite this government's more positive approach and the changing attitude of managers. Commenting on the process of how organisations can subvert attempts to address racism, Neil Dhruev (2002: pp 26–7) writes, 'The real process is clear: first, ensure the racist action is covert; second, silence the evidence. The twist comes in designing systems that appear to help, while maintaining the racist hierarchy.' Arguing for support for Black and Ethnic Minority Networks, he suggests:

> We need to find ways to preserve and develop humanitarian values that go beyond an individualistic approach to patient/client care. These values need to inform the implementation of strategic change, the operational management of services, and the daily relationships that enable our professional and clinical practices.

▶ Getting the needle: health and safety

As we shall see later in this chapter, nursing is now arguably the most dangerous job in Britain. But nurses' physical and mental health has long been jeopardised by their work. For example, it was estimated that back injuries cost the NHS

1.5 million working days every year, costing approximately £50 million (Smith and Seccombe, 1996). Millions of pounds are also being paid out in compensation to nurses who have damaged their backs in accidents at work (RCN, 1996). Stress is an even more costly problem. Trade unions have long fought for reforms in health and safety for the workforce and, following the landmark Health and Safety at Work Act, 1974, employers were legally bound to establish systems of work which, as far as was reasonably practicable, would be safe and without risk to health. Trade union representatives were given real clout when it came to dealing with health and safety matters, as well as guaranteed rights to time off for both education and training and attending meetings. They could issue enforcement notices and, if they were not acted upon, bring in the Health and Safety Executive (HSE). The Act allowed for trade union representatives to sit on recognised health and safety committees, alongside management, that each side had a statutory responsibility to facilitate. Further legislation and policy built on the 1974 Act. Some was general, some more specific, such as the manual handling guidelines issued by the HSE in 1992.

Nonetheless, in the workplace, use of legislation and policy was highly variable, depending on trade unions' presence and influence through a well-organised local branch. The arrival of the internal market with its new managerial culture, coupled with the decline of NHS trade unionism in the workplace, all made the monitoring and implementation of health and safety policies more difficult.

The range of potential hazards has risen with the increase of technological equipment, toxic substances and agents, infection risks and the general working environment. Policy decisions also have an impact. Fewer domestic staff – who tend to be expected to work shorter shifts, often spread across more than one ward, with less generous terms and conditions – are the norm as this is how commercial companies who take over domestic services can under-bid their competitors and win contracts. Frequency of cleaning schedules is lessened and, because of the conditions, staff turnover tends to be quite high. All these factors increase the risk of infection and pose a greater risk to staff.

Sometimes technological innovations fail to make the expected impact. For example, although moving and handling equipment should be standard, lack of training, lack of space, shortages of the correct type of equipment and a 'general mistrust on the part of both nurses and patients' are preventing specified safe procedures for lifting being followed (Rogers *et al.*, 1999).

It is probably a mix of poor practice, ignorance, or the hope that there won't be a bad accident within their area necessitating a big compensation pay out, that encourages trusts and their managers not to invest properly in health and safety. It is also a costly business and trusts don't have a health and safety budget. Thus, repair work may be viewed as essential by staff, and even their manager, but the estates' department team not directly affected by these concerns, may not authorise it.

Low expectations of the work getting done may put nurses off from actually informing their manager about potential or actual hazards, even though this may place others at risk. Trying to enforce repairs, essential or not, is time consuming and often unproductive. As with so many other things, risk becomes something nurses are tacitly expected to accept. So it is with needlestick injuries, of which there are an estimated 100,000 sustained by UK health workers every year. With the risk of contracting HIV after a needlestick injury at 0.3 per cent and hepatitis C transmission between 0.44 per cent and 3 per cent, the view of some decision makers is that it is not worth investing in safer needles that could reduce the risk of injury by 80 per cent. A trial in West Lothian Healthcare NHS Trust proved safer needles could be introduced. However, its director of nursing 'concluded that the £176,000 needed to introduce safer needles throughout Scotland was not justified by the relative risk' (Munro, 2001b: p 12). Health and safety legislation, enacted at a local level in committees and overseen by shop stewards and health and safety representatives, was a beacon to health workers in their attempts to keep their employers' practices in check. It gave them confidence through their legitimised power, organisational rights and authority. Moreover, it cost the employer money and circumscribed their right to manage. It had to be constrained. And so it was as the internal market was rolled out.

▶ Whistleblowing

Few people could have predicted the culture of fear and intimidation that was introduced into the NHS in the early 1990s. If the UKCC's role really was to protect the public, it should have been doing a lot more to protect nurses who were placing their careers at risk to do just that. Given the radicalism of the late 1980s, when nurses were talking to the media in droves about what their job meant to them, about the difficulties in caring for their patients and the experience of being seriously undervalued, it was perhaps all the more astonishing to discover that, just a few short years later, very few nurses would answer even the most anodyne questions unless they had the express permission of their manager. Of course, one was the consequence of the other.

Whistleblowing involves acting against the vested interests of those who have abused their position of power, by publicising that abuse. For this is an issue which involves the overt use of power and conflict, with those who control the system controlling the flow of information as an essential part of that process. Whistleblowers from the 1970s were subsequently praised. In the 1980s, individual or group abuse of patients was far less common. Nurses were now talking to the press far more openly, with the encouragement, support and protection of their trade unions, about the systematic failings of their own institutions and the NHS due to staffing shortages, cutbacks to the service and ward closures. However, the new management teams of self-governing trusts, with the blessing of the government, took a far harder line about staff talking to anyone outside their organisation. Staff were superficially encouraged to talk to line managers and complaints departments. Any deviation from this left them open to disciplinary action.

Whistleblowers, arguably, have their own issues for going outside recognised structures, even when there is a reasonable likelihood they can be utilised effectively. But what were nurses to do in this new climate? There were moral and ethical issues to be considered by individual nurses up and down the country. Trying to raise these issues through the proper channels risked being punished and bullied. If the organisation wasn't responding, through its line management structure or complaints system, options were limited. Nurses could get on with the work and make the best of it, move on and hope the situation would be better elsewhere, leave nursing altogether, try and get their union to address the problem or speak up themselves.

The key problem was the sense of corporate loyalty and identification that managers were trying to load into the accountability balance sheet they realised was laid before them by the UKCC. This was not something nurses were signed up to, however. They wanted to oppose both the newer ideological and clinical changes that were being foisted upon them but, if they weren't able to do that, wanted to tell the public about what was happening. This breakdown of consensus *within* NHS trusts was about the change of focus and purpose of the service. Given the highly vocal opposition to the plans for self-governing trusts, both within the health service and among the wider public, there was a recognition that potentially damaging stories about cuts, difficulties or poor patient care would be blamed on the new organisations, with the public inevitably siding with nurses and other clinicians. With workplace trade unions in decline, individuals had to speak out and carry the responsibility instead of a branch secretary or representative with the protection that can be afforded by their position. The situation was then further exacerbated when trusts started introducing 'gagging' or confidentiality clauses into people's contracts, making it a disciplinary offence to publicly divulge anything about the 'business' of the 'organisation'. So powerful was this, with a whole series of stories relating to nurses and other health workers being victimised and/or sacked, that even if nurses were not subject to such a clause they kept their mouths shut.

It is to New Labour's credit that, given its obsession with 'spin' and centralised control, it has introduced the legislation the Conservatives baulked at concerning whistleblowing, providing people with legal protection under the Public Interest Disclosure Act, 1998 if they divulged information about activities that are criminal, fraudulent or dangerous or may contravene health and safety. A 'reasonableness test' must be satisfied, in that it must be clear that the employee took every opportunity to utilise existing channels to deal with the issues of concerns – unless s/he feared this would lead to victimisation. Breaches of patient confidentiality or confidence would be likely to fail such a test. If victimised by their employer or sacked in breach of the Act they can be awarded uncapped compensation.

Undoubtedly, the safest way to raise such concerns, however, is through an established trade union. While this is much harder than it once was, that is still very much part of a union's role and affords a whistleblower with far more protection than anyone acting alone. This is probably the only way that individuals will regain the confidence to talk publicly about issues of concern in their workplace. For the consequence of such oppressive management during the 1990s is, in some ways, an even more sophisticated use of power: a legacy of self-censorship borne out of fear.

▶ Bullying

Bullying is not a new phenomenon for nursing. The term was not always in common currency but the practice was very much in evidence from the earliest days of organised and hierarchical nursing structures. It became headline news because of the breakdown in consensus within nursing and the NHS. Managers no longer had the active consent of many of their workforce for some of the things they were having to implement, yet were now working in a more rights' conscious culture where nurses had established a sense of their identity and independence. If change that was not welcomed by nurses was to be achieved, this would have to be broken down, even though it was unlikely to be easy. Almost two-thirds of Unison members surveyed in 1997 had either witnessed or experienced bullying in their workplace, with the manager being the person responsible in 83 per cent of cases. In 73 per cent of the cases in which the bullying was reported to a manager, s/he ignored it. For the purposes of the survey and its subsequent report, Unison defined bullying as, 'offensive, intimidating, malicious, insulting or humiliating behaviour, an abuse of power or authority which attempts to undermine an individual or group of employees and which may cause them to suffer stress'.

It can occur in a number of ways. These include:

- Making life difficult for staff who might be more competent than the bully;
- Constantly criticising or ridiculing staff;
- Removing responsibility and giving staff trivial work to do;
- Refusing to delegate work;
- Shouting, being abusive – either verbally or physically;
- Persistently picking on staff;
- Insisting on having things done in a particular way;
- Blocking promotion;
- Overloading people with work and reducing deadlines. (Unison, 1997).

This was not confined to management working under a Conservative government. An RCN survey of 4500 nurses, conducted in 2001, found that 17 per cent had been bullied in the previous twelve months. However, that number rose to 29 per cent of nurses from minority ethnic backgrounds.

When trusts were set a target of reducing their sickness absence rates by 20 per cent by 2001 and 30 per cent by 2003, the government not only ignored all the evidence on sickness absence but also the advice of the experts with whom it consulted. This advice was to set a target of an absence rate of not more than 5 per cent. Critics of the government's targets warned 'trusts may have to adopt a punitive approach' to meet them or 'get rid of staff, which is already happening in some trusts' (Agnew, 1998: p 5). Now, not only could bullying make nurses sick but also they could find themselves being threatened with the sack if they took too much time off sick as a consequence. Just to make matters worse, Helen Smart, project manager for leadership in south-east England, acknowledged that (New Labour's) changes in the NHS and pressure on managers to 'get results' had increased an already huge problem (Shamash, 2002: p 8).

Is there any particular link between nurses, nursing and bullying? In many respects, no. Bullying is widespread in British working life and undoubtedly a consequence of a particular aspect of British industrial relations. However, the qualities ascribed by Tim Field, an expert on the subject, to the victims of bullying make interesting reading. Field states that they are often kind, caring, empathic, sensitive, honest and trustworthy, conscientious and reliable, 'people focused'. They are willing to help, want to please, are selfless, tolerant and committed to service. Lacking assertiveness, they are deferential, put other's needs first and seek approval because of their need to feel valued (Field, 1996). Comparing those qualities to those sought in the 'suitable women' required to 'professionalise' and improve the nursing workforce reveals a startling overlap. Thus, within nursing, the bully and victim might be drawn to one another, recognising something familiar. However, unless the circumstances permit, often nothing will happen. But when there is pressure on the service, tacit approval, or an unwillingness to rein in bullying managers, they will impact on junior staff or peers. This closeness also offers a suggestion as to why nurses then mimic the behaviour of bullying senior nurses when they themselves gain promotion or a position of some power – and of why nurses talk so disparagingly of one another when they see apparent 'weakness' in their colleagues, convinced, or willing to convince themselves, that the characteristics they dislike are not their own and that it is the fault of individuals if they are being bullied rather than an organisational problem that can be tackled.

▶ Stress

Stress in nursing is arguably a social construct to explain the physical and psychological reaction experienced by people facing one insoluble problem after another. That volumes have been written about it only serves to legitimise stress as an individual experience or as an internal reaction, an inability to cope. It is as if these are separate from the reality that is created within an organisation, working environment or relationships. Working in the NHS is undoubtedly 'stressful' and nurses usually figure amongst the top occupational groups suffering from it. But it is, again, the individualisation of an organisational and structural experience.

Being under some degree of pressure is natural, can be stimulating and help improve performance, but stress is something more. The HSE have produced guidelines about it, defining it as 'a natural reaction to excessive pressure'. Noting that it is not a disease, it points to the fact that if stress is excessive and prolonged it can lead to mental and physical ill health (HSE, 1999). A survey of 12,000 NHS staff found 28.5 per cent of nurses had minor mental health problems, using the general health questionnaire (Borrill *et al.*, 1996). A government commissioned survey found that nurses are 40 per cent more likely to suffer stress than other groups of comparable workers (Health Service Manager Briefing, 1999). Undoubtedly, the worst case in recent years was that of Richard Pocock, an RMN who committed suicide when he was convinced he was going to lose his job as his hospital closed. Temporarily placed in a management position when already not coping, he reported to his manager all the classic symptoms of stress but was subjected to 'an "oppressive, ruthless and macho style of management"' which 'turned a blind eye to his worsening condition' until he killed himself. His family won an out of court settlement of £25,000 (Payne, 1998: p 15).

If the nature of a problem is not properly identified, it is impossible to work out a solution. What are the difficulties facing nurses that could be described as 'stressful'? Some are common to people working in different occupations, some unique. These include:

- Boring or repetitive work, increasing workload and shortened deadlines;
- Inflexible or unpredictable work schedules or shift patterns;
- Lack of control over workload;
- Lack of communication and consultation;
- A blame culture;
- Lack of support;
- Too little or too much training;
- Confusion about role;
- Managing others;
- Poor relationships with colleagues, bullying and/or harassment;
- Hazardous work;
- Staffing shortages.

More explicit to nursing are:

- Abusive and/or violent patients;
- Inter-disciplinary rivalry;
- Balancing academic requirements with maintaining a good work performance;
- Low wages and poor conditions of service;
- Insufficient time to provide emotional support to patients;
- Working with people badly injured, distressed and/or disturbed, suffering with illness or disease and/or dying.

Given that this list almost constitutes an index for this book, it is little wonder that nurses are told they are stressed. Teaching people stress management techniques or increasing the provision of stress counselling – often put forward as a solution – is unlikely to help do anything more than assist nurses to tolerate the conditions they find themselves in. Moreover, given the numbers affected, it is not something individuals can address in isolation from their colleagues and supportive organisations such as their trade unions, for most of the issues listed above require an organisational or political solution. Even small things, like shortened handover periods and the loss of the afternoon overlap between shifts, have their own impact, making communications harder and the opportunities for working together, education and training and arriving at a shared sense of the problems nursing teams grapple with more difficult. And, perhaps, for many nurses the biggest stressor is saying, 'No', both in the clinical situation and politically.

The Nuffield Trust Report, *Improving the Health of the Workforce* (1998), cited poor management being associated with staff ill health and a predictor of absenteeism. One simple response to dealing with problems that cause stress is for managers to do their job properly. Employers have a clear duty in law to make sure that employees aren't made ill by their work and, whether or not stress is a social construct, people's health does suffer if they are not managed properly and face the same unresolved problems day in, day out. Strategies to resolve it are not costly, and quite straightforward:

- To relieve boredom at work, rotate tasks, give people more – but manageable – levels of responsibility and increase the scope of the job;
- Encourage peer support and collective ways of working;
- Prioritise tasks, cut out unnecessary work and give warning of upcoming urgent deadlines;
- Help staff define individual roles and teams to identify their focus;
- Identify a clear focus to the work of the individual and/or team, thus allowing for
- some limit setting and an understanding of the parameters to the service, even if there is then an acceptance that some flexibility may be required;
- Use appraisals positively, to help staff identify strengths and weaknesses, agree objectives and responsibilities and structure their work and development;
- Provide good quality education and training to help staff develop the appropriate levels of knowledge and skills for the work required of them;
- Make training in communication and interpersonal skills an integral part of pre- and post-registration nurse education;
- Prevent bullying, abuse and harassment by introducing effective educational packages, as well as monitoring and managerial systems;
- Promote flexible working and family friendly policies that actively promote a healthy work–life balance for all, including managers;[9]

---

[9] Such programmes as this can often exclude managers. Not only is this patently unfair and impairs their ability to work effectively, it also makes it far less likely they will champion them for their staff in the way that is often necessary.

- Provide adequate control measures for the management of health and safety and to combat hazards;
- Use appropriate and agreed policies for consultation and negotiation through recognised unions, good communications systems and, wherever possible, means of involving staff in all decisions affecting their work;
- Introduce good support mechanisms, such as reflective practice groups, clinical supervision for all staff (and separate to managerial supervision, which should also be provided).

It is, of course, in the interests of the employer to observe for the types of behaviours people display when stressed, such as more erratic behaviour, deteriorating relationships with colleagues, anxiety, poor time keeping, irritability, indecisiveness, absenteeism, reduced level of performance, experiencing somatic symptoms and, in some cases, excessive use of tobacco, alcohol and illicit drugs. That managers and trusts cannot prevent the levels of stress permeating health services suggests either the most chronic case of incompetence imaginable or, far more likely, irreconcilable problems which managers are not empowered to resolve, as we shall explore below.

▶ Violence

Recent figures indicate that 75 per cent of nursing staff have been subjected to violence while at work and 85 per cent have experienced verbal abuse or been threatened with violence, suggesting nursing is the most dangerous job in the United Kingdom (Gournay, 2002).[10] Despite the government making the eradication of violence against nurses and other health workers one of its priorities, it has got nowhere near achieving the targets it set for reducing attacks on nurses. Indeed, the targets for psychiatric units were declared unachievable by Professor Kevin Gournay, after 850 nurses had been surveyed for the UKCC, because of lack of training for nurses and a lack of support from trusts (Mulholland, 2001a: p 9). 'Zero Tolerance' campaigns, setting trusts targets to reduce the number of incidents have all met with failure. The reason is pretty simple: they are the wrong targets. Violence doesn't occur in a vacuum. It had increased in the wider society for a range of complex reasons. Increased levels of alcohol and illicit drug consumption undoubtedly play their part, while any rise in levels of violent behaviour in society

---

[10] Mental health and learning disability is the most dangerous area of nursing, with twenty-four incidents per month per 1000 staff, with acute the least violent, with three incidents per 1000 staff per month. The Department of Health has, however, confirmed widely held suspicions that violence is underreported or 'swept under the carpet by "weak" management practices' (*Nursing Times*, 20 October 1999: p 9).

will inevitably be mirrored in the NHS.[11] Moreover, New Labour's famous 'joined up' government has also failed, with the criminal justice system only making matters worse. The police are too often ambivalent or refuse to act when nurses are assaulted in the line of duty. When convictions have been sought, magistrates have ruled that the threat of violence is part of a nurses' job.

Yet, the factors which influence violence against nurses could almost all be addressed. Violence in psychiatric settings occurs partly because of the concentration in wards of more acutely disturbed patients, many of whom have severe and enduring mental health problems, with a reliance on agency and bank nurses to make up a large part of the shift complement, thus making teamwork, consistency and containment harder. Moreover, nurses report that if it is a nurse being assaulted, the medical profession can be slow to respond, but this changes dramatically if a doctor is the victim. Too often, the criminal justice system won't act because of a patient's mental health problems, even though these may have little, if anything, to do with the violent behaviour. The same is often true in A&E departments and it is almost certainly no coincidence that both clinical services sustained dramatic cuts in the 1980s and 1990s before seeing levels of violence rise.

The government did all it could to heighten the expectation of what the NHS could achieve, creating an image of an NHS that could fix just about every social and physical ill imaginable, and then made a habit of announcing substantial increases in funding, staffing levels and just about every benchmark possible. Demand for services thus grows. In A&E departments, particularly, this meant that longer waits for triage and assessment, as well as treatment and admission were met by an angrier response.

These are key factors in understanding the context of violence. A number of practical measures can be employed to reduce violence, such as:

- Regular risk assessments to identify staff groups at risk and potential risk situations, then carrying out staff training to address these, while remedying risks within the environment;
- Developing a strong relationship with the local police, who can provide a pro-active presence in a hospital, in the A&E department especially. Employers can encourage the police and Crown Prosecution Service to take an unambiguous stance on violence towards healthcare staff and, with staff affected, initiate prosecutions when necessary;
- Regular and effective training in the prevention and management of violence, breakaway techniques and de-escalation strategies, for all potentially at risk staff;

---

[11] Nor is it only in the NHS that the problem emerges. More than 350,000 people a year are subject to violent attacks at work and many more go unreported (TUC, 1997).

- Creating waiting areas that are as calm and pleasant as possible, with material to relieve boredom;
- Ensuring there are up-to-date alarm systems;
- In the community, the use of mobile 'phones, personal alarms and clear safety procedures for conducting home visits, working on estates that are known as high risk and 'out of hours' should all be routine, with nurses working in pairs if visiting clients who are potentially at risk, and even with police support if necessary;
- Agreeing clear guidelines and policies locally is essential if staff are to behave consistently and safely, as well as protocols for categorising the severity of an incident, reporting it and action that is to be taken as a consequence.

Good staffing levels are fundamental to the process of preventing and managing violence. It is not just about having a sufficient number of bodies in situ. Staff groups should be working together for sufficiently long periods of time to get to know one another well, form stable, coherent and consistent teams and feel confident in working with their patient group, even in the most difficult circumstances. Moreover, they should have opportunities to develop an understanding of the client group with which they are working and what might prompt abuse and/or violence.

Nor is the problem of dealing with violence unrelated to the other practical problems facing contemporary nurses. Already 'stressed out' staff are not well equipped to deal with what are, by definition, highly stressful and hazardous situations. Spotting and defusing potentially dangerous situations in their early stages of development is made more difficult, as is summoning up the necessary calmness, concentration, and full use of a mindful approach, establishing boundaries in a clear and unequivocal manner. Regular training in de-escalation and breakaway techniques has to be utilised. In mental health nursing, safe restraint methods should also be taught. Moreover, staff who are frightened of being criticised, humiliated or punished for being seen as unable to 'cope' may spend too long trying to contain a potentially dangerous situation before seeking assistance.

Thus, the links in a dysfunctional organisation can be seen. Whistleblowing – or forms of dissent – are suppressed by bullying. Bullying prevents problems being resolved and staff become stressed. Stressed out staff are less able to deal with violence. Other combinations can be extrapolated but all are strands in the web of control that managers sought to spin around nurses in the new culture of the NHS but which, in turn, have impacted upon nurses, their performance and the effectiveness of the service.

▶ No place like home – what makes accommodation affordable?

Housing for public sector and other low paid workers is a major issue shared by nurses – in the south-east particularly, but also in cities right across the

United Kingdom. It is also linked with the nursing deficit in the NHS. Partly the result of successive governments forcing local councils to offload all of their housing stock, it is also due to the demise of affordable social housing as grants to housing associations have ended. The NHS was required to sell as much property as possible by the Tories in the 1980s. The current crisis is made all the worse, however, by the fact that billions of pounds worth of what could be affordable housing are still owned by the NHS, while NHS buildings that could be converted into accommodation units lay empty, despite trusts having to pay capital charges on them – back to the government. Meanwhile, much of government thinking – certainly in the Treasury – is focused on making accommodation available to buy, rather than exploring the merits of revitalising the social housing sector and rented accommodation. Is the issue one of increasing affordable accommodation, paying supplements to staff in areas of high cost housing or simply paying nurses a wage that allows them to compete with everyone else?

Trusts are selling off accommodation to housing associations, which then repair them and rent them out to nurses. The government has introduced cost of living supplements (COLS) as well as initiatives that enable nurses to take a part mortgage in a house or flat. However, these strategies show little sign of resolving the problem. The COLS initiative has been widely criticised. The unions fear it is the beginning of a re-introduction of local pay and are fiercely antagonistic to anything like this, despite a flat rate national wage meaning that nurses in London and large parts of the south-east are, in effect, vastly lower paid than colleagues in other parts of the country. Nurses dislike them because they are viewed as arbitrary and unfair. For example, West Sussex nurses received a supplement but those in East Sussex got nothing. Moreover, they still hold the view that they should receive a basic salary that will allow them to choose where they live. Yet, the problem of nurses literally being unable to afford a roof over their head is symptomatic of the long-term problems they have endured of low wages, serving others and being taken for granted.

▶ Case study 7: Agenda for change – a genuinely radical improvement in nurses' pay or more of the same?

The cost of staging nurses' pay rises since the mid-1980s – to each nurse – has been approximately £2000. For government, it has represented a saving of approximately £100 million – not even loose change out of government expenditure during that period. Since the beginning of New Labour's first administration, the promise of a 'fairer' pay system has been the carrot dangled in front of the unions. Yet, as much as they have chomped, they have still to taste the rewards. Five years on, *Agenda for Change* was still on the negotiating table.

Agenda for Change has had an interesting genesis, arising out of the debacle of local pay, with a single pay spine for all health workers being informally floated by interested parties from both the management and trade union side. Its principal supporters were the unlikely bedfellows of Unison and the NHS Confederation. The latter wanted it because it would simplify the pay process, particularly the PRB and Whitley Council structures. They saw it as means of agreeing a core of national terms and conditions which could then be expanded upon by local negotiation as well as re-introducing the notion of productivity into pay negotiations. Unison saw it as an opportunity to address a wide range of anomalies experienced by both its nursing and non-nursing members, using job evaluation schemes and looking at comparisons between different groups. Unison was proposing that this would enable the NHS to pay staff for the work they did rather than according to their job title. The RCN was bitterly opposed, arguing that it would foster generic working and multi-skilling, promoting the work of healthcare assistants and undermining the role of the registered nurse. Unison, in turn, was delighted to be in the driving seat on a policy that would attract government support and consolidate its hoped for alliance with New Labour and reputation as a union with which government could 'do business'. There was, within Unison, a recognition that the BMA would never allow itself to be placed on the same salary scale as other health workers and would negotiate a separate deal but the hope that the RCN, in sticking to its position of keeping nurses in a different category, would isolate itself and lose credibility. That was 1997, but when government proposals eventually emerged in 1999, Unison was deeply disappointed, for there were three spines, not two. The doctors and dentists' review body would remain as was; a single new negotiating council for all Whitley groups would be introduced; with a separate spine for nurses and the professions allied to medicine (PAMs). Moreover, there were hints that annual increments would give way to performance-related pay along with a 'fairer' national framework for determining pay increases. The RCN would later suffer a significant setback when its attempts to get at least ten pay bands were thwarted and the government imposed a limit of eight.

The government then set a tight timetable for consultation, wanting to move things forward quickly. More than a year later, the negotiations were mired in the detail. The unions walked out as new arrangements were being made for doctors outside those negotiations. The original April 2001 deadline for implementation was delayed by a year. That deadline came and went. Discretionary points – a system of additional points at the top of the pay scale for grades F–I, for which nurses could apply to their managers – introduced in 1998, had failed, with only 13 per cent of nurses gaining any additional points and tiny numbers gaining the maximum three points. The downgrading of nursing posts was continuing. Both the PRB and department pointed to *Agenda for Change* as the solution to all nurses' problems. However, later that year there were further problems in negotiations as the Treasury clamped down and made it clear that nothing could be agreed until it was clear how much money would be available from the government's spending review the following summer.[12] This was reminiscent of the Treasury interference that wrecked any chance of clinical grading – the system *Agenda for Change* was being designed to replace – being successful. So, too, was the notion of job evaluation as a means of allocating staff to pay bands. Sixteen different factors were identified to help this process, including knowledge skills and experience, the physical and mental effort required to do the job and the emotional impact the job had. This is obviously extremely complex and could only realistically be achieved by interviewing each staff member about their work and, in some cases, conducting corroborating interviews with managers and/or colleagues. However, this was actually to be done by comparing job descriptions with job profiles prepared at national level. These of course, barely capture anything of the work many nurses do. Moreover, job descriptions for large numbers of staff, e.g., 'E' grade nurses working on a medical ward or community nurses at 'G' grade, would then be 'grouped' within their trust. The re-writing of job descriptions was to be undertaken by senior nurses, managers and human resources staff, with no definitive process agreed or identified for ensuring proper consultation and staff involvement. This is not the procedure many nurses expected, imagining instead that the work they did, their individual skills, knowledge and experience would be the key factors in seeing them placed not only on the appropriate band but one which would reward them suitably. This would almost certainly have been the process RCN nurses thought they were voting for when they supported the College's aggressive call for a 'Yes' vote for *Agenda for Change* at a time when no one had seen the hard detail of the scheme, and despite having only a below inflation increase for the first year of a three year deal that could not be re-opened for negotiation.

---

[12] War has always had profound effects on healthcare provision. The outcry when it was discovered that 30 per cent of recruits for the Boer War were unfit led to profound changes in public health and, particularly health visiting. It became inevitable after the First World War that women would at last get the vote. The consequent changes to the status of women had as profound an effect on nursing as anything in the twentieth century. The events of the Second World War, and the changed attitudes of the British people who went on to give Labour a landslide election victory in 1945, contributed to the establishment of the NHS. The fallout is still settling from Tony Blair's support for George W. Bush's military adventurism in Iraq. At the time of writing, the only weapons of mass destruction found have been in the United States and New Labour's grounds for taking the country to war appear either very misjudged or something more sinister. In the run up to war, with international markets jittery, public spending was being carefully scrutinised. The government sat on the *Agenda for Change* proposals, assessing the financial cost of war. Post war, the government has lost several ministers and tested the support of even some of its most loyal backbenchers, which may make it all the more difficult to push through unpopular policies on foundation hospitals and the like.

With the deadline for full implementation now put back to April 2004 at the earliest, the unions could do no more than put a brave face on it. The doctors, far more aggressive in their negotiating tactics, had long secured the concessions they were seeking. Moreover, when consultants were offered a pay rise of 20 per cent for 2003, which could relate to an annual salary of more than £90,000 within three years, in return for contractual changes, they felt themselves to be in a strong enough position to overwhelmingly reject it in England and Wales although, interestingly enough, their Scottish and Northern Irish counterparts were in favour of acceptance. Milburn huffed and puffed and made a bullish declaration that this was the only contract on offer. The government was clearly more confident about taking on the firefighters, who vetoed a similar proposal of contractual changes in return for a 4 per cent pay rise. The strategy with the doctors, however, was to try and implement the new contracts on a trust-by-trust basis (Butler, 2002). Before long, the government was back at the negotiating table, promising doctors even more say in the future direction of the NHS (Wright, 2003).

This was only one more blow to nurses whose anger over pay had been steadily mounting. Inevitably, it was not only the government who were the target, as they wondered just what was being negotiated in their name and why it was not delivering any material gain.

As the gap between public and private sector pay widened, so comparable earnings within it changed. Soldiers, police officers, teachers and junior doctors all saw their pay increase more than nurses. Indeed, a 'D' grade nurse's pay rise in 2001 was 300 per cent less than that of a junior doctor. The starting salary for a nurse consultant was marginally more than a police sergeant and significantly less than an inspector. A police constable with fourteen years service would earn as much as a senior 'H' grade nurse.

Holding out hope that *Agenda for Change* will, of itself, deliver fundamental change to nurses' pay is to see angels where there are clouds. Despite an ability to achieve some degree of wealth re-distribution through stealth, Gordon Brown's Treasury Department epitomises New Labour philosophy by demonstrating that siding with those who are economically powerful will be the overwhelming factor in his financial strategy. It was perfectly understandable that this government was going to stretch the process out for as long as possible and secure the best deal it could – not for nurses but the government. As the unions continued to negotiate in isolation from their members, using no external pressures, it became impossible to imagine that nurses were not going to get dumped on in the final outcome. If the government had, contrary to every other decision it has made, abandoned caution and resolved to lavish a generous scheme on nurses and other health workers, it would have done so much earlier and gained the political kudos from it – the money is there to be handed over, as we shall see below.

In fact Alan Milburn announced at the 2002 RCN Congress that the new pay system was to be a 'Something for something arrangement', with more pay only coming as a result of nurses taking on new roles and responsibilities, adding, 'Investment in pay ... has to pass our "acid test" – it must contribute to expansion in NHS capacity, it must bring about increases in NHS productivity and deliver improved NHS performance.' In so doing he was only emphasising that *Agenda for Change* is essentially an old-fashioned productivity deal, with the carrot – but not the promise – of redressing age-old grievances. He made no mention of why nurses increased 'productivity' hadn't been substantially rewarded in the previous five years of his government.

Again, analysing *Agenda for Change* is impossible at this stage. It will undoubtedly have a number of twists and turns before it is finalised. Nonetheless, the way in which the final offer from government was announced again tells us about those key relationships between New Labour and the unions, as well as those of the unions and their members. On the day of the announcement that nurses were getting a 10 per cent pay rise spread over three years, amid a flurry of national media activity, Beverly Malone had to declare that she couldn't comment on the detail of the agreement as she wasn't aware of it. Unison's Karen Jennings said her union couldn't begin consultation with its members until the fire fighters' dispute was settled.[13] How, one was left wondering, could the unions have 'agreed' to anything when they were unaware of the detail and couldn't consult with their members? Neither Ms Malone nor Ms Jennings denounced the government for a premature announcement or said that there was no deal at that time. It was clear that at least part of the government's agenda was its desire to embarrass the Fire Brigade's Union and force them back to the negotiating table. Indeed, senior ministers had been saying all along that, were the fire fighters to get a big pay rise then it might be necessary to give the nurses something similar.

The firefighter's dispute offered a stark contrast to the position nurses found themselves in. The union's membership was involved in both setting its own claim (for 40 per cent, which equated to a basic wage of £30,000 for most fire fighters)

---

[13] The Fire Brigade's Union was in the middle of a bitter dispute that, at times, threatened to spill over into high farce, as the local government employers first offered a 16 per cent deal with no strings attached and then had to withdraw it upon objection from the government. Then, after a series of strikes, with another offer of 16 per cent apparently ready to be agreed, John Prescott, the deputy prime minister was accused of being unable to get out of bed to ratify it (although it was far more likely that Gordon Brown and his Treasury team had already vetoed it). The dispute quickly turned into a 'no win' situation for the government. On the one hand, it had decided it couldn't accede to the FBU's demands but could not afford to be seen to lose to the strikers. Yet, dealing a crushing defeat to such a high profile and respected group would inevitably dent its popularity with the public and, coupled with the government's determined refusal to listen to its own party or the public over Iraq, could be the last straw for unions that have stayed loyal to Blair and New Labour.

and then deciding a strategy for achieving it. Shortly before Christmas 2002, with many within the TUC and New Labour worried that the dispute could prompt a complete schism within the wider movement, the independent arbitration service, ACAS, stepped in and further strikes were put on hold as both parties again sought a negotiated settlement. This was shortly after the *Agenda for Change* announcement, which heralded the 'victory' for nurses and other health workers (doctors, of course, excluded) of a 3.33 per cent increase for the next three years. Yet, even this was not straightforward. The *Nursing Times* announced, 'The waiting is over and final proposals for the new pay system for the NHS have been issued.' So it was puzzling to find, in the same article, that 'unresolved issues' included, 'Agreement on exactly where nurses will sit on the pay bands....' Just as worrying was the statement that, 'Proper agreement on the concept of equal pay for equal value across the professions will need to be ironed out but is under debate while consultants and GPs remain in discussion over new contracts' (O'Dowd, 2002a: pp 23–5). So that's clear: everything is settled except how much nurses will be paid and nothing has particularly changed: nurses are kept waiting to be told what they get while the doctors negotiate.

Within a week, Unison's general secretary Dave Prentis was taking a much harder line against the government, himself linking the government's announcements about *Agenda for Change* with attempts to break the FBU and siding with the latter, re-emphasising that Unison would not consult while the fire fighter's dispute was ongoing. Prentis was clearly doing no more than reflecting the mood of nurses polled by the *Nursing Times* (Waters, 2002: pp 10–11). Of the 1117 who took part, 61 per cent stated a willingness to strike over pay.

Agenda for Change certainly marks the first time in the history of the NHS that unions have negotiated for staff to work longer hours, as would be the case for PAMs and many admin and clerical workers, most of whom are women. This clearly doesn't fit with the image of promoting family friendly policies and a healthier work – life balance. Moreover, it also began to emerge that as many as one in six health workers could be financially worse off under the proposals, although the Department of Health tried to limit this to one in twelve – still around 100,000 people. The suggestion of those staff having pay frozen rather than taking a pay cut would mean up to five years without a pay rise. In the period leading up to its special consultation conference, Unison's health service group executive still did not have enough information to resolve questions about job profiles or other 'technical' aspects of the proposed deal, thus composing two, contradictory motions to place before their members. One senior regional official summed it up as, 'A shambles...you couldn't make it up.' In many ways, the outcome of the consultation process was no longer the issue: the 'happy family' was more dysfunctional than ever before and the process for *Agenda for Change* was an extraordinary one for any group of unions to have agreed to. For the government, however, it may be the end of a long, hard road that will have solved the misery of the annual tribulations of the nurses' and health workers, pay round while finally ditching the unwieldy and outdated Whitley system. Getting the unions to actually campaign for a three year deal with a below inflation increase in the first year, at least, was probably beyond its wildest dreams.

Yet, there might still be a sting in the tail. A three year pay cycle moves the issue of terms and conditions way down the nursing agenda, which will certainly suit the College, which was unlikely to ever build the large activist base required to build a 'bottom up' pay campaign. Indeed, the radical involvement of nurses in any campaigns with their unions is looking less and less likely. Which will leave a huge vacuum which the College can easily fill with its professional agenda, thus consolidating its grip on nursing even further. One thing is certain: nursing trade unionism will not be the same once *Agenda for Change* is established – even if foundation hospitals only use it as a staging post for more aggressive bargaining tactics on weakened unions.

▶ PFI and the private sector – making money out of illness

One of the most misjudged claims to fame is that of New Labour's Deputy Prime Minister, John Prescott, insisting that the PFI was his original idea, although it was actually introduced by the Tory government in the 1992 budget. Call it the Private Enterprise Funding Initiative or Profit-based Funding Initiative and people will see it very differently. The word 'private' suggests something intimate, individual and personal. It is far from that. It is about money and – inevitably, as a bottom line for any commercial company with shareholders – profit. And the money that is to be made has to be from ill health. In the long term, apart from the effect on the individual hospitals built under the PFI scheme, it will distort the overall health economy once big business has its teeth into profit from illness and there is a serious risk that any emphasis on health promotion and health prevention will be severely undermined.

Doubts about PFI were raised from the outset. The policy meant that capital was rented, or leased, from private contractors by the government for the building of new hospitals. No 'up front' money was required of government, which meant it could stick to self-imposed spending limits, but the trusts that would rent the new hospitals were committed to re-paying the fees out of revenue allocated by government, over periods varying between twenty-five, thirty or even sixty years. Given that it is vastly more expensive for the private sector to borrow money than the government, the interest payments are such that PFI built hospitals end up costing far more than would be the case had government financed their building. The private enterprise firms involved in PFI lose out financially if the building is not finished on time or the heating system packs up after five years but can sue for 'loss of profit' and charge 'punitive interest penalties' if, for any reason, the NHS trust cannot make its monthly payments. Moreover, if the private consortium went bust, the NHS would have to pick up the entire cost. Historically, whenever money has been tighter than expected, trusts have cut back on non-clinical services, but won't have that flexibility under the terms of the new contracts and will have to look to clinical areas for savings.

How money is dictating the pace of change can be seen from the example of the Norwich PFI scheme. The NHS trust chairman at the time of the deal, Malcolm Stamp, was also the former chairman of Norwich Union, the private health insurance company which had a 33 per cent stake in Innisfree, a private investment fund putting £50 million into ten PFI hospital schemes and expecting a 15 per cent return for their money – a cool £7.5 million of taxpayers' money. The city centre site for the hospital was abandoned for a greenfield site that was less accessible, particularly for those with health and mobility problems, and would require a 30 per cent reduction in beds. University College London Hospital is being rebuilt at a cost of £160 million, with the money coming from private enterprise companies. 'But for the next 30 years the hospital trust will have to shell out almost £30 million a year to the developers. In other words, the taxpayer is obliged to pay nearly £900 million for something that would have cost £160 million. *And at the end of those 30 years, the hospital will belong to the private consortium*' [my emphasis] (Wheen, 1999). The scandal of the whole enterprise doesn't end there. The trust is tied to the hospital and its structure for the entire period of the lease or until a review. In Norwich's case, this isn't for thirty years into its sixty-year lease, which means that the local community reliant on the hospital, as well as those working in it, will get a fixed form of service provision that won't allow for any changing priorities in healthcare.

There is also the possibility that PFI is actually signalling a far greater policy shift than first appears, as big as that is. Top civil servants have an undeclared policy to use PFI to 'downsize the NHS to 60 publicly funded hospitals'. Some estimate the 'plan' is to reduce bed numbers by as much as 30–50 per cent and help, in the process, reduce spending 'whatever the real needs of patients'. With 'capacity in NHS hospitals already stretched to breaking point', this will leave private hospitals to profit (Durham, 1998: p 22). With more than £5 billion of taxpayers' money already committed to going into the pockets of private consortiums over the next thirty years, no one can accuse New Labour of not doing its bit for private enterprise:

> The 'build now, pay later' hospital schemes were promoted by Conservative think tankers as a way to dismantle the NHS by setting up 'downsized', semi privatised hospitals. In 1994, Tory guru David Willets looked forward to clinical staff joining porters and cleaners as commercial employees in what he called the 'unbundled' NHS hospital (Leigh, 1997).

Scotland's first health minister, Sam Galbraith, was always at pains to emphasise that clinical services would not be managed by the private sector. '"The core values which bind together the NHS must not be eroded. Clinical services should be a public resource provided by the NHS," he said' (Wright, 1997: p 9). This exposes the hypocrisy and confusion of the government's position. If the private sector is good enough to run every other aspect of healthcare provision more efficiently, why not clinical services?

When the Institute of Public Policy Research recommended that the private sector not only design, build and manage new hospitals but also run nursing and medical services, one might have thought this was a conservative group following David Willets' thinking. It included Claire Perry, director of change management at the UKCC, and Ruth Kelly, a Labour MP close to Chancellor, Gordon Brown. In fact, nurses and other health workers have everything to fear from PFI. Reducing bed numbers by 30–50 per cent will not allow any savings unless nurse numbers drop at the same rate. Nurses at Hereford Hospitals NHS Trust were informed that they would be downgraded from 'E' to 'D' because of a 'surplus' of 'E' grades when three hospitals were due to merge under a new PFI scheme. Northumbria Healthcare NHS Trust also started downgrading senior nursing posts *in preparation* for its PFI hospital opening. It was only at this point that the RCN went on record as arguing for a 'suspension of PFI schemes until ministers carried out a robust evaluation'. Its opposition has remained based on that issue rather than the economics or any recognition of the inevitability of falling nurse numbers. Senior RCN members involved in the concordat signed by Alan Milburn with the private sector, which allowed trusts to send NHS patients to private hospitals for treatment when there were no NHS beds, were altogether more positive about PFI and private sector involvement (Akid, 2001: p 4).

The Private Finance Initiative does have a logic of its own. But this does not stand up to scrutiny. It made ideological sense to a Tory government, which had a track record of commercialisation. New Labour's opposition to it when it was first announced quickly dissipated and driving the policy forward now makes no sense. Unless it is New Labour giving over the clearest message possible that it has completely re-modelled itself as the party of business. It has adopted this position because it is big business that will, in the eyes of the government, do most to help them retain their parliamentary power. This is not about any great intellectual leap forward, nor a logical process of rational, evidence-based decision making. It is about the ideological use of power. But blaming Blair for finding as many ways as possible to put money into the hands of entrepreneurs and private enterprise is almost like blaming him for the fact there are seven days in the week. Almost. But not quite. The government responds to pressure, power and political initiatives. In this respect, Unison finds itself in a real bind. It doesn't want to fall out with the government and jumps on any small concession it is able to wrest from it. Nonetheless, it knows that New Labour is ploughing on, regardless of all the opposition of the unions, confident that none of them will take the ultimate step on the road to serious opposition.

Massive sums of public money are being lost to NHS patients and the staff who want to care for them. NHS patients are now being transported to other countries for treatment, as well as occupying private beds in the United Kingdom. This matters because it is money that could have been invested in NHS buildings and staff – nurses included. As it is, New Labour's concordat with the private sector, along with proposals for foundation hospitals and PFI, have taken British health-care further down the road of commercialisation than the Tories ever managed to. That is not, however, enough for the private firms involved. Their profit margins demand fewer beds, fewer staff and lower overheads and this will set the parameters for healthcare in Britain for half a century. Yet, nurses could change the equation. If they took concerted action, they could halt PFI schemes. Assume they have no mutual interest with the cause of non-clinical staff and the process will continue unabated. But going along with the prevailing ideology will ultimately further disadvantage them. They won't be able to oppose PFI in isolation. It will require pushing their unions into a new and uncomfortable position. If nurses don't address this issue in the very near future, and PFI's detractors are proved to be right, nursing will be fundamentally and irrevocably changed, with many working in a shrunken, largely privatised service seriously distorted by commercial concerns and priorities and decisions. The lesson from the private sector for nurses is that they will certainly not be any better off than they are in the NHS. The privatisation of ancillary services and early PFI schemes suggests that, when they have a local monopoly, commercial companies will cut wages and conditions of service.

The area of nursing where privatisation has already had a vast impact is, of course, through agency working. Linked as it is to recruitment and retention problems resulting in poor staffing levels, the NHS can be said to be the author of its own downfall in this area. But the cost is enormous. An Audit Commission report showed that bank and agency staff cost the NHS £810 million in 2000–01, accounting for 10 per cent of the nursing workforce, with one in ten NHS trusts spending over 20 per cent of its wage bills on temporary staff (Mullholland, 2001b: p 4). This was an example of nurses recognising their interests, as they chose to work for agencies paying, in some cases, more than five times as much as the average bank shift.[14] The cost to the NHS, however, went a lot further than the money spent. The Audit Commission study found, inevitably, that standards of care were severely compromised, morale was lowered by a reliance on temporary staff. Registration and police checks were not carried out by employers. Nurses were missing out on training and were thus less able to meet the demands of the job.

---

[14] So nurses effectively withdraw their labour from the NHS, taking what is, in effect, individualised industrial action, using the market to sell their labour back at a more attractive rate.

As with PFI, there is no real logic to this absolute waste of public money. It has to be remembered that the Audit Commission has also estimated it costs an average of £5000 for every 'E' grade nurse recruited. The problems stem from the inability to retain nurses in the workplace, not a new problem but one that successive governments have not tackled. It is now costing more money than ever for a government that both prides itself on its prudence and re-states its determination to turn the NHS into one of the finest healthcare systems in the world. Is it a devilishly fiendish conspiracy or simply a confederacy of dunces?

Imagine what the NHS would look like if the government built the PFI hospitals itself and diverted the remaining cash into resolving the issue of nurses pay, training, education and outstanding grievances over conditions of service. As the money wasted on temporary staff was saved and re-invested in nursing, imagine how the service would be transformed.[15] The maths is relatively simple. Of course, the government would point to its reputation with the City and need for financial prudence. If it was honest, it would also admit its concern about the inflationary pressures on the economy that it feared would arise were health workers substantially better paid. It would worry that increasing nurses' pay would set off a competition, not just with other groups in the health service but also the public sector. If that wasn't contained, their fear would be that private sector workers would demand more, with a major inflationary spiral undermining both its economic credibility and industrial relations strategy – even though many leading economists would rebut such fears as completely unfounded.[16]

Managing a competitive wage economy is the job of government, which should recognise that a low wage economy is incompatible with the skills, knowledge base and the new technology revolution it is trying to engineer. Stability would be brought to the NHS if its largest staff group was more settled, working consistently and cohesively and able to develop itself without the diversions of staffing crises, unplanned change and the interruptions to the core task of nursing that go with them. Yet, if the current system and ideology are accepted, this reads like some kind of utopian idyll that will never be achieved. And it is, as yet, not articulated by anyone charged with, or who has taken on, the role of leading nurses, yet another

---

[15] It also has to be remembered that the private sector so admired by Tony Blair and Alan Milburn doesn't train or educate any of its staff but attracts them from the NHS, only adding to the vicious spiral of costs.

[16] In fact, economic predictors for 2003 were that 'Britain's economy is set for accelerated growth as it continues to outperform the US and Europe. GDP growth is expected to be close to government predictions of 2.5 per cent, underpinned by an increase in government spending of between 3 and 4 per cent.' Although inflation was expected to stay above the government's targets of 2.5 per cent, it would be public spending that would underpin the country's economic recovery (Islam and Morgan, 2002: p 20).

example of the unhealthy, exclusive, 'politically correct' consensus that exists between the government, senior nurses and trade unions and which has so alienated nurses.

▶ Trade unions and nurses: act local, think global?

Both the RCN and Unison have straightforward, if different choices. For the RCN, it is whether or not to support nurses or the cause of nursing in serving 'the needs of the service', i.e., government. Most of its members and staff have probably never even considered it in these terms before. But the College cannot do both without damaging the interests of its members. Given that, barring a seismic shift in politics that would be unparalleled even by the events of 1997, New Labour are going to be in government until 2009 at least, the choice for Unison is whether or not to cut itself off from a Party that has signally failed to deliver on key issues and redirect the millions of pounds Unison members have paid into New Labour towards campaigns to promote their concerns. It could then develop a far healthier relationship with the government based on recognising areas of mutual benefit and genuine difference.[17] A 'modern' agenda can be radical and the unions can also be a serious force, seeking new alliances and relationships, free of their past.

The same is true, in respective terms, of the GMB and other unions but it is unlikely, however, that the broader leadership of any of the unions will change unless they have to. The great difficulty is that, for all the organisations concerned, an enormous institutional shift in thinking is required, since all associate their current position as being the one that gives them power, rather than truly believing that their power as an organisation is derived from the membership.

This being the case, it is nurses who are facing the biggest choice. How can they change the situation to their advantage? Can their unions be reformed by a membership which, to some extent, has been increasingly disenfranchised and is now less involved than ever before? Trying to work within their structures has not been effective so far. If nurses are to make genuine progress on an agenda that is over a century old, there needs to be a recognition of mutual need alongside a greater tolerance of difference. Yet, unity within a pluralistic tradition has eluded nursing throughout its history. Bob Abberley, then Unison's head of health, has talked of

---

[17] It is almost certain that the hundreds of thousands of Unison members working in healthcare don't realise that they can opt out of the union's affiliated political fund which places the money directly in New Labour's pocket, simply by signing a form available from their branch representatives. Their political donation then goes into the non-affiliated political fund, which is used to finance general political campaigns on behalf of the union and its members, rather than funding New Labour campaigns.

the need to realign members and functions, even going so far as to suggest that all registered nurses be represented by the RCN while Unison represents all healthcare assistants (Cole, 2001: pp 24–7). As was to be expected, this view was slammed by some leading Unison activists, who interpreted it as being borne out of a defeatist attitude rather than any genuine bi-partisanship. Moreover, while Abberley's view failed to recognise the growing mutuality of these two groups and the blurring of boundaries as more HCAs see their role develop or are able to access pathways that bring them into registered nurse training, it was barely acknowledged as a serious idea by the College, which went on to take HCAs into membership. Similar ideas about the ways in which to bridge this fundamental gap, such as the RCN taking on the 'professional' role, allowing Unison to concentrate on terms and conditions or even a full-scale merger, have never made a serious bid to get on the negotiating table.

Those who work in large organisations rarely reform themselves willingly and this is just as true of our trade unions. Trade union mergers have largely been about consolidating resources and enabling them to cling to some vestige of power rather than being driven by members' desires for change and a new, invigorated relationship between union and members. This is despite the genuinely visionary and benevolent aspirations of some of those involved in the planning of such mergers and determination to create a new, effective organisation after the merger has been effected. Some will genuinely see no need for change. Others will simply feel that, given the size, ideology and structure of the system, it is inevitably monolithic, while others still have their own vested interest in maintaining the status quo. Individuals and groups will also have a good relationship with members and vice versa. Nurses have accepted that the relationship with their unions is as it is, impervious to their, admittedly often unstated, needs or desire for change.

The managerialist culture in the RCN means that any effective change is going to have to be agreed, and driven, by Council and the general secretary.[18] In Unison, it will mean that the competing vested interests within its national executive

---

[18] The RCN has one new and significant factor in its favour if the argument for change is to be made, and that is its general secretary, Beverley Malone. She has taken every opportunity to stress that the College needs to strengthen its organisational base in the workplace, recruiting more stewards and activists, and that British nurses must become far more politically active, even if this involves working in small cadres, with individuals taking on varying roles and levels of activity that they are comfortable with. She is aware of the impact this will have, not only on nursing but also her own organisation. The measure of her success in this strategy will inevitably be based on how she manages to take her Council with her, but is a profound change from earlier leaders and philosophies. Moreover, if successful, every other healthcare union will need to completely re-think its own strategies.

committee, national conference, regional committees and councils, health groups at national and regional level and other service groups, as well as its bureaucracy, will have to agree a way forward. But current union structures are extremely difficult for nurses to utilise. They remain highly bureaucratic, unresponsive, alienating to the inexperienced, inflexible and hierarchical despite attempts at reform. They are clearly not engaging the vast majority of their members. The key is how these obstacles to participation can be overcome while improving on democratic safeguards and egalitarianism.

If nurses want greater unity, they will have to forge it for themselves by making their will known and using their power to express it. Being moved into the community not only fragmented nurses' work experience but also a sense of their own community and identity that had developed from the hospital. Communications were more difficult at every level. Holding together union branches that had once operated on one site became virtually impossible as staff were spread across literally dozens of workplaces. Things have changed now. The internet offers a potent means of communication that almost all nurses are familiar with and the telecommunications revolution offers a variety of means for organising and remaining in touch. Nowhere was this seen more clearly than when farmers and truck drivers staged their protests against the government in the fuel dispute in 2000. Some suspected a well-rehearsed strategy to attack the government and take advantage of sensitive issues for these two groups, developed by allies of the Conservative Party. This might explain why it coincided with the announcement of further increases in public expenditure on health and education. But what propelled it was almost secondary to the means by which those who genuinely bore a grievance maintained their onslaught from isolated rural outposts. Interpreting Ani DeFranco's observation that any tool is a weapon if used correctly, they turned mobile 'phones and computers into the tools of revolution. Setting simple and achievable objectives and using regional co-ordinators, a group of 2500 protesters brought the country to a standstill. The same methods have been used by anti-capitalist protesters.

Nurses could utilise these tools to advertise their views and communicate, either from union branch to union branch or through independent websites. Nurses' networks are developing across Britain in all kinds of ways, usually focusing on clinical special interests, but could just as easily be used to reflect and facilitate debate on issues fundamental to the future of nursing and nurses. These could then be used as a far more powerful vehicle of change, allowing nurses to participate more meaningfully in their unions and policy making. Model resolutions could be drafted, circulated to different groups and taken to key meetings, with nurses from across union regions agreeing which they would target. In hospitals, old-fashioned word of mouth, notices and meetings can be used. One of the reasons nurses don't give up the little time they have for union meetings is because they don't find them relevant. Ongoing committees, which sit to work through the same agenda, month in, month out, have a similar effect. If the issues are focused and 'right', i.e., if they connect with the concerns of nurses, they will be attended.[19] Using modern telecommunications can enable nurses to agree their own strategic objectives, locally, within their region, e.g., on issues such as London weighting, and nationally. If the unions think it is acceptable to ask for 'a little more than last time' as a pay claim on behalf of their members, there is no reason why nurses cannot organise, take a leaf out of the fire fighters' book, make clear their own demands and take those into union meetings – whatever their union – as a legitimate demand.

Starting afresh is never easy but it has been done before, and in conditions far more adverse than those we are experiencing now. When Thora Silverthorne formed the Association of Nurses in 1937 she was vilified in the nursing press, attacked and condemned by the College of Nursing. Employers and matrons intimidated those nurses who had, or wished to, join it. She and the radical nurses who supported her had little money and the most primitive resources. Yet, they exerted far more influence than could ever have been imagined at the time. Ultimately, given widespread dissatisfaction with the super-unions that have become so dominant, it would appear to be no more than a matter of time before a group of nurses somewhere break away and form a local union, with or without other health workers. This would inevitably raise all sorts of problems but none that would be insurmountable. There have already been breakaways from the College and Unison. The latter lost an ambulance branch, which formed itself into a separate union and eventually gained TUC recognition. If the use of new technology makes it more likely that some form of local organisation could be sustained now, the economics support it as well. The level of union membership density within an average NHS trust is estimated to be somewhere in the region of 60 per cent, although in some this is obviously a major exaggeration. However, a local union that came out of a trust that employs 1200 nurses could generate more than £70,000 in annual income if it were able to attract that percentage of members, paying lower subscription fees than both the RCN and Unison. That figure could obviously be increased if nurses allied themselves with other health workers and/or were able to recruit more nurses. A branch could then easily buy in administrative

---

[19] In this sense, the American Psychiatric Nurses Association, which broke away from the American Nurses' Association, offers an interesting template. It has deliberately kept its bureaucracy small yet is an expanding organisation, targeting the Congressional and legislative agenda in a sharply focused way, as well as making effective use of the Web and its journal. It sets up working groups to tackle particular issues and then disbands them and doesn't have a roster of standing committees. Each state chapter, or branch, has a high degree of autonomy but feeds into the national organisation, which comes together annually for a clinically focused conference.

support, specialist training, expert legal and campaigning support if required, as well as anything else needed, and produce its own, high quality publicity. Given that it would be negotiating with the local employer on local issues, driven by a locally driven agenda that was arrived at democratically and owned by the staff, attracting members would be unlikely to pose a problem. Other branches, whether or not they broke away, would easily be able to share their own support and communications infrastructure. The average Unison branch only retains approximately 20 per cent of members' subscriptions. Increasingly, activists are unable to see to what use the remaining 80 per cent is put. Full-time officials' roles are being 'redefined' in relation to individual representation and their role is meant to be less 'hands on' and more 'facilitative'. But, as branches receive less assistance with individual or collective representation some are concluding that they are doing 95 per cent of the work while controlling only 20 per cent of the cash. With the levels of dissatisfaction towards their union expressed by RCN members working alongside members of other unions, there is every possibility that a once unlikely alliance could occur. It is almost certainly the only way nurses – and hopefully with other health workers – will ever find real unity.

It is not a question of advocating that nurses should not be a member of a trade union – far from it. There is overwhelming evidence that nurses can gain immeasurably from membership and, whatever their shortcomings, twenty-first century nurses are far better off being union members than not. But it is a question of what nurses can do to organise themselves in order to get their existing organisations to seriously address their needs – and what they can do if those organisations don't respond. This is the challenge facing the unions now and one they have to take seriously. Branches 'opting out' certainly would be the catalyst that would smash the complacent façade and be the required impetus for change. It would impact upon the national bargaining machinery and prove the biggest shake up in industrial relations at all levels of the NHS. In almost all respects, it is far from desirable, given the potential that could be realised within the existing infrastructure. It won't, of itself, resolve nurses' problems. Nurses are going to have to do that. However, were those branches to be successful in clearly articulating their members' needs, uniting them in support of their objectives and negotiating an improved deal for them, how many more would follow? Ironically, Unison has experienced something akin to this process as the Scottish region in health has developed greater autonomy and established a different, harder edged identity from much of the rest of the national union. This has enabled it to form a relationship with the Scottish Executive based on a recognition of both mutual interests and areas of difference, with a willingness to face one another across the negotiating table – and even on opposite sides of a picket line – yet maintain a working relationship

Nurses will never be *fully* united – there are too many, with too many divergent interests, but some core values and interests shared can be signed up to when necessary, even if only on a short-term basis. And nurses can be organised to agree to support or, at the very least, not obstruct the pursuit of those legitimate aims.

For nurses need to be organised to thrive. There is no soft option or alternative. They won't be given what they want but can negotiate for it if they are prepared to bring a new dimension of support to that which they already give one another in the clinical arena. This involves taking a stand for what they collectively believe is right. Thinking globally but acting locally allows the connection with larger events but retains the focus on what can be influenced and achieved in the place that matters most to nurses – in their own workplace. If enough follow, wider change occurs and a new movement is born. For, in truth, local concerns *are* largely global concerns. It is not just about communicating successful strategies, success stories and issues of common concern. These are all ways of validating and articulating nurses' experiences and spread progress. It is in the act of doing, or practice, that change is created until, ultimately, the act of determining one's own destiny becomes liberating in itself.

▶ What work will nurses do?

The pace of change has grown exponentially as we have rolled into the new millennium and perhaps one of the big failings in nurse education has been to ignore this – not insignificant – factor both in acknowledging it and preparing students for it once they qualify. Some of the changes focused on within this book reflect global health and economic trends. There are others that have impacted upon the work nurses do: the growing numbers of older people, new and emerging diseases – it is easy to forget that AIDS is still a relatively new phenomena – resistant organisms, the effects of poverty, rising numbers of displaced peoples and refugees and shifting social roles for men, resulting in higher morbidity and suicide rates among the male populations of European countries, particularly in the old Eastern bloc since the fall of Communism. There is yet another attempt to put place health promotion and preventative measures in place that will reduce the pressure on our over-stretched health services while attempts to address social exclusion, poverty, deprivation, housing shortages, unemployment and the problems caused by a transport system in a state of collapse all have an impact on health and nursing.[20]

---

[20] Speculating on the future, technological change, largely through the microchip, will fundamentally change not only the nature of illness and disability but how people receive treatment, with life expectancy for the affluent continuing to expand until – possibly within a century – microchip implants finally transform the nature of humanity itself. The gap between those who have and have not is likely to be even wider than it is now. This is the subject of a chapter in itself at the very least but begs a profound question. With machines increasingly taking the place of people, it is possible that even nursing will succumb to the whirr of the computer programme, but what of the current reliance on human contact and relationships?

Current attitudes to health, the self, religion and spirituality have also changed significantly. With increasing leisure and recreational opportunities for those with sufficient money, they have responded to arguments emphasising individual responsibility for health, 'lifestyle' choices – and the decline of the NHS – by joining health clubs, taking out private healthcare insurance and utilising 'new age' or alternative therapies. In part, this 'consumerisation' of health is nothing more than a means for making profit; but it also hints at something else, a way in which people are dissatisfied with the experience of visiting GPs, A&E departments and large, impersonal healthcare settings.

Alternative therapies, once vehemently opposed by the BMA, which accused its supporters and practitioners of a flight from science, are more in demand than ever and have found a degree of respectability even within the NHS. 'Wacky' has given way to 'alternative' which, in turn, has become 'complimentary'. Whatever the strengths and weaknesses, or problems around a lack of an evidence base, undoubtedly one of the reasons for the popularity of 'alternative' approaches to healthcare is the very simple aspect of care that is encapsulated within them. Most practitioners of alternative therapies spend time talking to their patients, letting the patient tell her/his story and placing their health problems within the context of their past and current situation. Many therapies involve some kind of 'laying on of hands' or touch. The care is often genuinely holistic in a way that nursing rarely is these days and medicine and surgery never have been. Ironically, this has not strengthened nurses' hand in the argument about sustaining a caring component to their role. Rather, alternative therapists have flourished outside of any dialogue with nursing and, if anything, attracted some nurses who have found the lack of opportunity to develop relationships with their patients within the traditional healthcare setting too frustrating.

At the opposite end of the spectrum, genetics is offering nursing an enticing pathway into the scientific community. Genetics is the study of heredity. Many diseases have a genetic component by which the disease is passed from one generation within a family to the next. An understanding of basic genetics is a necessary part of a nurse's education, particularly in relation to understanding the role of genes in disease and inherited conditions. However, the decoding of DNA and more and more genetic links to disease and the human condition being claimed are prompting the possibility of change to healthcare on a revolutionary scale, which could undermine the psychosocial model of nursing and pull it back to the biological straightjacket from which it has fought for so long to escape, with genetic and biological explanations being put forward as a scientific and indisputable explanation for all kinds of human behaviour, illness processes and disease, particularly in mental health and, being strongly linked with it, criminal and anti-social behaviour.

Evidence-based practice has adopted the language of science and has become central to nurse education and training, even though critical analysis of exactly what and whose evidence base is being used is not always rigorous. It has been around since the Briggs Report (DHSS, 1972). Like so much in science, its proponents put it forward as a neutral, objective mechanism for seeking a broader truth that will be of benefit. Of course, this is not always the case. Gathering evidence around practice and disseminating findings from research is used to garner more monies and secure ongoing funds for both future research projects and clinical services. It is logistically more difficult for nurses to involve themselves in valid research or even audit projects because they have no time routinely dedicated for it. As explored earlier, those aspects of nursing which are far harder to quantify, measure and evaluate are, in the eyes of many policy makers and managers, discredited, while research and practise that has a solid evidence base can be sold as scientific – which is valued in a masculine culture like that of the manager-doctor led NHS – cost effective and productive. 'Value for money' is the small print on some research proposals or reports on evidence-based practice. There is also the perceived need of many practitioners within the field to debase and undermine that nursing practice which does not fit the template. Close analysis of some evidence-based practice reveals that, in fact, there is very little evidence that links with outcomes about practice; in other cases the evidence is highly disputable and in others the conclusion of very costly research projects is either to confirm something that was absolutely obvious at the outset or deduce that further research is necessary before any clear conclusions can be reached.

The desirability of developing a wider evidence base and helping nurses make use of it is important: the slavish 'worship' of an adherence to an apparent evidence-based practice above all else in nursing can be highly detrimental.

Taking on more of the doctor's role is, in some circles of nursing and government, still high on the agenda. Nurses have long taken blood and administered intravenous drugs, but now perform coloscopies, endoscopies and male catheterisation. They run Walk In Centres, specialist clinics in GP practices, carry out their own assessments, with admission and discharge rights in liaison psychiatry teams, and have taken on highly specialised work in all areas of in-patient and community work. The process of agreeing what and how nurses can prescribe, is still making slow progress. Two hundred prescription only medicines (POMs) for fifty conditions are being added as an extension to nurse prescribing. The option to all nurses, including those in A&E and secondary care, to become prescribers from the earlier restriction of district nurses and health visitors has been added, with two layers to the prescribing cake. Independent prescribers will be able to prescribe all POMs while supplementary prescribers will prescribe POMs related to specific conditions. The difference will be determined by choice, training and supervision. In most cases doctors will be the mentors. With £24 million pledged by government to train 20,000 nurses, it might seem a prime example of government supporting nursing – until it is recognised that the same amount of money would train a mere 120 GPs.

There are far more radical possibilities for change in the future, however, with some particular branches of nursing having more cause for concern than others. The number of nurse consultant posts continues to rise, although by nowhere enough to really make an impact across NHS trusts and in practice across large clinical areas. Although popular mythology has it that Tony Blair dreamt up the idea of nurse consultants while walking up the stairs at 10 Downing Street as a means of having a positive statement about nursing and deflecting criticism away from that year's pay offer, the post actually had its origins in the innovative work pioneered by those like Kim Manley, a lecturer-practitioner at St George's Hospital in Tooting (Parish, 2000: p 13). A survey of the 160 nurse consultants in post in February 2001 found that 54 per cent were hospital based. About 65 per cent either had a PhD or MSc. The average salary was £34,000 (with a salary range of £24,000–£45,000). Only 25 per cent reported adequate resources and management support, although this was balanced by 80 per cent finding they had high levels of autonomy and control in their jobs. High levels of job satisfaction were reported by 83 per cent and 70 per cent thought the posts would help retain experienced staff. Consultants reported they were engaged across all four aspects of their role – expert practice professional leadership and consultancy, training and education, and research and development – 'with the highest involvement in leadership and the lowest in expert practice. They rated their most important activities to be concerned with leadership followed by aspects of expert practice' (Guest *et al.*, 2001).

Health visiting, as has been seen earlier, had a major fight to remain in existence, along with its public health remit, with the question of how closely it remained tied to its nursing roots unresolved. To an extent, midwives are still struggling to pull themselves from the wreckage of clinical grading. The RCM has found that, although there are 99,000 midwives eligible to practice, more than 60 per cent choose not to. Of those working, 51 per cent are actually part time. Reasons midwives had stopped practising were, unfortunately, very familiar, including increasing workload, staff shortages, bullying, poor management and a lack of control over their workload. Their desire to work as midwives was not enough to outweigh their unwillingness to practice 'the type of midwifery that was demanded of them in the modern NHS' (Mullholland, 2002: p 11). Mental health nursing is facing a new onslaught from two directions. First, there is the proposal that Britain should follow many European states and America in adopting a generic model of training – a move that would have major repercussions for nurses in all speciality branches, given that 'generic' training would be mostly focused on extending the adult branch. This arose out of *Fitness for Practice* (UKCC, 1999), which considered the pre-registration training needs for nurses. One recommendation was that nurse training become generic, with specialist programmes being taken after a general qualification is attained. However, this contradicted another key recommendation, which was that student nurses needed to spend longer in specialist branch programmes. *Fitness for Practice and Purpose* (UKCC, 2001) built on the earlier document and proposed six options, only one of which maintained the status quo, with three proposing combinations of generic training. Considering these proposals is one of the earliest priorities of the new NMC.[21] Multi-disciplinary education that puts nurses with staff from other disciplines is known to be effective and to break down the barriers between different occupational groups. It can be achieved through shared modules and could be introduced with little effort, allowing knowledge, skills and experiences to be shared, roles to evolve and, where appropriate, overlap. Importantly, it also allows for staff to understand the differences in their roles and respect the things that mark them out.

Many mental health trusts have been busy integrating with social services over the latter part of the 1990s, with varying degrees of success, both in the level of actual integration as opposed to staff sharing a building and developing clear roles that all disciples are not only comfortable with but also equipped to do. Ministers have also floated ideas about recruiting generic mental health workers, creating a workforce comprising teams rather that 'professional tribes'. The prime purpose behind such thinking is, again, to create a workforce that can deliver the nation's healthcare needs – in this case through policies like the National Service Framework for Mental Health and the raft of other initiatives announced with little consultation by the government (Munro, 2000b: p 12). However, supporters of such proposals ignore the essential facts. Practitioners need to be highly skilled and properly educated – but also require the necessary managerial and clinical support structures as well as suitable rewards. These can be produced through nursing as well as any other system. Moving away from nursing is an admission of failure only on the part of the policy makers. The unwritten objective of those in government is to be able to expand the workforce with less skilled and trained nurses who will be cheaper to employ. However, rather than actually trying to resolve the problems, it represents an attempt to sidestep them, whether or not the work is done by nurses, generic workers or any other occupational group the government cares to name.

This is not to diminish the role and opportunities for expanding the role of 'untrained' nurses and healthcare assistants. They are prime examples of the potential of non-academic nurses to fulfil a key caring role for patients who, when push comes to shove, don't mind whether or not the person nursing them has a diploma, degree, National Vocational Qualification (NVQ) or certificate in painting

---

[21] There are endless possibilities for reforming nursing structures and other health disciplines. Indeed, all governments since the 1960s would probably have liked to undertake a complete overhaul of the NHS workforce had it been politically possible. However, the failure of Project 2000 as the definitive attempt to finally professionalise nursing has undoubtedly strengthened the hand of civil servants and politicians who want to make fundamental changes to nursing – although those who support them should beware.

and decorating if they know what they are doing, do it well and are able to establish a relationship and care for them.

For the emotional labour of nursing has not changed, a fact worth considering by those attempting to get new people to undertake it. Pam Smith (1992) concluded in her study of the subject 'that "caring" does not come naturally. Nurses have to work emotionally on themselves in order to appear to care, irrespective of how they personally feel about themselves, individual patients, their conditions and circumstances. They can also be taught to manage their feelings more effectively'. Recognising that caring is work in itself could not be underestimated, she wrote, 'if this most essential ingredient of what nurses do is to be recognised and valued ... supported educationally and organisationally in the institutions where nurses work and learn and by the political and economic structures within society' (p 136). Smith notes that some of the most difficult work nurses do is related to death, and being with the dying as they make that last journey. In a variety of ways, she notes, we learn from it, learn from the experience of watching more experienced nurses and listening to what they say to the terminally ill. Some nurses described carrying out the last offices as an act of 'closure', one last duty that can be performed for a patient to whom they felt close. Other patients watch how one of their number is nursed in those final days or hours, as well as the relatives. On occasions like that, nurses really are close enough to touch people's lives – that is always going to be the key moment of caring which won't change, for it has to be done, and if for no other reason, is why we should value nurses, whatever their grade or background.

▶ Patient involvement

The relatively recent arrival of patient, or user, groups contrasts with the decline of organisational strength within nursing. Traditionally it had been the middle classes who organised themselves to protect a valued service or lobby for something new, be it specialised care for themselves or a relative, a ward at their local hospital or health centre, or improved breast-screening programmes. Indeed, this has been an integral part of Tudor Hart's inverse care law (1971), which has seen those most in need get less service. However, by the 1970s, communities were forming local campaign groups, often made up of working-class men and women, and joining forces with trade unions to try and keep local hospitals open, such as the South London Hospital for Women in Clapham. Others went even further, forming groups under the umbrella of health while addressing wider environmental issues such as housing, transport and employment in the recognition that they seriously impact upon the health not just of individuals but whole communities (Mitchell, 1984).

Nowhere has the growth of user involvement had more of an impact than in mental health. Virtually excluded from institutional, legislative, political and functional structures, people using mental health services had to force their way into a society that had successfully marginalised them for decades. In the early 1970s, they began to emerge from a world of shadows as the asylums were at last closing, just as wider social movements were establishing themselves. Women, people from black and other minority ethnic groups, gays and lesbians were all fighting to establish a public identity, attain improved civil rights and establish an agenda for change. Mental health user movements were already established in the United States, where the now highly influential Clubhouse movement originated as early as 1944, quickly spreading to Canada and the Netherlands. Britain's user movement took on a peculiarly homespun, somewhat anachronistic form when it became increasingly well established in the 1980s. It complemented the political philosophies of the other groups of 'dispossessed' at the time, in that it was libertarian, collectivist, non-hierarchical, anti-authoritarian and anti-bureaucratic, while being grounded in a radical agenda. It was also made up of diffuse groups and groupings who did not necessarily share identical aspirations or goals but were able to work together because of their non-sectarian approach, allying themselves to particular causes and then moving on. Equally, they were not bound to a tradition of seeking change through parliamentary procedures or bureaucratic negotiations. Their success, in part, lay in their willingness to take direct action, use more idiosyncratic lobbying techniques and/or protest than a more traditional campaigning group, political party or trade union might be comfortable with, and seek alliances outside the narrow confines of their own movement.

Paradoxically, the Thatcherite promotion of the consumer helped, but mental health user groups went well beyond this narrow agenda, as outlined earlier. It was also a matter of right time, right place. They connected, both with the mood of the times and with a less easily defined sense that the injustices and inconsistencies they had endured for so long needed remedying. Most importantly, user groups also benefited from the unlikely alliance they forged with some general managers, who responded to the government's overt insistence on consumer choice and, a less overt agenda to introduce service changes and break the dominance of the medical profession and, to a much lesser though still significant extent, the trade unions.

Many of those groups are now well established and have joined the mainstream. MIND is actually a service provider, as are other groups, including the Clubhouse movement, receiving statutory funding for projects. Consultation exercises are undertaken with the public, many trusts routinely include people with a background of using services on interview panels for staff and planning committees and user involvement is an essential part of any Commission for Health Improvement (CHI) visit. Advocacy projects are now more the norm than the exception. Effectively managed and organised education services have recognised that people who use health services can make a key contribution to both helping with curriculum design and the actual education of students. PCGs signalled a major advance in the involvement of service users in consultation and planning of services, although this is still in its infancy. This has led, in better PCGs and PCTs, to a far greater commitment to developing a true public health agenda, although the danger remains that an articulate, affluent minority dominate the public agenda and consultative process.

In the government's drive towards integration of health and social services, there is a similar recognition that addressing people's health needs collectively is a far more cost effective and better means of achieving a healthier nation than by piling more and more money into the kind of health – or, actually, illness – factories that big district general hospitals have become. When New Labour recognised the Black Report on Inequalities in Health (Townsend and Davidson, 1982), this reversed the official government position established by the Conservative government, who had sat, squirming, on the report like a hen on an egg it never wanted to lay, until it lost the general election fifteen years after the report's original publication. Professor Black's group found that, 'If the mortality rates of occupational class I (professional workers and members of their families) had applied to classes IV and V (partly skilled and unskilled manual workers and family members) during 1970–72, 74,000 lives of people aged under seventy-five would not have been lost'. The report concluded that, despite more than thirty years of the NHS and an expressed commitment to equal care, 'there remained a marked class gradient in standards of health' and 'present social inequalities in health in a country with substantial resources like Britain are unacceptable'. Although this was largely due to factors outlined earlier and out of the control of the NHS, there was still a marked disparity between usage of services and need (*op. cit.*: pp 15–16). Little has changed, and many benchmarks of inequality have worsened, despite the avowed commitment to eradicate it. There are now more children living in poverty than when New Labour came to power and a wide range of indicators that the problems for the poor have worsened. The murder of another young black boy, Damilola Taylor, threw up a number of exceptionally uncomfortable truths for British society when the door was thrown open to life on estates such as those in Peckham, revealing:

> ... hundreds of children like the controversial Witness Bromley and the boys acquitted of Damilola Taylor's murder. Children so neglected and brutalised that they run wild through the estates of South London. For whom violence is just background noise to everyday life.
>
> Evidence is growing that they are living through a social disaster, brutalised at home or on the street by older versions of themselves (Wynne-Jones, 2002).

News reporters wrote about 'feral' children running riot as if they had discovered a new breed of animal. If any of those children looked through their history books they would recognise themselves from the poor, disadvantaged and dislocated from Victorian Britain and earlier. And like so many who are the 'victims' of social policy, they found the call that rang out from many commentators was for vengeance to be wreaked upon those same children, the platitudes having dried up, politicians no longer visiting the estates, the hand ringing at an end. For the poor there are often fine words and announcements of new initiatives. New policies, about which they've had no say, will make their lives better, they are told. If the policies don't work, it's the fault of the individual's and their lifestyle choices, not the policy makers or politicians.

For nurses trying to work in difficult circumstances, with communities where people experience themselves as being isolated and having nothing in common with others, the work goes a long way beyond the normal parameters of nursing, as exemplified by Jane Deville-Almond, a practice nurse and public health specialist in Walsall. She was given the task of improving the health of people in Moxley, on the border of Walsall and Wolverhampton. It had a population of 4000, with more than 60 per cent in local authority housing and 26 per cent unemployed and higher than average rate of major illness. The GP facilities had one consulting room, no hot running water and a small waiting room, which often had to accommodate patients for two hours before they were seen. Services such as cervical smears were only available one hour per week and there was no practice nurse. The services at the nearest health centre, although only two miles away, were inaccessible to more than 50 per cent of Moxley families, who did not own a car. Central to Ms Deville-Almond's success in transforming the healthcare of the local population were a range of factors:

- Money from the local health authority – but also its willingness and support to let her develop policy and practice semi autonomously;
- An incredible amount of energy and commitment to go with creative practice – organising men's health checks in pubs and betting offices, for example;
- Addressing wider health issues as part of the work, such as improved street lighting and adequate street crossings.

Fundamental to its success, however, was the work done with the people of Moxley, involving them in thinking about what was needed – not just wanted – planning how these could be delivered and taking ownership in as many projects as possible (Deville-Almond, 1998). Inherent in her account of her work is a fundamental recognition of the difference between good nursing care and a biological approach to illness. The latter seeks to impose an external cure, in effect, providing food for the hungry man. The former offers the opportunity to explore the nature of the problem and seek a solution that comes from the internal resources of the 'patient', similar to learning to grow one's own food and feed oneself.

User involvement is never easy. There is an inherent tension between service providers and users. Often, policy makers, managers and clinicians want – or have – to be able to say that they have consulted but don't like the results, as they either contradict accepted views or cannot be accommodated in plans which are already underway. It takes time and creates serious problems when, for good reason, the service cannot accommodate deeply held views – such as may well be the case in mental health where there is a clash between the rights and autonomy of the individual and clinicians' views on safety, the need for treatment and wider public and political concerns. However, if the dialogue is open, honest and transparent, such differences can often be tolerated, understood and adapted. It has brought needed reform as well as clinical innovation and a 'humanisation' of many approaches to healthcare. On a macro level, this mirrors how nurses work most effectively with their patients, recognising the 'expertise' the patient has about their own health and self, offering advice and assistance and acting as an agent of change through working with, and providing care for, a living person experiencing trauma and difficulty rather than 'doing to' a passive, uninformed patient receiving treatment. There may be disagreement. But out of that, and its resolution, the patient is empowered.

Through this process, both at a micro and macro level, another possibility arises. Nursing has been at its best when it has recognised its common cause not just with its patients but the community from which they have come. This was true in the days of the Poor Law, when nurses started advocating for those forced into destitution, wholly dispossessed and not just marginalised, but locked out of sight. The asylum workers understood this when they stood side by side with their patients at the Battle of Radcliffe. It was there in the struggles to keep services open in the 1970s and 1980s. The people who form the majority of patients in the twenty-first century are the same as they were in the nineteenth, the elderly, children, the poor, socially disadvantaged and chronically sick. There is also much that nurses can learn from patients' movements, which have maintained democratic principles as their foundation but minimised bureaucracy and hierarchy. Admittedly, this is easier in single-issue politics but that is not so different from nurses' concerns. True empowerment of patients can only come through having an empowered workforce and, with nurses making up the vast majority of that, it is essential for nurses to take the necessary steps on that road. One of the reasons patients always support nurses' protests, even to the point of industrial action, is a basic – if unarticulated – understanding of that premise. Nurses have yet to make that connection.

The contemporary political process might seem impervious to nurses' and patients' influence, but is actually extremely vulnerable. Anyone who doesn't understand this has ignored some very simple mathematics. The ability of community politics to shake the national system was seen at Wyre Forest, in Worcestershire, during the 2001 general election, when Richard Taylor, a retired doctor took on the might of the New Labour machine and won. The issue was PFI and the closure of the local hospital. The 'Save Kidderminster Hospital' campaign saw sixteen district and six county councillors elected, as well as Dr Taylor.

Thousands of nurses live in each marginal constituency up and down the United Kingdom, with the potential to throw out sitting MPs through determined effort if relatively small bands of nurses organised them, with their patients, to vote in a particular way. That is a very powerful position to occupy and, again, modern telecommunications and the internet make the task a lot easier. It also makes the task of getting politicians to focus their attention on a health agenda a lot more likely.

▶ Genuinely making a difference – shared governance and a new type of nursing

We are not powerless. One nurse on her own often is. But nurses together are powerful and have often proven this in the most dramatic ways. Yet, life is made up of the mundane, the ordinary, where drama is difficult to disentangle from the everyday experience because we do not always see the impact of apparently isolated events or actions. One ward sister or charge nurse who takes 'her problem' to her manager is perpetuating a system that works against her interests. If she talks through an issue affecting her unit and/or team with three, four, five of her peers, it is likely they will either have experienced something similar or be grappling with the same thing. If, collectively, they can't resolve it when they attempt to do so but present it to the manager as an issue that is having a strategic impact on the service it is a very different matter.

Shared governance was developed in the United States and has featured in much of the UK government's literature and policy documents about NHS reform, notably *Shifting the Balance of Power* (Department of Health, 2001). Different systems have been applied under its broad heading although most involve staff within an organisation, participating in small groups or committees that have direct input into decision making, often being subdivided into special interest sections. These are usually referred to as councils. The difference between these and the more traditional committees that exist in organisations is the participation of 'shopfloor' staff, who have equal status with managers. The group focus also differs from those like joint staff committees, which involve managers and trade union representatives. Rather than being oppositional, these are forward looking, concerned with planning and developing ideas within a forum that is open, where information is shared and the focus is on problem solving.

In some trusts this idea gained currency in the latter part of the 1990s, with nurses having their own councils. Clinical practice, professional development and quality were common themes. Outcome studies from the United States cite improvements in patient care, improvements to morale, lower sickness and absence levels and a sense of 'professional' purpose (Gulland and Payne, 1997: pp 14–15). Some went further. Bob Abberley of Unison and Gordon Best from the King's Fund brought their organisations together with a small number of trusts, while the Tories were still in power, to nurture a project called 'Crafting a workforce for the 21st Century.'

It was a far more radical vision of shared governance which offered staff not just an opportunity to be involved with clinical initiatives but decisions that lay at the very heart of their trust. In some cases the trusts had a very poor history of industrial relations. Others simply didn't have much of a relationship. Facilitated by Best and colleagues from the King's Fund, Abberley and national officers from Unison brought special expertise in industrial relations. In some cases, short-term pressures, particularly around finances, proved too much and trusts dropped out. At its most effective, the project enabled staff and managers to develop a dialogue about working together on problem solving, the importance of developing and sustaining relationships, teamwork, learning how to change together and openness. Wider staff empowerment was in evidence with upwards of 100 staff attending meetings about local projects, putting forward ideas that were then developed by local project teams. Chief executives who supported the project found that uncomfortable middle managers had to be 'helped' through the early stages but that levels of participation, interest and involvement were high, with consequential improvements in morale, a much better understanding of the problems facing the NHS and greater willingness to embrace change.

This, of course, fitted with New Labour's agenda and Bob Abberley was quickly established as one of the key people in national projects in staff involvement, which drew heavily on the work of the task force Unison and the King's Fund had piloted (Department of Health, 1999). *The Report of the NHS Taskforce on Workplace Involvement* recommendations included:

- Encouraging good leadership;
- Promoting good industrial relations;
- Local statements of rights;
- Monitoring performance and progress;
- Improving communications;
- Investing in personal development; and
- Conducting attitude surveys.

A year later, John Denham, then a minister within the health team, oversaw the release of *The Action Plan to Implement the Recommendations of the NHS Taskforce on Staff Involvement* (Department of Health, 2000). It covered training and performance indicators for things the minister 'expected to see at a national level' as well as three pages of action points for 'making staff involvement a reality'. Among these was developing and issuing a framework agreement on staff rights and responsibilities for local implementation as well as getting staff involvement at the policy development stage. Developing leadership was another key area.

Along with the proposals for *Making a Difference* (1999) and *Investment and Reform for NHS Staff* (2001), nurses should have experienced a profound change in their working culture. Yet, as late as April 2002, five years after shared governance was being hailed as a turning point for the NHS and five years after New Labour took office, 74 per cent of 1455 nurses surveyed were saying that the NHS was not safe in the government's hands, 76 per cent stated they had acquired more responsibility, 97 per cent were enjoying the job less than when they started their career as a trained nurse, 61 per cent would leave if they could find a job that paid the same and 77 per cent would not encourage their children to go into nursing. As many as 86 per cent identified 'more staff and more pay as key to improving their working lives (Radcliffe and Crouch, 2002: pp 26–9).

How could a development that has garnered such positive reviews not now be part of mainstream thinking? Partly, it is because decision makers cannot square the circle and agree to give up power, while nurses and other disempowered groups within healthcare have not had the opportunity to do more to get their hands on it. Partly, it is because valuable pearls get lost in the welter of initiatives constantly falling like hailstones out of the New Labour sky. Moreover, as highlighted in Chapter 6, governments that are determined to set a centralised agenda inevitably foul up any attempt to enable staff locally. But, fundamentally, the government has demanded more productivity while failing to deliver the flexibility and rewards it promised.[22] Only about a third of the NHS workforce enjoys flexible working time. 'Innovations' like self-rostering are almost unknown. Recruitment initiatives have only been developed in approximately 25 per cent of trusts. Less than 25 per cent of staff has access to child care facilities. Bullying and violence remain high. Nobody is even bothering to measure staff involvement in decision making.

If shared governance is really going to make a difference it has got to go a lot further than enabling nurses to decide on standardised nursing forms and 'ensuring best practice', the kind of things they are being allowed to at the moment. It would need to embrace the principles of republican management and become established alongside new forms of managerial structures, as outlined in Chapter 6. The principles identified by the NHS taskforce on staff involvement would need to be made a priority. Councils, involving staff and their trade unions, would have to be organised for every aspect of a local organisation's work. This would mean that nurses would not expend useful energy making decisions, around 'best practice' or anything else, that will never be enacted because they are blocked elsewhere. As we have seen, nurses have much in their tradition, the nature of their work and the aspects of themselves that they bring to that work that would, in a different structure, equip them to be good leaders and team workers. The skills are there, as is the

---

[22] It is telling to note that, in a supplement about work–life balance produced by the Department of Trade and Industry and *The Observer*, the NHS did not feature in any of its case studies (*The Observer*, 3 March 2002).

potential and capability, willingness and vision. Such a new 'triangle', tough yet flexible, creative yet firm in its boundaries, empathic yet clear in its focus, could actually deliver a new kind of health service, the one for which Tony Blair claims New Labour is striving. How change is managed becomes far less of an issue because, largely, the process is shaped by those it will affect the most, making it easier to achieve.

In summarising the nature of the problems many nurses are grappling with, it becomes possible to see how shared governance could play its part in resolving them. The problems include:

- Lack of role clarity;
- Lack of control over very difficult and demanding work;
- Lack of appropriate training or support for an evolving role in a continually changing service;
- Policy overload – with varying degrees of involvement in policy formulation;
- Increased hours, responsibility, workload and stress;
- Perceived inequalities in terms of work, value and pay;
- Little opportunity for (particularly clinical) career development;
- Limited opportunities to organically develop clinical initiatives;
- Poor leadership;
- Little work–life support;
- Low morale.

The research into successful change and management amply demonstrates that it is not so much a case of *what* change occurs within a workplace; rather, it is *how* that change process is managed. Thus, the most important change required within an organisation is ideological, but is complicated by:

- Continuing 'top-down' initiatives;
- A changing middle-management group and their lack of involvement with actual clinical services;
- The uncertainty of middle management about organisational direction;
- Lack of clarity around decision making;
- Poor decision making;
- Workforce instability and reliance on temporary staff;
- Nurses partially disengaged from the managerial process – and often not seen as a resource;
- Short termism;
- Inadequate resources;
- Weak trade unions and lack of a representative voice.

It can immediately be seen why shared governance has yet to make an impact on the health service and the difficulty New Labour is going to have with it. There is no single formula for shared governance because its agenda must be generated by the workforce. Nonetheless, elements of its composition in the NHS would need to include:

- Identifying appropriate means for communications for different areas and staff groups;
- Identifying key areas for information giving, consultation, negotiation and devolved decision making – and sticking with the process and results;
- Creating a culture of employee rights, with performance indicators for managers and human resources staff about how they were ensuring staff involvement is taking place;
- Identify local rewards and performance incentives;
- Minimising the policy agenda to key performance areas, with a degree of local autonomy, monitored from the centre, for meeting simplified, broader and more realistic targets;
- Creating forums for staff involvement and leadership on pertinent issues;
- Developing new decision-making models and a problem-solving approach;
- Developing openness, critical thinking and well-managed risk taking;
- Developing leadership and role modelling through mentorship, with specialist training and people-management skills for leaders at all levels in the organisation;
- Succession planning;
- Personal development planning;
- Continuing education and training programmes;
- Creative application of equal opportunities.

The policy issue obviously generates further problems. However, if the government allowed trusts to organise themselves more autonomously and spend the necessary time regenerating clinical services, they would be able to reap the benefits of an evolving, deeper rooted, organically generated change rather than constant disruption. Creating an environment that is shaped by shared governance takes time, can be costly and means the powerful have to lose a degree of control. It raises anxiety, leaves vulnerabilities exposed and highlights areas of conflict. It requires total commitment if it is going to work but empowering nurses can, of itself, create a change culture and enable them to help empower their patients. It can help the government meet its targets on sickness absence rates, recruitment and retention, as well as improved performance and patient care.

Most importantly, it is a viable alternative, because maintaining a demoralised, crushed workforce is not a viable option in the twenty-first century. Nonetheless, the costs may be perceived as being greater than the benefits and managers may not wish to participate in such a process. This doesn't mean nurses, whether it be within their own teams or across units, large or small, can't apply these principles. Eventually, it becomes difficult, if not impossible, to stop people having good ideas about how to resolve ongoing problems and organising ways in which they can be enacted.

► Conclusions: the value of nurses and nursing

At this stage of the book, I'm reminded of the ending of an episode of *The Simpsons* TV series, in which Homer plaintively says to Marge, 'I'm not sure if this is a good ending or a bad ending.' Without turning a hair of her fabulous blue bouffant, Marge replies, 'It's an ending, Homey, and that's all there is'. This is an ending, not of the story but of this book. As mentioned earlier, it is a story that evolves, with new layers of ideology being placed onto those already existing, with new ideas, structures, participants and influences. Life goes on.

Nursing and nurses have come a long way. It has been an epic journey in every respect, and not just 150 years of modern and post-modern history. Clinical practice, the work that nurses do, has changed beyond all recognition, although something at its core has survived, sometimes against all the odds. In other ways, not much progress has been made. Yet, one statistic from the *Nursing Times* survey (see page 294) not mentioned so far is that 65 per cent of the nurses surveyed said they had felt proud to be a nurse at some point in the month prior to the survey. In this there is hope. As difficult as the job is, something holds nurses to nursing and holds nurses together. And it is upon this that resistance against the tyranny of old ideologies and failed traditions must be built. The old radical tendency in nursing has graduated on to become the gardening tendency with no direct replacements. Younger radical nurses are battling for animal rights, human rights, for the environment and against capitalism. Yet, there is as important a struggle closer to home.

There are any number of ways that nurses can effect change. A summary of so many issues discussed in this book is difficult, but includes:

- A reformed education and training system, both pre-and post-registration, incorporating new ways of educating nurses, broadening out the opportunities for non-academic nurses, such as HCAs, to complete a training for registration and far more multi disciplinary education and training. It will be an educated, rather than 'trained' workforce that will advance the cause of both nursing and nurses;
- Nurses should have rights to ongoing time off for research and training as is the case with medical staff;
- Ending the bursary system, bringing student nurses back into salaried, NHS employment;
- Resolving staffing shortages by either establishing policies for the ongoing recruitment and retention of a nursing workforce that can meet the demands being placed upon it or re-defining the work for the numbers available to carry it out;
- Ensuring there is sufficient affordable accommodation for nurses and public sector workers in London, the south-east and other metropolitan areas;
- A new system of pay that provides nurses with competitive rewards for the work they do, on an equal footing with colleagues in other disciplines and recognises – and rewards – the value of nonclinical staff. A single pay spine is almost essential to this;

- New managerial structures and adopting the principles of republican management;
- Shared governance;
- Genuinely implementing the strategies identified in policies such as the *Report on Staff Involvement, Shifting the Balance of Power* and *Improving Working Lives*. There is also a need to enforce more progressive policies on equal opportunities, health and safety, preventing bullying and violence;
- Both increasing funding still further and freeing up the funding allocations to trusts to enable them to deliver locally driven services and involve their staff properly, without having to jump through policy hoops that actually either prevent the money reaching its targets or result in inappropriate, centrally driven services;
- Longer term, rebuilding the social infrastructure of the nation and place more emphasis on public health, through affordable housing, more employment schemes, a better, publicly funded transport system and a return to free education, that will, overall, improve the health of the nation;
- Dump PFI and use the money productively *within* the NHS;
- There is an urgent need to reform the trade unions or for nurses to begin re-organising themselves in new unions if they are to even begin tackling such an agenda.

If nurses develop and use an understanding of nursing, power and wider political processes they will, as a consequence, empower themselves in the workplace. The development of critical thinking can enable them to begin to reflect upon why things are as they are. Moreover, they can imagine how they could be different and develop a modern alternative to professionalism and status – which have always held them back – building a renewed sense of pride and purpose, recognising the importance of caring in a pluralistic culture. Nurses' flexibility and adaptability to change will always be a necessary and continuing strength in the world of health-care, which will be in a perpetual state of evolution. In this, the gender base of nursing, the ways in which women learn, can draw upon emotional intelligence, work together and communicate is key. Ultimately, if the NHS or any other health-care organisation is going to be successful, nursing needs to be at the centre of deci-sion making given that it accounts for the largest part of the workforce and is key to the delivery of care. Sooner or later this government, or the next, or the one after, is going to have to accept that. Attempts to introduce new grades of staff, generic workers or 'reform' the existing disciplines will all be trying to resolve the age old problem that has confounded governments since the early twentieth century – how to get more work from the people who care for patients for less pay and yet retain a stable workforce. But nurses do not have to wait passively. Now is as good a time as any for them to bring together theory and practice, thought and action. To bring about change.

In this, they will be returning to the work of their predecessors, particularly in the late 1970s and 1980s. These were ministering angels but also angels who had seen Jericho and were ready to consign sinners – or managers and government ministers, at least – 'into the furnace of fire'. In this sense the analogy between nurses and angels is more accurate than was previously assumed. Nurses have enormous potential to fight on behalf of what they believe to be right, which clearly frightens a lot of people in positions of power, not just in government and the civil service, but in management, education, trade unions and nursing itself.

Throughout all the difficulties, most nurses retain their aspirations for altruism, a willingness to do the right thing, caring, fostering compassion, a willingness to be with people when they are in pain, at their most distressed and vulnerable, holding onto hope when all seems lost. When nursing is at its best, this is what nurses do. These are noble and admirable intentions. In this, without any analysis of what they are doing or why, nurses aspire in a very ordinary way to something heroic. Ironically, given their pre-occupation with such matters, this is not about status or elitism. Nor do they always make it. Often we get lost in the day to day grind of the work, are crushed by cruel and insensitive managers or colleagues, our own failings and anxieties, simply overwhelmed by the demands and needs of too many patients, until we are unable to empathise, understand or help. There are times when nurses cannot care or act as if they are caring. But there is something that runs through the work that we do like a river that flows through a parched land, carrying hope when we feel we've lost it in ourselves. It carries the enduring characteristics of generations of nurses, who have sought the best for their patients, and carries new life deep within its currents. Our inherited imagination floats on it, with a desire for something different, something better.

The message for nurses everywhere is a simple one, encapsulated in the excerpt from Belloc's poem, because it is a message for *nurses* rather than *nursing*: keep a hold of one another, for it is in recognising a collective strength, the things that are common to all, the threads that link us together rather than ties that bind, that can enable this more pluralistic culture to breathe *within* nursing. Then a concerted effort can be made to address the problems both within and outside it. In his poem, 'To Althea From Prison', written in 1649, Richard Lovelace reminds us of the power of inherited imagination:

> Stone walls do not a prison make,
> Nor iron bars a cage;
> Minds innocent and quiet take
> That for an hermitage;
> If I have freedom in my love,
> And in my soul am free;
> Angels alone, that soar above,
> Enjoy such liberty.

For, finally, it will be a triumph of nurses' imaginations, thought and actions that will help create an answer to the dilemmas arising out of practice, power and politics.

▶ Further reading

Beardshaw V (1981) *Conscientious Objectors at Work*. London: Social Audit: this small book contains vivid accounts of the role of whistleblowers whose complaints initiated inquiries in large psychiatric and learning disability institutions.

Beishon S *et al*. (1995) Nursing in a Multi-Ethnic NHS. London: *Policy Studies Institute*.

Coker N (ed) (2001) *Racism in Medicine – An Agenda for Change*. London: King's Fund.

Field T (1996) *Bully in Sight*. Oxfordshire: Success Unlimited.

Finlayson L and Nazroo J (1998) *Gender Inequalities in Nursing Careers*. London: *Policy Studies Institute*.

Hardt M and Negri N (2001) *Empire*. MA: Harvard University Press.

Macpherson W (1999) *The Stephen Lawrence Inquiry*. London: The Stationery Office.

Mitchell J (1984) *What is to be Done about Illness and Health?* London: Penguin.

Rogers A and Pilgrim D (1996) *Mental Health Policy in Britain: A Critical Introduction*. Basingstoke: Macmillan: contains a useful chapter on consumerism and mental health.

Rogers R, Salvage J and Cowell R (1999) *Nurses at Risk: A Guide to Health and Safety at Work*. 2nd edition. Basingstoke: Macmillan.

Smith A and Russell J (1991) Using critical learning incidents in nurse education. *Nurse Education Today*, 11, 284–91.

Solomos J and Back L (1996) *Racism and Society*. Basingstoke: Macmillan.

Townsend P and Davidson N (1982) *The Black Report: Inequalities in Health*. Harmondsworth: Pelican

Williams B (2001) Developing critical reflection for professional practice through problem based learning. *Journal of Advance Nursing*: 43(1), 18–26.

▶ Useful websites

The range of Department of Health policy documents referred to in this chapter can be accessed through its website: *www.doh.gov.uk*.

More information about nursing policy documents from the UKCC and NMC can be accessed through the NMC website: *www.nmc-uk.org*.

www.unison.org.uk

www.rcn.org

References

Abel-Smith B (1960) *The History of the Nursing Profession*. London: Hutchinson

Agnew T (1998) Sick nurses face the sack, *Nursing Times*, **94**(48), 5 (2.12.1998)

Ahmed K and Hinsliff G (2001) Huge NHS underspend threatens reforms, *The Observer*, p. 2 (2.12.2001)

Aitken I (2000) New Labour might not like us but it needs our money, *The Guardian*, 26.4.2000

Akid M (2001) RCN call to put PFI on hold, *Nursing Time*, **97**(42), 4 (18.10.2001)

Akid M (2002a) Closure of 13,000 beds fans crisis, *Nursing Times*, **98**(22), 4

Akid M (2002b) Number of students need to double, *Nursing Times*, **98**(11), 7

Alexander and Dewjee (eds) (1984) *The Wonderful Adventures of Mrs Seacole in Many Lands*. Bristol, Falling Wall Press

Allison G T (1971) *Essence of Decision*. Boston: Little and Brown

Andrain C F and Apter D E (1995) *Political Protest and Social Change*. Basingstoke: Macmillan

Anonymous (1997) I pray for the day I don't have to wear my uniform again, *The Observer*, p. 18, (12.12 1997)

Asbridge J (2002) *NMC News*. London: Nursing and Midwifery Council

Audit Commision (1997) Finders Keepers. London: Audit Commission

Audit Commission (1999) First Assessment: A Review of District Nursing Services in England and Wales. London: Audit Commission

Baggot R (1994) *Health and Health Care in Britain*. Basingstoke: Macmillan

Baly M (1986) Nightingale nurses: the myth and the reality. In: Maggs C (ed.) *Nursing History: The State of the Art*. Kent: Croom Helm

Barker P and Reynolds B (1996) Rediscovering the proper focus of nursing: a critique of Gournay's position on nursing theory and models. *Journal of Psychiatric and Mental Health Nursing*, **3**, 75–80

Barker P *et al.* (1998) The Wounded Healer. In: Barker P and Davidson B (eds) *Psychiatric Nursing: Ethical Strife*. London: Arnold

Barker P (1999a) Our flexible friends need backing, *Nursing Times*, **95**(5), 24 (3.2.1999)

Barker P (1999b) Growing from experience, *Nursing Times*, **95**(33) (18.8.1999)

Barr N, Glennerster H and Le Grand J (1989) Working for Patients? The Right Approach? *Social Policy and Administration*, **23**(2)

Beardshaw V (1981) *Conscientious Objectors at Work*, London: Social Audit, 84–9

Beishon S *et al.* (1995) *Nursing in a Multi-Ethnic NHS.* London: Policy Studies Institute

Bellaby P and Oribor P (1980) The history of the present – contradictions and struggles in nursing. In: Davies C (ed.) *Rewriting Nursing History.* London: Croom Helm

Belle-Fortune B (1999) The final reckoning, *Nursing Times*, **95**(42), 37 (20.10.1999)

Bingham S (1979) *Ministering Angels.* Osprey: London

Blait J (2002) E-Learning: a virtual challenge for educators, *Nursing Times* **98**(31), 34–35 (30.7.2002)

Borrill C, Haynes C and Carter A (1996) *NHS Workforce Initiative: Phase 1 Final Report – Summary.* Institute of Work Psychology: University of Sheffield

Bosanquet N (ed.) (1979) *Industrial Relations in the NHS – The Search for a System.* London: Croom Helm

Bradley M (2002) Vision of the future, *Nursing Management*, **8**(9), 6–10

Bradshaw Y (1997) Perspectives. In: North N and Bradshaw Y (eds) *Perspective in Health Care.* London: Macmillan, pp. 9–19

Bray J (1998) Psychiatric nursing and the myth of altruism. In: *Psychiatric Nursing: Ethical Strife*, Barker P and Davidson B (eds). London: Arnold

Briggs Report (1972) *Report of the Committee on Nursing.* London: Department of Health and Social Security

Brindle D (1988) Nurses threaten indefinite strike, *The Guardian* (18.8.1988)

Brindle D (1998a) Sick leave costs the NHS £700 m a year, *The Guardian* (25.3.1998)

Brindle D (1998b) Sceptics query NHS recruitment pledges, *The Guardian* (17.7.1998)

Brindle D (1998c) Depth charge, *The Guardian* (11.3.1998)

Brindle D (1999) Labour admits NHS in crisis, *The Guardian* (9.1.1999)

Brook H (1997) Mayday pays more for redundancy than medical equipment, *Croydon Advertiser* (12.9.97)

Buckley M (1998) Death rights, *Nursing Times*, **94**(25), 26–32 (24.6.1998)

Buerhaus P *et al.* (2000) Implications of an ageing registered workforce, *Journal of the American Medical Association*, **283**, 2948–54

Burgess P (1998) In the letters pages of the *Nursing Times*, **94**(47) (25.11.1998)

Burnard P *et al.* (2000) When the pressure's too much, *Nursing Times*, **96**(19), 28–30 (11.5.2000)

Buswell C (1997) What do you pay to work? *Nursing Times*, **93**(38), 24

Butler P (2002) Milburn aims to sidestep consultants' vote, *The Guardian* (31.10.2002)

Byrne D L, Asmussen T and Freeman J (2000) Descriptive terms for women attending ante natal classes: mother knows best? *British Journal of Obstetrics and Gynaecology*, **107**, 1233–6

Calder J M (1971) *The Story of Nursing.* Methuen: London

Caldwell K *et al.* (1998) *The Envy of the World.* London: NHS Support Federation

Carlisle D (1990) Racism in nursing, *Nursing Times*, **86**(14), 25–9 (4.4.1990)

Carlisle D (1995) Huge vote to ditch rule 12, *Nursing Times*, **91**(27), 5–6 (5.7.1995)

Carpenter M (1980) Asylum nursing before 1914. In: Davies C (ed.) *Rewriting Nursing History*. London: Croom Helm

Carpenter M (1987) *Working for Health*. London: Routledge

Carpenter M (1991) Nurse Subordination in Health Care: Towards a Social Divisions Approach (Unpublished paper) p. 9

Carter R (1998) *Mapping the Mind*. London: Phoenix

Carvel J (2002) Racism 'rife' in NHS merit awards to consultants, *The Guardian* (7.11.2002)

Cassidy J (1996) Divided we stand, *Nursing Times*, **92**(18), 20 (1.5.1996)

Caulkin S (2000) No laughs for staff, *Observer Business supplement*, p. 9 (20.2.2000)

The Catholic Bishop's Conference of England and Wales (1996) *The Common Good and the Catholic Church's Social Teaching*. London: The Catholic Bishop's Conference of England and Wales

Cervi B (1996) Anger greets consultant attack on rise in nurse practitioners, *Nursing Times*, **92**(19) (8.5.1996)

Chapman P (2000) Unknown factor, *Nursing Times*, **96**(6), 28 (10.2.2000)

Charmley J (1996) *A History of Conservative Politics*. London: Macmillan

Clarke J (1988) Striking attitudes. *Nursing Standard*, **3**(20), 11

Clarke et al. (2001) Best of British ... *Community Practitioner*, **74**(7), 246–50

Clay T (1989) *Power and Politics*. London: Heinemann

Clewes G (2000) Walk in centres, one step at a time, *BMA News Review*, pp. 18–20 (27.5.2000)

COHSE (1991) *Recruitment Strategy for the 1990s*. Banstead: COHSE

Coker N (ed.) (2001) *Racism in Medicine – An Agenda for Change*. London: King's Fund

Cole A (2001) Divided they'll fall, *Health Service Journal*, 24–7 (1.2.2001)

Coombes R (1996) UKCC report will slam managers, *Nursing Times*, **92**(43) (23.10.1996)

Coombes R (1999a) Skill mix report attacks 'autocratic' trust bosses, *Nursing Times*, **95**(42), 7 (20.10.1999)

Coombes R (1999b) Unions clash over move to bring students back into NHS employ, *Nursing Times*, **95**(48) (1.12.1999)

Coombes R (2000a) Nurses still back Blair, *Nursing Times*, **96**(4) (27.1.2000)

Coombes R (2000b) Fears for patient safety as nursing students 'regularly left in charge', *Nursing Times*, **96**(36) (7.9.2000)

Cowell B and Wainwright D (1981) *Behind the Blue Door. The History of the Royal College of Midwives*. London: Bailliere Tindall

CPHVA (1997) *Public Health: The Role of Nurses and Health Visitors, CPHVA Position Statement*. London: CPHVA

Cresswell J (1993) London's hospitals fight for survival with a price war, *Health Service Journal*, 4 (14.10.1993)

Crouch D (2002) New year, new image, *Nursing Times*, **96**(1) (6.1.2000)

Cullen J (1998) *Born in the USA: Bruce Springsteen and the American tradition*. London: Helter Skelter

Dangerfield G (1966) *The Strange Death of Liberal England*, 2nd Edition. London: Palladin

Davies C (ed.) (1980) *Rewriting Nursing History*. London: Croom Helm

Davies C (1996) Cloaked in a tattered illusion. *Nursing Times*, **92**(45), 44–6

Davies N (1994) The casualty still in Ward Four, *The Guardian* (12.2.1994)

Davin A (1978) Imperialism and motherhood, *History Workshop Journal*, 5

Davis C (2002) Divided we fall. *Nursing Times*, **98**(14), 14

Department of Health and Social Security (1983) *The NHS Management Inquiry*. London: HMSO

Department of Health and Social Security (1986) *Neighbourhood Nursing: A Focus for Care*. London: HMSO

Department of Health (1990) *Working for Patients*. London: HMSO

Department of Health (1993) *Making London Better*. London: HMSO

Department of Health (1995) *Building Bridges*. London: DoH

Department of Health (1997) *The New NHS: Modern, Dependable*. London: DoH

Department of Health (1998) *A First Class Service: Quality in the New NHS*. London: DoH

Department of Health (1999a) *Mental Health Nursing: Addressing Acute Concerns*. London: DoH

Department of Health (1999b) *Report of the Committee of Inquiry into the Personality Disorders Unit, Ashworth Special Hospital, Vol 1*. London: DoH

Department of Health (1999c) *Making a Difference*. London: DoH

Department of Health (1999d) *Report of the NHS Taskforce on Workplace Involvement*. London: DoH

Department of Health (1999e) *Report of the Committee of Inquiry into the Personality Disorders Unit, Ashworth Special Hospital, Vol 1*. HMSO: London

Department of Health (1999f) *Saving Lives: Our Healthier Nation*. London: DoH

Department of Health (2000a) *The Action Plan to Implement the Recommendations of the NHS Plan*. London: DoH

Department of Health (2000b) *Taskforce on Staff Involvement*. London: DoH

Department of Health (2000c) *The NHS Plan*. London: DoH

Department of Health (2001a) *Improving Working Lives*. London: DoH

Department of Health (2001b) *Investment and Reform for NHS Staff*. London: DoH

Department of Health, Social Services and Public Safety (2002) *Developing Better Services*. Belfast: DHSSPF

Deville-Almond J (1998) Power points, *Nursing Times*, **94**(36) (9.9.1998)

Dhruev N (2002) Not just skin deep: how systems sustain racism. *Nursing Times*, **98**(23), 26–7

Dingwall R, Rafferty A M and Webster C (1988) *An Introduction to the Social History of Nursing*. London: Routledge

Dinsdale P (2002) Across the divide, *Nursing Standard*, **16**(49), 12

Doyal L (1979) *The Political Economy of Health*. London: Pluto Press

Doyal L (1985) Women and the crisis in the National Health Service. In Ungerson C (ed.) *Women and Social Policy*. Basingstoke: Macmillan

Duffin C (2000) Waiting game, *Nursing Standard*, 7(3), 12

Duggan M *et al.* (1997) *Pulling Together: The Future Roles and Training of Mental Health Care Staff*. London: Sainsbury Centre for Mental Health

Durham M (1998) Nice new hospital but will it have patients? *The Observer*, p. 22 (12.7.1998)

Eden J (1998) Facing cancer, *Nursing Times*, **94**(46), 32–3 (18.11.1998)

Editorial (1996) How long must we wait? *Nursing Times*, **92**(47), 3 (20.9.1996)

Editorial (1997) Life bans take a lifetime, *Nursing Times*, **93**(4) (22.1.1997)

Editorial (2000) Mr Brown's healthy brew, *The Guardian* (15.3.2000)

Editorial (2000) Head banging tendency can't stop march of time, *Health Service Journal* (23.3.2000)

Edwards, S (1996) Are nursing's 'extraordinary' moral standards unrealistic? *Nursing Times*, **92**(43), 34–5 (23.10.1996)

Edwards S D (ed.) (1998) *Philosophical Issues in Nursing*. Basingstoke: Macmillan

Ersser S and Tutton L (eds) (1991) *Primary Nursing in Perspective*. Middlesex: Scutari

Evans D and Allen H (2002) Emotional intelligence: its role in training, *Nursing Times*, **98**(27), 41–2

Fabricus, J (1999) The crisis in nursing, *Psychoanalytic Psychotherapy*, **13**(3), 203

Fergy S (2001) *Reconceptualising Nursing for the New Millennium: The duvet and the Sardine can*. Unpublished PhD Thesis

Field N (1998) Small comforts, *Nursing Times*, **94**(25), 28 (24.6.1998)

Field T (1996) *Bully in Sight*. Oxfordshire: Success Unlimited

Finlayson B *et al.* (2002) Mind the gap: the extent of the NHS nursing shortage, *British Medical Journal*, **325**(7363), 538–41

Finlayson L and Nazroo J (1998) *Gender Inequalities in Nursing Careers*. London: Policy Studies Institute

Flockhart S (2001) Could this man's musings change your life? *Sunday Herald*, p. 7 (27.5.2001)

Foucault M (1961) *Madness and Civilization*. London: Tavistock

Fox L (2001) *The Health We Deserve*: A speech by Dr Liam Fox MP to the Society of Apothecaries, London: Conservative Policy Forum (20.2.2001)

Freedland J (2002) Reaching for power, *The Guardian*, p. 19 (20.11.2002)

Friedman N and Friedman R (1981) *Free to Choose*. Harmondsworth: Penguin

Fulop *et al.* (2002) Process and impact of mergers of NHS trusts: multicentre case study and management cost analysis, *British Medical Journal*, **325**(7358), 246–9

Furlong S and Glover D (1998) Confusion surrounds piecemeal changes in nurses' roles, *Nursing Times*, **94**(37) (16.9.1998)

Gamarnikow E (1978) Sexual division of labour, the case of nursing. In: Kuhn A and Wolpe A (eds) *Feminism and Materialism: Women and Modes of Production*. London, Routledge and Kegan Paul

Gamarnikow E (1991) Nurse or woman: gender and professionalism in reformed nursing 1860–1923. In: Holden P and Littlewood J (eds) *Anthropology and Nursing*. London: Routledge

Garavelli, D (2002) Ghost of Christmas past rises from the shopfloor, *Scotland on Sunday*, p. 22 (10.11.2002)

Gardner H (1989) Multiple intelligences go to school. *Educational Researcher*, **18**(8)

Gaze H (1990) Dangerous economies, *Nursing Times*, **86**(14), 19 (4.4.1990)

Glover D (1999) Self-regulation: apply within, *Nursing Times*, **95**(43), 30–1 (27.10.1999)

Gomm R and Davies C (eds) (2000) *Using Evidence in Health and Social Care Settings*. London: Sage

Gooch S (1989) White paper whitewash, *Nursing Standard*, **3**(28) 42

Gough I (1975) State expenditure in advanced capitalism, *New Left Review*, **I**, 92, July–August 1975, 53–92

Gould D, Kelly D, Goldstone L and Maidwell A (2001) The changing training needs of clinical nurse managers: exploring issues for continuing professional development, *Journal of Advanced Nursing*, **34**(1), 3–6

Gould M (1998a) Promising start but must try harder, *Nursing Times*, **94**(17), 32–3 (29.4.1998)

Gould M (1998b) March of the midwives. *Nursing Times*, **94**(43) (28.10.1998)

Gould M (1999) Trust finds patient death linked to staff shortages, *Nursing Times*, **95**(33), 8 (18.8.1999)

Gournay K (1996) Schizophrenia: a review of the contemporary literature and implications for mental health nursing theory, practice and education, *Journal of Psychiatric and Mental Health Nursing*, **3**, 7–12

Gournay K (2002) *The Recognition, Prevention and Therapeutic Management of Violence*. London: UKCC

Gramsci A (1971) *Selections from the Prison Notebooks*. London: Lawrence and Wisehart

Griffiths R (1983) *NHS Management Inquiry*. London, HMSO

Guest D *et al.* (2001) *A Preliminary Evaluation of the Establishment of Nurse, Midwife and Health Visitor Consultants*. London: King's College

Gulland A (1998a) Evolutionary thoughts, *Nursing Times*, **94**(33) (19.8.1998)

Gulland A (1998b) Congress says no to RCN members, *Nursing Times*, **94**(17), 5 (29.4.1998)

Gulland A (1998c) Figures show sickness absence costs NHS a mint, *Nursing Times*, **94**(2) (14.1.1998)

Gulland A (1999a) Dead men's shoes, *Nursing Times*, **95**(43) (27.10.1999)

Gulland A (1999b) Hunt is on for chief nurse after Moores bows out, *Nursing Times*, **95**(19) (12.5.1999)

Gulland A and Payne D (1997) Daisy chain power, *Nursing Times*, **93**(34) 14–15 (20.8.1997)

Gulland A and Porter R (1997) Brown pressed for NHS cash lifeline, *Nursing Times*, **93**(27) (2.7.1997)

Hale G (2000) Should students be employed by the NHS throughout their studies, *Nursing Times*, **96**(4) (27.1.2000)

Ham C (1992) *Health Policy in Britain*, 3rd Edition. Basingstoke: Macmillan

Ham C (1996) Diagnosis in dispute. *The Guardian* (4.12.1996)

Ham C and Hill M (1993) *The Policy Process in the Modern Capitalist State*, 3rd Edition. New York: Harvester

Hamblin R, Harrison A and Boyle S (1998) The wrong target, *Health Service Journal*, **108**(5598), 28–31

Hardt M and Negri A (2001) *Empire*. Massachussetts: Harvard University Press

Hart C (1994) *Behind the Mask: Nurses, their Trade Unions and Nursing Policy*. London: Bailliere Tindall

Hart C (1995) The great divide, *International History of Nursing Journal*, **1**(3) London: Nursing Standard Publications

Hart C (1999) Keeping teams together, *Nursing Times*, **95**(37), 48–9

Hassan G and Warhurst C (2002) *Anatomy of the New Scotland: Power, Influence and Change*. Edinburgh: Mainstream Publishing

Hayward M (1998) Time to fight, *Nursing Times*, **94**(45) (11.11.1998)

Haywood S and Alazewski A (1980) *Crisis in the Health Service*. London: Croom Helm

Haywood S and Hunter D J (1982) Consultative processes in health policy in the United Kingdom: a view from the centre, *Policy Administration*, **69**, 152–4

Health Education Authority (1995) *Health at Work in the NHS: Key Indicators*. London: Health Education Authority

Health and Safety Executive (1999) *Help on Work Related Stress: A Short Guide*. London: HSE

Health Service Manager Briefing (1999) No 48, Surrey, Croner

Healy P (1997) Trust claims staff on local terms are earning too much, *Health Service Journal*, 6 (14.8.1997)

Held D and Keane J (1984) Socialism and the limits of state action. In: Curran (ed.) *The Future of the Left*. London: Polity Press

Helgesen S (1990) *The Female Advantage: Women's Ways of Leadership*. New York: Doubleday

Hogwood B W and Gunn L A (1984) *Policy Analysis for the Real World*. Oxford: Oxford University Press

Holt J (1998) The unexamined life is not worth living. In: Edwards S D (ed.) *Philosophical Issues in Nursing*. Basingstoke: Macmillan

Hugman R (1991) *Power in Caring Professions*. Basingstoke: Macmillan

Hutton W (1996) Fool's gold in a fool's paradise, *Observer Review*, 1–2 (2.6.1996)

Hutton W (1999) The NHS has caught a cold. But who will cure it? *The Observer* (10.1.1999)

Illich I (1977) *Disabling Professions*. London: Chapman & Hall

Income Data Services (1998) *Public Sector/Labour Market Survey*. London: IDS

Institute of Health Services Management (1994) *Creative Career Paths in the NHS; Report No 1: Top Managers. A study by IHSM Consultants for the NHS women's unit*. London: IHSM

Islam P and Morgan O (2002) UK to grow faster in 2003, *The Observer*, 20 (29.12.02)

JM Consulting (1999) *Review of Nurses' Midwives' and Health Visitors' Act*. Bristol: JM Consulting

Kellner P (1998) Time unions broke away as Labour leaves 'paymasters' out of pocket, *The Standard* (22.5.1998)

Kellner P (1999) £40 billion is not enough for us to feel good, *The Standard* (1.2.1999)

Kenny C (1998) Nurse MPs 'out of touch', *Nursing Times*, **94**(19), 12 (13.5.1998)

Kenward G and Hodgetts T (2002) Nurse concern: a predictor of patient deterioration, *Nursing Times*, **98**(22), 38–9

Kerr A and Waddington J (1998) *Unison Membership Survey*. London: Unison

Kinnell HG (2000) Serial homicide by doctors: shipman in perspective, *British Medical Journal*, **321**, 594–8

Klein R (1989) *The Politics of the NHS*, 2nd Edition. London: Longman

Kutz I (2000) Job and his 'doctors': bedside wisdom in the book of Job, *British Medical Journal*, (**23–30**) 1613–15 (December 2000)

Lashmar P (1997) Death by hospital, *The Guardian* (22.10.97)

Le Grand J (1982) *The Strategy of Equality*. London: Allen and Unwin

Le Grand J and Robinson R (1984) *The Economics of Social Problems*. London: Macmillan

Legge A (1998) Nurse-led hospital service takes on GPs' night calls, *Nursing Times*, **94**(2) (14.1.98)

Leigh D (1997) Dobson's choice is what the Tory doctor ordered, *The Observer* (3.8.1997)

Leigh D *et al.* (1997) Patient care to suffer as hospitals try to pay private finance bills, *The Guardian* (3.8.1997)

Lewis J (1998a) Action man, *Nursing Times*, **95**(22), 32–3 (2.6.1998)

Lewis J (1998b) Miracle worker, *Nursing Times*, **95**(25), 30–1 (23.6.1998)

Lewis P (1989) Reasons for training and subsequent career paths. In: Wilson-Barnet, J (ed.) *Directions in Nursing Research*. London: Scutari Press

Lindblom C E (1959) The science of 'muddling through', *Public Administration Review*, **19**

Lipley N (2000) Unfilled potential, *Nursing Standard*, **14**(52), 20–1

Lister J (1988) Cutting the Lifeline. London: Journeyman

Lister J (1997) *Response to the Independent Inquiry into London's Health Services*. London: Unison Greater London Region

Lister J (1999) *Better Mental Health Services*. London: Unison

Littlewood R (1991) Gender, role and sickness: the ritual psychopathologies of the nurse. In: Holden P and Littlewood (eds) *Anthropology and Nursing*. London: Routledge

London Health Emergency (1999) Capital's trusts face extra wage bill, *Health Emergency*, **49**, 1

Lukes S (1974) *Power: A Radical View*. London: Macmillan

MacDonell H (2003) SNP attacks increase in NHS bureaucracy, *The Scotsman* (8.1.2003)

Mackay L (1989) *Nursing A Grievance*. Milton Keynes: Open University Press

Macpherson W (1999) *The Stephen Lawrence Inquiry*. London: The Stationery Office

Mahoney M (1998) Caution re-ignites prescribing row, *Nursing Times*, **94**(31) (5.8.1998)

Marsh D (1992) *The New Politics of British Trade Unionism*. Basingstoke: Macmillan

Masterton G and Mander A (1990) Psychiatric emergencies, Scotland and the World Cup Finals, *British Journal of Psychiatry*, **156**, 475–8

McCarthy W (1976) *Making Whitley Work*. London: HMSO

McCullough A and Ashburner L (1997) Primary Dolours. *Health Service Journal*, 22–3 (28.8.1997)

McDonald A (1996) Responding to the results of the Beverly Allitt inquiry, *Nursing Times*, **92**(2) (10.1.1996)

McDonald I (1994) *Revolution in the Head*. London: 4th Estate

McLelland S (2002) Health policy in Wales – distinctive or derivative? *Social Policy and Society* **1**(4), Cambridge: Cambridge University Press

McSmith A (1997) Dobson in mass purge of NHS Tories, *The Observer*, p. 1 (29.6.1997)

Meikle J (2001) Inflexible NHS 'holds back' women doctors, *The Guardian* (27.6.2001)

The Mental Health Act Commission (1999) *Mental Health Nursing: Addressing Acute Concerns*. London: Department of Health

Mental Hospital and Institutional Workers' Union (1931) *The History of the MHIWU*. Manchester: MHIWU

Menzies I E P (1970) *The Functioning of Social Systems as a Defence Against Anxiety*. London: Tavistock

Milburn A (2002) Speech to the New Health Network (15.1.2002)

Miller G (1962) *Psychology*. Harmondsworth: Penguin

Minford P (1984) The role of the social services: a view from the New Right. In: *The State or the Market?* London: Sage

Mitchell J (1984) *What is to be Done About Illness and Health?* Harmondsworth: Penguin

Mohan J (1995) *A National Health Service?* Basingstoke: Macmillan

Moore M (2002) *Stupid White Men*. London: Penguin

Moore W (1995) Is the 56-hour week good for you, your family, or the NHS? *Health Service Journal*, 24–7 (13.7.1995)

Morgan K O (1992) *The People's History: British History 1945–1990*. Oxford: Oxford University Press

Morton I (1999) *Person Centred Approaches to Dementia Care*. Oxon: Winslow

Mullholland H (2001a) Inquiry says PREP is 'just a piece of paper', *Nursing Times*, **97**(30) (26.7.2001)

Mullholland H (2001b) 'Chaotic' staff cover costs NHS £810m a year, *Nursing Times*, 97(36), 4 (6.9.2001)

Mullholland H (2001c) Violence targets 'unachievable', *Nursing Times*, 97(37), 9

Mullholland H (2002a) RCN says NHS needs 115,000 more nurses, *Nursing Times*, 98(8) (21.2.2002)

Mullholland H (2002b) Birth of a new breed? *Nursing Times*, 98(20) 11

Munro R (2000a) 'Last chance' for NHS, *Nursing Times*, 96(14), 5 (6.4.2000)

Munro R (2000b) Back-door route to generic nursing, *Nursing Times*, 96(30), 12 (27.7.2000)

Munro R (2001a) Two-thirds of nurses struck off are men, *Nursing Times*, 97(46) (15.11.2001)

Munro R (2001b) Solving the needlestick nightmare, *Nursing Times*, 97(24) 12 (14.6.2001)

Munro R (2002a) What we need from Gordon Brown's millions, *Nursing Times*, 98(22), 10–13

Munro R (2002b) Professions unite to slam reforms, *Nursing Times*, 98(10), 8

Munro R (2002c) Ringing endorsement, *Nursing Times*, 98(15), 10–11

Munro R (2002d) Death threats spark protest, *Nursing Times*, 98(33), 8

Naish J (1998) Friend or foe? *Nursing Times*, 94(15), 26–8 (15.4.1998)

The National Assembly for Wales (2000) *Realising the Potential: A Strategic Framework for Nursing, Midwifery and Health Visiting in Wales into the 21st Century*. Cardiff: The National Assembly for Wales

The National Assembly for Wales (2001) *Creating the Potential*. Cardiff: The National Assembly for Wales

National Health News (2000) *Staff are 'Cornerstone' of Radical Plans for NHS*. Leeds: Department of Health

Navarro V (1979) *Class Struggle, the State and Medicine*. London: Martin Robertson

Navarro V (1986) *Crisis, Health and Medicine: A Social Critique*. London: Tavistock

Neenan T (1999) A hole lot more, *Nursing Times*, 95(2) (13.1.1999)

News Item (no author) (1997) National pay doesn't mean more pay, warns Abberley, *Health Service Journal*, 14 (3.7.1997)

News Item (no author) (1999) BBC's Casualty star is voted top TV nurse, *Nursing Standard*, 13(33), 5 (5.5.1999)

News Item (no author) (1999) Risk of violence depends on where you work, *Nursing Times*, 95(42), 9 (20.10.1999)

News Item (no author) (2000) Send students back to NHS, *Nursing Times*, 96(4) (27.1.2000)

News Item (no author) (2001) Unions demand 'quite a bit more' than last year, *Nursing Times*, 97(37), 4 (13.9.2001)

News Item (no author) (2002) Malone faces push for a vote of no confidence, *Nursing Times*, 98(25), 5

News Item (no author) (2002) The real Charlie Fairhead resigns, *Nursing Times*, 98(37), 7

News Item (no author) (2002) Vice-president claims Malone turned down her offer to resign, *Nursing Times*, 98(44), 6

NHS Federation (1996) *NHS Matters*. London: NHS Federation

NHSScotland (2000) *Scottish NHS Plan*. Edinburgh: NHSScotland

NHSScotland (2002) *Caring for Scotland: The Strategy for Nursing and Midwifery in Scotland*. Edinburgh: NHSScotland

Nolan P (1993) *A History of Mental Health Nursing*. London: Chapman & Hall

Nolan *et al.* (1998) Getting to know you. *Nursing Times* 94(39) (30.9.98)

Nolan *et al.* (1999) Brainstorming the role of the mental health nurse, *Nursing Times*, 95(46) (17.11.1999)

Norman A (1998) Speaking out, *Nursing Times*, 94(49) (9.12.1998)

O'Connor J (1973) *The Fiscal Crisis of the State*. New York: St Martin's Press

O'Dowd A (1998a) The urbane fox, *Nursing Times*, 95(30) (28.7.1998)

O'Dowd A (1998b) Wake up to nurse power, *Nursing Times*, 94(27) (8.7.1998)

O'Dowd A (1998c) Pay: it's us against them, *Nursing Times*, 94(38) (23.9.1998)

O'Dowd A (2000) Young, gifted and black? *Nursing Times*, 96(40), 5

O'Dowd A (2001) Malone ranger shoots from the hip, *Nursing Times*, 97(31), 10–11 (2.8.2001)

O'Dowd A (2002) 'Dickensian' staffing found in Scots trusts, *Nursing Times*, 98(51), 4

O'Dowd A (2002a) Setting the new agenda, *Nursing Times*, 98(49), 23–5

O'Dowd A (2002b) Union success in push for regrading, *Nursing Times*, 98(28), 5

O'Dowd A (2002c) Fewer than 100 nurses recruited in a year, *Nursing Times*, 98(6) (7.2.2002)

O'Farrell J (2000) The secret life of a bald Labour mole, *The Guardian* (4.10.2000)

Owens P and Glennerster H (1990) *Nursing in Conflict*. London: Macmillan

Parish C (2000) Early consultation, *Nursing Standard*, 14(35), 13

Parry R (2002) Delivery structure and policy development in post-devolution Scotland, *Social Policy and Society*, 1(4), 315–24

Paton C *et al.* (1997) Counting the costs, *Health Service Journal*, 24–7 (21.8.1997)

Payne D (1996) Delegates warned to 'get their act together', *Nursing Times*, 92(19), 23 (8.5.1996)

Payne D (1998) Stressed to death, *Nursing Times*, 94(10), 9 (11.3.1998)

Pettigrew A, McKee L and Ferlie E (1988) Understanding change in the NHS, *Public Administration*, 66

Poole J (2000) Thirst to be equals, *Nursing Times*, 96(1) (6.1.2000)

Pownall M (1988) Working on, *Nursing Times*, 84(5), 18

Pyne R H (1982) The General Nursing Council. In: Allen P and Jolley M (eds) *Nursing, Midwifery and Health Visiting Since 1900*. London: Faber and Faber

Radcliffe M and Crouch D (2002) 'Don't take us for granted', *Nursing Times*, 98(16), 26–9

Radcliffe M and Munro R (1999) Murders by disordered offenders half 1979 rate, *Nursing Times*, **95**(2)

RCN Bulletin (2003) *Record Numbers of Nurses join RCN*. London: RCN

Reid T (1993) Kill or cure? *Nursing Times*, 89(39), 41–5

Revill J (1998) One bereaved daughter for whom the NHS stands for the Neglect and Humiliation Service, *Evening Standard* (30.1.1998)

Revill J (1999a) We train nurses then they disappear, *Evening Standard* (25.1.999)

Revill J (1999b) Hospital is forced to close children's beds, *Evening Standard* (5.8.1999)

Revill J (2002a) NHS gets better all the time, *The Observer* (8.12.2002)

Revill J (2002b) Revealed: one in four health employees is now a bureaucrat, *The Observer*, 6 (13.10.2002)

Revill J (2003) Whistleblower reveals NHS culture of secrecy, *The Observer*, 4 (26.1.2003)

Rild C W, Hayes D, Ames D J (2000) Patient or client? The opinion of people attending a psychiatric clinic, *Bulletin*, **24**, 447–50

Ritter S (1997) Taking stock of psychiatric nursing. In: Tilley S (ed.) *The Mental Health Nurse*. Oxford: Blackwell Scientific

Rivett G (1998) *From Cradle to Grave: 50 Years of the NHS*. London: King's Fund Publishing

Robinson R *et al.* (1997) Cracks in the evidence, *Health Service Journal*, 26–9 (4.9.1997)

Robothom M (1997) Nurse or midwife? *Nursing Times*, **93**(38) (17.9.1997)

Robotham M (1999) What you think of doctors, *Nursing Times*, **95**(2) (13.1.1999)

Rogers R, Salvage J and Cowell C (1999) *Nurses at risk*. London: Macmillan

Rose R I (1986) *The Voters Begin to Choose*. London: Sage

Royal College of Nursing (1996) *Hazards of Nursing: Personal Injuries at Work*. London: RCN

Royle J A and Walsh M (1992) *Watson's Medical Surgical Nursing and Related Physiology*, 4th Edition. London: Bailliere Tindall

Ryan C (2000a) Milburn's pledges cheer delegates, *Nursing Times*, **96**(15) (13.4.2000)

Ryan C (2000b) Students demand salaries, *Nursing Times*, **96**(35) (31.8.2000)

Salvage J (1999) Do you have faith in Eileen Drewery? *Nursing Times*, **95**(7), 20 (17.2.1999)

Salvage J and Smith R (2000) Who wears the trousers? *Nursing Times*, **96**(15), 24 (13.4.2000)

Sethi S and Dimmock S (eds) (1982) *Industrial Relations and the Health Service*. London: Croom Helm

Shamash J (2002) NHS changes are causing bullying, *Nursing Times*, **98**(25), 8

Shamash J and Gallagher C (2002) No time to lose, *Nursing Times*, **98**(43), 20–3

Sherman J (1988) Strike threat by nurses at eight hospitals, *The Times* (3.2.1988)

Simpson S (2001) Near death experience: a concept analysis as applied to nursing, *Journal of Advanced Nursing*, **36**(4), 520–6

Smith A and Russell J (1991) Using critical learning incidents in nurse education, *Nurse Education Today*, **11**, 284–91

Smith G and Seccombe I (1996) In the balance: registered nurse supply and demand, *Institute for Employment Studies: Report 315*. London: Institute for Employment Studies

Smith K *et al.* (1999) Second among equals, *Nursing Times*, **95**(13), 54–5 (31.3.1999)

Smith P (1982) *A History of the RCN and Industrial Relations Within the NHS*. Unpublished dissertation

Smith P (1992) *The Emotional Labour of Nursing*. Basingstoke: Macmillan

Snell J and Gaze H (1991) Riding the wave, *Nursing Times*, **87**(33), 18–19 (25.9.1991)

Solomas J and Back L (1996) *Racism and Society*. London, Macmillan

South London and Maudsley Unison Branch (2001) *Unison Eyes*, **9**, 1

St George's Hospital Committee Minutes (1868) London: St George's Hospital Archive

St George's Hospital Committee Minutes (1887) London: St George's Hospital Archive

St George's Hospital Gazette (1948) London: St George's Hospital Archive

St George's Hospital Reports (1864–65) London: St George's Hospital Archive

Summers A (1988) *Angels and Citizens: British Women as Military Nurses*. London: Routledge & Kegan Paul

Synapse (2002) Pickled union, *Nursing Times*, **98**(14), 13

Syrett M and Lammiman J (1999) Forget IQ – it's brains that matter, *The Observer* (7.11.1999)

Taylor Gooby P (1986) Privatisation, power and the state, *Sociology*, **20**(2)

Tellis-Nyak M and Tellis Nyak V (1984) Games that physicians play: the social psychology of physician-nurse interaction, *Social Science and Medicine*, **18**(12), 1063–9

Thompson E P (1968) *The Making of the English Working Class*. Harmondsworth: Penguin

Timmins N (1995a) How three top managers nearly sank the reforms, *Health Service Journal*, 11–13 (29.6.1995)

Timmins N (1995b) *The Five Giants: A Biography of the Welfare State*. London: Harper Collins

Tomlinson B (1993) *Report of the Inquiry into London's Health Service, Medical Education and Research: Making London Better*. London: Department of Health

Tonkin B (1988) Strong medicine, *Community Care* (10.11.1989)

Townsend P and Davidson N (1982) *Inequalities in Health*. Harmondsworth: Pelican

Trades Union Congress (1997) *Hazards at work: TUC guide to Health and Safety*. London: TUC

Tudor Hart J (1971) The Inverse care Law. *The Lancet*

Unison (1993) *Evidence to the Pay Review Body.* London: Unison

Unison (1997) *Bullying at Work.* London: Unison

Unison (1998a) *Cause for Concern.* London: Unison

Unison/Opinion Leader Research Ltd (1998b) *Findings of a Programme of Quantitative and Qualitative Research among Active Members of the Unison Health Group.* London: Unison Health Group

Unison (1998c) Strategic review endorsed, *Unison focus,* **93** (11.12.1998)

Unison (1998d) *Unison Labour Link News.* London: Unison

Unison (1999) *First Class Team, Second Class Pay.* London: Unison

Unison News (20.1.03) www.unison.org

United Kingdom Central Council (1989) *Exercising Accountability.* London: UKCC

United Kingdom Central Council (1992) *The Scope of Professional Practice.* London: UKCC

United Kingdom Central Council (1992) *UKCC Code of Conduct.* London: UKCC

United Kingdom Central Council (1995) *PREP & You.* London: UKCC

United Kingdom Central Council (1998a) *Guidelines for Mental Health and Learning Disabilities Nursing.* London: UKCC

United Kingdom Central Council (1998b) *Guidelines for Records and Record Keeping.* London: UKCC

United Kingdom Central Council (1998c) UKCC Register 23, Spring 1998, London. UKCC

United Kingdom Central Council (1999a) *A Higher Level of Practice.* London: UKCC

United Kingdom Central Council (1999b) *Fitness for Practice.* London: UKCC

United Kingdom Central Council (2000) *Guidelines for the Administration of Medicines.* London: UKCC

United Kingdom Central Council (2000a) Register 33, UKCC, Autumn 2000

United Kingdom Central Council (2000b) Register 32, Summer 2000

Vaizey J (1984) *National Health.* Oxford: Martin Robertson

Vousden M (1988) A year to remember, *Nursing Times,* **84**(51) (21.12.1988)

Vousden M (1998) Nursing a grievance, *Nursing Times,* **94**(26) (1.7.1998)

Walsh N and Gough P (1997) From profession to commodity, *Nursing Times,* 93(30) (23.7.97)

Waters A (2002) Nurses say: its time to strike, *Nursing Times,* 98(14) 10–11

Weale A (1987) Why are we waiting? The problems of unresponsiveness in the social services. In: Klein R and Higgins I (eds) *The Future of Welfare.* London: Blackwell

Webster C (1969) *The Health Service Since the War: Problems of Health Care: The NHS Before 1957.* London: HMSO

Weiner J (1995) *Come Together, John Lennon in his Own Time.* London: Faber & Faber

Wheen F (1999) Cutting hospital corners, *The Guardian* (29.9.1999)

White R (1978) *Social Change and the Development of Nursing.* London: Henry Kimpton

White R (1985) *The Effects of the NHS on the Nursing Profession 1948–1961*. London: King's Fund

Whitston C and Waddington J (1993) *Recruitment & Organisation in a Changing Environment*. Banstead: COHSE

Whittington D and Boone J (1989) Competencies in nursing. In: Ellis R (ed.) *Professional Competence and Quality Assurance in the Caring Professions*. London: Chapman & Hall

Wilkinson G and Miers M (eds) (1999) *Power and Nursing Practice*. Basingstoke: Macmillan

Williams B (2001) Developing critical reflection for professional practice through problem based learning, *Journal of Advance Nursing*, **43**(1) 18–26

Williams S, Michie S, Pattani S (1998) *Improving the Health of the Workforce: Report of the Partnership on the Health of the NHS Workforce*. London: The Nuffield Trust

Wintour P (1996) Clarke's dodgy pass catches Brown offside, *The Observer* (1.12.96)

Wintour P (1999) Healthy, stealthy and wise, *The Observer* (14.3.1999)

Wolfe T (1997) Sorry, but your soul just died, *The Observer*, 6–10 (2.2.1997)

Wright C (1997) Minister gives PFI pledge, *Nursing Times*, **93**(38), 9 (17.9.1997)

Wright C (2000) MSPs condemn NHS for 'secrecy culture', *Health Service Journal*, 10 (23.3.2000)

Wynne-Jones R (2002) Betrayed by Britain, *Daily Mirror*, 8–9 (26.4.2002)

Fair Shares for All: The Report of the National Review of Resource Allocation for the NHS in Scotland (1999)

Health Which? (August 2000)

ICM state of the nation poll, *The Guardian* (8.10.1997)

Making the Connections (2002) www.scotland.gov.uk

Caring for Scotland: The Strategy for Nursing and Midwifery in Scotland (2002), Work-life balance, *The Observer* (3.3.2002)

Index

Pepsi-Co 188
Perkins, Ian 156
Perry, Clare 274
Personal Medical Services 104–05
Person centred approach to dementia
    care 17
Peterloo Massacre 38
Pinel, Phillipe 50
Pocock, Richard 261
Policy Studies Institute 26
Poole, Jo 105
Poor Law Act (1834) 39, 291
Poor Law hospitals 46, 49, 52–3, 61
Poor Law nurses [see also: Pauper
    nurses] 39, 49, 65
Poor Law Workers' Trade Union 8,
    48–9, 202
Power 177–181
Powys Healthcare NHS Trust* 228
Practice nurses 16, 106
Prentis, Dave 216, 223, 271
PREP 252–3
Prescott, John 270 (footnote), 272
Prescription only medicines 284
Primary Care Groups 19, 28, 104,
    288–9
Primary Care Trusts 3, 19, 104, 106,
    149, 289
Primary health care 17, 104
Primary nursing 71, 83
Private Finance Initiative [PFI] 134,
    136, 152, 217, 223, 238, 272–3,
    275–6, 298
  and nursing posts downgraded 274
  and policy to downsize NHS 273
  and Save Kidderminster Hospital
      Campaign 291
Privatisation [see also:
    commercialisation] 21, 70, 127,
    141, 146, 205, 209
Probationers [see also: student nurses]
    46, 53
Problem based learning 243
Problem solving 187, 242, 292, 296
Productivity 193
Professional Associations and
    industrial action 205
Professionalisation and nursing 63
Professionalism 7 (and footnote),
    8, 298
Professional organisations 10

Professions Allied to Medicine [PAMs]
    200, 267, 271
Project 2000 14, 19, 83, 93, 105, 122,
    146, 219, 239–242
Psychosocial interventions 144
Psychosocial model of nursing 93
Public Interest Disclosure Act
    (1998) 258
*Pulling Together: The Future Roles and
    Training of Mental Health Care
    Staff* 240

Q
Qualitative research 94
Quantitative research 94
Queen Elizabeth Hospital 135

R
Race and ethnicity 24
Racism 120
Radical Health Vistor's Association 230
Rafferty, Anne-Marie 36
Railtrack 177 (footnote)
Randomised Control Trials 94
Raphael 86
Rathbone, William 13, 44
Rationing healthcare 175
RCN Direct 232
Realising the Potential 167
Recruitment 141, 238
Redistribution of wealth 120
Redistribution of welfare 120
Reformation, The 37
Register 249
Registration Act 1919 48
Renal nursing 145
*Report of the NHS Taskforce on Workplace
    Involvement* 293, 298
Republican leadership 189
Research
  and value for money 282
Research Assessment Exercise 94
Retail Price Index 126
Retention 238
Revill, Jo 155, 191
Reynolds, Bill 96
Right brain 189
Risk assessment 264
Rolling Stones, The 63
Roman Catholic Church and social
    teaching 90